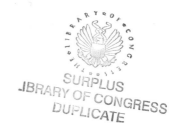
Corneal Topography in the Wavefront Era

A Guide for Clinical Application

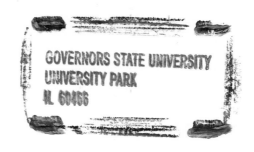
Corneal Topography in the Wavefront Era

A Guide for Clinical Application

Edited by Ming Wang, MD, PhD

Coordinated by Tracy Swartz, OD, MS

Wang Vision Institute
Nashville, Tennessee

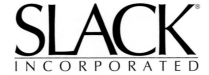

SLACK®

INCORPORATED

Delivering the best in health care information and education worldwide

ISBN-10: 1-55642-718-2
ISBN-13: 978-1-55642-718-3

Published by: SLACK Incorporated
                6900 Grove Road
                Thorofare, NJ 08086 USA
                Telephone: 856-848-1000
                Fax: 856-853-5991
                www.slackbooks.com

Corneal topography in the wavefront era : a guide for clinical application / edited by Ming Wang.
    p. ; cm.
 Includes bibliographical references and index.
 ISBN-13: 978-1-55642-718-3 (alk. paper)
 ISBN-10: 1-55642-718-2 (alk. paper)
 1. Corneal topography. 2. Cornea--Pathophysiology. 3. Cornea--Surgery.
 [DNLM: 1. Corneal Topography. 2. Cornea--physiology. WW 220 C81375 2006] I. Wang, Ming, MD.

RE336.C685 2006
617.7'1907545--dc22

                                    2006001901

Last digit is print number: 10   9   8   7   6   5   4   3   2   1

Dedication

To my dear friend and mentor, the late Professor Guy Chan, a humble and dedicated teacher of ophthalmology, and for all of his students from around the world.

Professor Chan, thank you for your patience, inspiration, and guidance. You exemplify the true essence and spirit of a teacher. We miss you.

This book is for you, Guy.

Contents

Section I: Basic Topographic Principles

Section II: Topographic Applications

Section III: Topography-Based Custom Treatment

Section IV: Specific Topographic Systems

Acknowledgments

My sincere appreciation goes to Dr. Tracy Schroeder Swartz for her profound dedication, organization, and project leadership in the process of editing for this book. Without Dr. Swartz, this book would not be possible.

I would also like to thank all of my professors from whom I have learned everything that I know about the cornea—professors at Harvard Medical School and MIT in Boston, MA, where I did my medical training; Claes Dohlman, Elliott Finkelstein, Jonathan Talamo, and Reza Dana; professors at the Wills Eye Hospital in Philadelphia, PA, where I did my residency in ophthalmology; Peter Laibson, Elizabeth Cohen, Christopher Rapuano, and Larry Donoso; professors at Bascom Palmer Eye Institute in Miami, FL, where I did my corneal fellowship; Richard Forster, William Culberson, Scheffer Tseng, Khalil Hanna, Carol Karp, Stephen Pflugfelder, Andrew Huang, Eduardo Alfonso, and Lori Ventura; professors at Vanderbilt University Department of Ophthalmology in Nashville, TN, where I was a junior faculty member; James Elliott, Spencer Thornton, and Dennis O'Day.

I would like to thank all of my colleagues and staff at Wang Vision Institute in Nashville, TN, particularly Dr. Helen Boerman and Dr. Shawna Hill for their assistance in editing. I would also like to thank Rong Yang, Lisa Flores, and Suzanne Gordon for their support; and my friends Carlos Gonzalez, Simin Soroush, Peng Liang, J. R. Davis, Charles Grummon, Alanna Napier, Polly Nichols, and Gene Angle for their assistance with corneal patients.

Many thanks go to my ophthalmology colleagues in China, Hong Kong, Taiwan, the U.S, and internationally: Jian Ge, Ren-yuan Chu, Jia-liang Zhao, Shi-yuan Zhang, David Liu, David Pao, Bao-song Liu, Michael Zhou, Wei-li Li, Zhu-guo Liu, Jun-ping Zhang, Jun-wen Zhen, Ray-Ann Lin, Ying-min Zheng, Jay Hsu, Ray Tsai, Fung-rong Hu, Arun Gulani, Ralph Chu, Terry Kim, Dimitri Azar, Jay Peppose, Noel Alpins, Trevor Gray, Gates Wayburn, Gary Jerkins, Peter Netland, Thomas Gettelfinger, James Freeman, Deborah Distefano, Natalie Kerr, Francis Munier, and Aleksandar Stojanovic, and to Bang Chen, who arranged the first Intralase LASIK procedure in China, which I performed.

I would like to thank my current and previous corneal fellows from whom I have learned as much as I have taught about the cornea: Drs. Shin Kang, Ilan Cohen, Uyen Tran, Walid Haddard, Mouhab Aljajeh, Keming Yu, Yangzi Jiang, and Lav Panchal.

Especially, I would like to thank Professor Guy Chan, my mentor and teacher, to whom this book is dedicated.

Additionally, I would like to thank my family—my father, Dr. Zhen-sheng Wang; my mother, Dr. A-lian Xu; and my brother, Dr. Ming-yu Wang, for their unfailing support and love in my life.

About the Editor

Ming Wang, MD, PhD, is a Clinical Associate Professor of Ophthalmology at the University of Tennessee, Attending Surgeon at Saint Thomas Hospital, and Director of Wang Vision Institute in Nashville, Tennessee, USA. He is also the Director of Refractive Surgery at the Aier Eye Hospitals, the largest private eye hospital system in China. Dr. Wang received his doctorate degree in laser spectroscopy and his post-doctorate fellowship from the University of Maryland in College Park, Maryland, and the Massachusetts Institute of Technology in Boston, Massachusetts, respectively. In 1991, he received his medical degree (graduating magna cum laude and receiving the award for the best thesis) from Harvard Medical School and Massachusetts Institute of Technology in Boston, Massachusetts, and the Harold Lamport Biomedical Research Prize from Harvard and MIT. After completing both a residency in ophthalmology and a fellowship in ocular genetics at the Wills Eye Hospital in Philadelphia, Pennsylvania, he completed a clinical fellowship in cornea and external disease and refractive surgery at the Bascom Palmer Eye Institute, University of Miami School of Medicine in Miami, Florida. In 1997, he became the founding director of the Vanderbilt Laser Sight Center and a full-time faculty member of the Department of Ophthalmology at the Vanderbilt University School of Medicine. He remained at Vanderbilt for 5 years before he went into private practice in 2002.

Dr. Wang's research career encompasses three distinctively different fields. From 1982 to 1987, he published as the first author of a dozen original papers in the leading physics journal, *Physical Review A*, describing the development of a novel experimental atomic physics technique that he developed with Professor John Weiner, a Doppler velocity-selected associative ionization process between sodium atoms. In 1987, Dr. Wang turned his inquisitive mind to the study of molecular biology at Harvard and MIT, and published as the first author of a major paper in the world-renowned journal, *Nature*, regarding a novel molecular biology technique that he invented with Professor George Church, a whole-genome approach to *in vivo* DNA-protein interaction and gene expression regulation. After research careers in experimental atomic physics and molecular biology, Dr. Wang then began yet another research career in 1992, this time in ophthalmology, ocular genetics, novel anterior segment reconstructive surgeries, and corneal topography. Working with Professor Larry Donoso, he cloned the first ocular melanoma-associated antigen. Dr. Wang made an original contribution to the field of corneal wound healing by publishing with Professor Scheffer Tseng the first paper in the literature regarding laboratory success in the reduction of corneal scarring and apoptosis with amniotic membrane transplantation. Dr. Wang holds a U.S. patent for his invention of the amniotic membrane contact lens, and he successfully made the first prototype. He was a former consultant to the U.S. Food and Drug Administration Ophthalmic Device Panel and a primary reviewer for the panel for the first U.S. LASIK approval by the FDA in 1999. Dr. Wang conducted the first large-scale clinical study and was the principal clinical investigator of the first 3-D stereo corneal topographer, AstraMax. He was the first surgeon from the U.S. to study a new, high frequency excimer laser and treatment-planning platform designed to treat post-LASIK complex eyes. Dr. Wang performed the first femtosecond laser-assisted artificial cornea implantation. He was a LASIK surgeon for ABC's national network reality show program, *Extreme Makeover*.

Dr. Wang is on the editorial board of *Cataract and Refractive Surgery Today*, and is a reviewer for *Ophthalmology*, *American Journal of Ophthalmology*, *Cornea*, *Journal of Cataract and Refractive Surgery*, *Journal of Refractive Surgery*, *Genome*, and *Investigative Ophthalmology and Visual Sciences*. Dr. Wang was the editor of *Corneal Dystrophies and Degenerations*, published by the American Academy of Ophthalmology. He offers the only fellowship in cornea and external disease and refractive surgery in the state of Tennessee. He has been invited to lecture around the world and is an honorary professor of ophthalmology at Xiamen and Zhongshan Medical Universities in China and Shanghai Aier Eye Hospital, where in 2005 he performed China's first Intralase LASIK procedure. Dr. Wang is the founding chairman of the Wang Foundation for Sight Restoration, a nonprofit organization that assists terminally corneal blind patients to undergo novel eye reconstructive surgeries performed free of charge by Dr. Wang. The foundation holds an annual fundraiser, the Eye Ball, each year in the fall. Dr. Wang is the recipient of numerous awards, including being listed continuously each year by Castle Connelly as one of the Best Doctors in America (an honor bestowed on less than 1 percent of U.S. physicians), a Fight for Sight Research Grant of the Research Division to Prevent Blindness, faculty research award of Vanderbilt University, and was a co-principal investigator of a RO1 grant from the National Institutes of Health.

Dr. Wang has a diverse interest in hobbies. He has a band with classical guitarist Mr. Carlos Gonzalez called Music for Sight, in which Dr. Wang plays the Er-hu, a Chinese violin. In Dolly Parton's new CD, *Those Were the Days*, he played his Er-hu to Ms. Parton's song "The Cruel War." In addition, Dr. Wang is an accomplished ballroom dancer and member of the U.S. collegiate champion Harvard University team. He is the president of the Music City Chapter of the United States Amateur Ballroom Dancers Association, and is ranked fourth in the United States in pro-am international ballroom 10-dance.

Contributing Authors

Amar Agarwal, MS, FRCS, FRCOphth
Dr. Agarwal's Eye Hospital
Chennai, Madras, India

Athiya Agarwal, MD, DO
Dr. Agarwal's Eye Hospital
Chennai, Madras, India

Sunita Agarwal, MS, DO
Dr. Agarwal's Eye Hospital
Chennai, Madras, India

Noel Alpins, FRACO, FRCOphth, FACS
New Vision Clinics
Cheltenham, Victoria, Australia

Guillermo Avalos-Urzua, MD
University of Guadalajara Mexico
Guadalajara, Jalisco, Mexico

Giuseppe Bellezza, MD
Rome, Italy

Michael W. Belin, MD
Albany Medical College Lions Eye Institute
Albany, New York

Helen Boerman, OD
Wang Vision Institute
Nashville, Tennessee

Megan Buliano, OD
Chu Laser Eye Institute
Edina, Minnesota

Ralph Chu, MD
Chu Laser Eye Institute
Edina, Minnesota

Ilan Cohen, MD
Fifth Avenue Eye Center
New York, New York

David Coward, OD
Wang Vision Institute
Nashville, Tennessee

Giuseppe D'Ippolito, DrIng
Taranto, Italy

Michael Endl, MD
Fichte-Endl Eye Associates
Amherst, New York

Claus Fichte, MD
Fichte-Endl Eye Associates
Amherst, New York

Arun C. Gulani, MD
Department of Ophthalmology
University of Florida
Jacksonville, Florida

Shawna Hill, OD
Wang Vision Institute
Nashville, Tennessee

Doug Horner, OD, PhD
Indiana University School of Optometry
Bloomington, Indiana

Bruce Jackson, MD
University of Ottawa Eye Institute
Ottawa, Ontario, Canada

Soosan Jacob, MS, FRCS, DipNB, FERC
Dr. Agarwal's Eye Hospital
Chennai, Madras, India

Nilesh Kanjiani, DipNB, DO, FERC
Dr. Agarwal's Eye Hospital
Chennai, Madras, India

Paul M. Karpecki, OD
Moyes Eye Clinic
Kansas City, Missouri

Stephen D. Klyce, PhD
New Orleans, Louisiana

Stephan Kröber
Augenzentrum Maus+Heiser, Köln, Germany

Ray-Ann Lin, MD
Taipei, Taiwan, ROC

Zuguo Liu, MD, PhD
Eye Institute of Xiamen
Xiamen University
Xiamen, China

(Continued)

Naoyuki Maeda, MD
Osaka University Medical School
Department of Ophthalmology
Osaka, Japan

Vincenzo Marchi, MD
Roma, Italy

Renzo Mattioli, PhD
Optikon 2000 S.p.A
Rome, Italy

Mathas Maus, MD
Augenzentrum Maus+Heiser
Cologne, Germany

Marc Michaelson, M.D.
University of Alabama
Birmingham, Alabama

Sergey Molebny, MS
Houston, Texas

Rejean Munger, PhD
University of Ottawa Eye Institute
Ottawa, Ontario, Canada

Tom D. Padrick, PhD
Houston, Texas

Roberto Pinelli, MD
Instituto Laser Microchirurgia
Brescia, Italy

Dan Z. Reinstein, MD
London Vision Clinic
London, England

Mario G. Serrano, MD
Centro de Cirugia Refractiva y Catarata
Bogotá, Colombia

Ariadna Silva-Lepe, MD
University of Guadalajara Mexico
Guadalajara, Jalisco, Mexico

Ronald H. Silverman, PhD
London Vision Clinic
London, England

George Stamatelatos, BscOptom
New Vision Clinics
Cheltenham, Victoria, Australia

Charles Wm. Stewart, OD
Lake Mary, Florida

Aleksandar Stojanovic, MD
Synslaser Clinic, Eye Department
University Hospital North
Tromsoe, Norway

John Sutphin, MD
Dept of Ophthalmology
University of Iowa
Iowa City, Iowa

Tracy Swartz, OD, MS
Wang Vision Institute
Nasvhille, Tennessee

Gustavo E. Tamayo, MD
Centro de Cirugia Refractiva y Catarata
Bogotá, Colombia

Nancy K. Tripoli, MA
Department of Ophthalmology
University of North Carolina at Chapel Hill
Chapel Hill, North Carolina

Joe S. Wakil, MD
Houston, Texas

Xiao Yang, MD
Zhongshan Ophthalmic Center
Guangzhou, China

Keming Yu, MD, PhD
Wang Vision Institute
Nashville, Tennessee

Mei Zhang, MD, PhD
Zhongshan Ophthalmic Center
Guangzhou, China

Zhenpin Zhang, MD, PhD
Zhongshan Ophthalmic Center
Guangzhou, China

Jason Zornek
Fichte-Endl Eye Associates
Amherst, New York

Preface

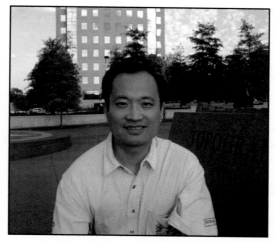

What is the role that corneal topography plays in the era of wavefront technology today? Is there a need for a new comprehensive textbook on corneal topography? What are the new diagnostic capabilities of modern corneal topography, and how should one integrate corneal topographic and wavefront data to improve clinical outcome? At the annual meetings of the American Academy of Ophthalmology (AAO) and the American Society of Cataract and Refractive Surgery (ASCRS) in the past several years, I have been the principal instructor of the advanced corneal topography course. Based on the tremendous amount of interest shown by ophthalmologists attending the course, who were eager to keep abreast of the latest developments in modern corneal topography, I realized that there is indeed a need for an updated comprehensive textbook on this important subject.

Although wavefront sensing technology has offered us a new dimension of knowledge about the eye, an understanding of corneal topography remains indispensable for the following reasons:

1. The cornea is the most powerful refractive structure of the eye.

2. The cornea is what we alter surgically in the dominant surgical approach to correcting refractive error today.

3. Modern corneal topographic technologies offer powerful new capabilities not available in traditional Placido disk-based technology, such as the measurements of posterior corneal surface, pachymetry, and surface elevational changes. These have become indispensable clinically, as exemplified in the detection and prevention of keratoectasia.

4. There are some intrinsic limitations of wavefront sensing technology, such as lack of information of the location of aberration (cornea vs. lens), areas outside the pupil, and accommodative dependence of the data.

5. The 21st century may usher in a new era that calls for a combined and integrated approach to anterior segment surgery using both corneal topography and wavefront sensing. It will give us the unprecedented ability to truly approach supervision.

In order to write an updated and comprehensive textbook on corneal topography, I assembled a group of experts from around the world. My guiding principle in directing the writing of this new topography textbook is to elucidate the scientific principles underlying various modern topographic technologies and offer a comprehensive and useful guide for clinical applications. Whenever possible, generic names are used that denote the type of technology being discussed (eg, Placido disk-based versus slit scanning-based) rather than manufacturer's trade names, thus maximizing the understanding of the underlying scientific principles, while minimizing commercial promotion of any particular instrument.

The result of the collective work of this team of research scientists and physicians is *Corneal Topography in the Wavefront Era: A Guide for Clinical Application*, a comprehensive, updated, and excellently illustrated textbook on corneal topography.

The book begins with Section I: Basic Topographic Principles. The anatomy, physiology, and optical principles of the cornea are discussed, and the history of corneal topography is reviewed. Classification of various topographic technology principles and all maps are presented, as well as the keratometry scales and topographic conventions used. This section provides the reader with a solid foundation of the science behind modern topographies, classification systems, and all representative maps.

In Section II: Topographic Applications, we present topography in normal and diseased corneas, in pre-refractive surgery evaluation and post-refractive surgery complication management. Emphasis is placed on the most important clinical issues such as the identification of forme fruste keratoconus and the proper examination of new topographic capabilities, such as posterior corneal surfaces, elevational changes, and pachymetry. This section provides the reader with an in-depth discussion and presentation of clinical guidance when approaching important issues encountered in refractive surgery, such as the detection and prevention of keratoectasia.

Section III: Topography-Based Custom Treatment presents new technologies for an integrated approach to refractive and corneal surgery by combining corneal topography with wavefront sensing. Relationships and clinical correlates between corneal topography and wavefront sensing data are presented, as well as representative methods for designing treatment based on a combined data set of corneal topography and wavefront sensing. The goal of this section is to provide the readers with a fresh understanding of this new integrated approach, scientific principles, and a guide for clinical application in using topography- and wavefront-guided custom treatment.

Section IV: Specific Topographic Systems presents the principles and applications of the representative corneal topographic systems on the market today. Each chapter describes one commercially available corneal topography system, and its unique attributes and guide for clinical use. Ample clinical examples are provided in this section for each system, which give the reader a complete list and easy searching ability for references and clinical examples.

This book serves as a comprehensive clinical guide for not only the traditional corneal topographers such as the Placido disk systems (Humphrey Atlas, Magellan Mapper, Tracey-EyeSys, Optikon, Tomey, and Topcon) and the elevational and optical slit-scanning systems (Parks and Orbscan), but also the latest topographic technologies such as ultrasonic topographic system (Artemis), 3-D checker board topography (AstraMax), and the more recent Scheimpflug 360 rotational slit scanning systems (Pentacam and Precisio).

The book concludes with a chapter that looks into the future of corneal topography. It suggests that through a combined approach of all available imaging systems, we may truly approach the "holy grail" of vision surgery: optimizing vision in our patients without introducing surgically induced aberrations.

It is my desire that *Corneal Topography in the Wavefront Era: A Guide for Clinical Application* will serve as an important and useful desk reference for all ophthalmologists and optometrists from around the world in their medical and surgical ophthalmic care of their patients.

SECTION I

BASIC TOPOGRAPHIC PRINCIPLES

Chapter 1

History of Topography

Tracy Swartz, OD, MS; Renzo Mattioli, PhD;
Nancy K. Tripoli, MA; Doug Horner, OD, PhD; and Ming Wang, MD, PhD

The interface of air with the tear layer on the human cornea accounts for approximately two-thirds of the eye's refractive power. The typical cornea is responsible for 43 of the 60 diopters (D) of the refractive power of the eye. The average radius of curvature, 7.8 mm, generates the majority of the refractive power of the cornea (about +48.00 D). The posterior surface, with its concave shape and stromal index similar to that of the aqueous, contributes about –5.00 D. In addition, the majority of astigmatism originates from the corneal shape. It is not surprising that great effort has been put forth to measure this surface of the eye.

A normal cornea is not spherical but rather *aspherotorical*, vaguely like a bell with flat sides that have been slightly "squeezed" vertically. "With-the-rule" (wherein the vertical axis is steeper and horizontal axis flatter) corneal astigmatism from around 0.50 D to 1.00 D is usually compensated by the natural tilt of the crystalline lens. The central 6 to 7 mm "apical cap" is ellipsoidal, with nearly constant curvature only at its apex. The surrounding periphery is considerably flatter. And finally, in some corneas, a small steep junction to the limbus (like the bell's edge) can be found.

Corneal curvature measurement has been the subject of study since Father Christoph Scheiner's works on the human eye (in 1619). Ophthalmologists have tried to measure corneal topographic characteristics for over 150 years, when A. Placido designed the keratoscopy target still in use today.

Two techniques, *keratometry* and *keratoscopy*, were used during the last century before merging into the present-day computer-assisted video keratography or, as it is commonly called, *corneal topography* (CT). A comprehensive review can help us understand the real meaning of keratometric readings and topographic color maps.

HISTORY OF KERATOMETRY

In 1796, Ramsden created a telescope to magnify images reflected off the cornea to measure corneal curvature. Magnification of the reflected images also magnifies the normal instability of eye movements that become a serious issue in making accurate measurements. Ramsden is credited with developing a doubling device that eliminates the problems arising from normal instability of eye movements.

Not until 1839 was another such instrument used, when Kohlrausch used a telescope with adjustable mires. In 1881, Javal and Schiotz improved the instrument by using mires that were adjustable in size, and this model is still used clinically as the Haag-Streit ophthalmometer (Haag-Streit USA Inc, Mason, OH). The modern configuration is shown in Figure 1-1. Since this and similar instruments measure the curvature and astigmatism of the cornea, they were retitled "keratometers." Bausch & Lomb improved on the keratometer in 1932 by adding a Scheiner's disk to improve focusing mechanisms, circular mires, and the ability to measure two meridians simultaneously. This model essentially remains unchanged in current Bausch & Lomb and Reichert models. Such instruments are designed to measure the size of an image reflected off a convex surface using illuminated mires, a magnifying telescope, and a doubling prism.

Keratometry measurements are typically written in diopters. However, keratometers do not actually measure refractive power. They measure radius of curvature of the central 3 mm of the cornea. The formula for calculating the corneal radius treats the cornea as a spherical reflecting surface:

$$\frac{h'}{h} = \frac{-f}{x}$$

where *h'* is the linear image size; *h* is the linear object size, *f* is the focal length and *x* is the distance from mires to the convex mirror focal plane. Note that focal length, *f*, of a spherical refracting surface is *r/2*, and the equation then becomes:

$$\frac{h'}{h} = \frac{-r}{-2x}$$

where *r* is the mirror radius of curvature. The distance from the mires to the image approximates the distance from the mires to the focal plane of the spherical convex mirror (*x*), resulting in the following formula:

$$\frac{h'}{h} = \frac{-r}{-2d}$$

The distance *d* is fixed in most instruments. For example, it is 75 mm for the Reichert keratometer (Reichert Ophthalmic Instruments, Depew, NY). In Reichert and similar keratometers, the mire separation (*h*) is constant, and the size of the image (*h'*) is measured. Microscopic eye movements make this measurement problematic, so a doubling system is employed. A moveable prism is used to form a doubled image of the mires such that one image is displaced from the other, and then manually aligned. The distance required to align the images is equal to the size of one image (*h'*), allowing calculation of *r*. Eye movements are minimized because they affect both mires equally.

The radius to diopter conversion requires the following equation:

$$F = \frac{(n'-n)}{r}$$

where *F* is the corneal surface power in diopters; *n'* is the corneal index of refraction; *n* is the refractive index surrounding medium (for air, *n* = 1.0), and *r* is the corneal radius of curvature in meters.

Javal's index of 1.3375 has become the standard corneal refractive index used. Note that the anterior tear film surface index is closer to 1.376. Because the Javal ophthalmometer as well as Bausch & Lomb keratometer were designed to measure the total corneal power, this reduced index accounts for the negative power contribution of the posterior corneal surface.

Keratometers acquire data from a central annular zone of the cornea, which may vary in size depending on the curvature and instrument. In the Reichert keratometer, the annulus is approximately 0.1 mm wide, and the diameter varies from 2.8 mm (in a 48.00 D cornea) to 3.5 (in a 37.00 D cornea). It is important to remember the following assumptions related to keratometry[1]:

1. The formula used is based on spherical geometry. The cornea however is not spherical but is a prolate (flattened) ellipsoid. Thus, the central radius is slightly steeper than actually measured.

2. Keratometry is based on four data points within the central 3 mm of the cornea. It provides no insight

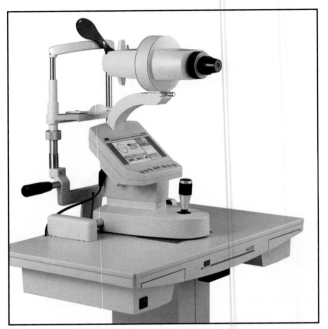

Figure 1-1. Haag-Streit ophthalmometer.

into the area inside or outside of the 3 mm ring.

3. Keratometry theory assumes paraxial optics. While the approximation may be clinically acceptable for fitting contacts or estimating corneal astigmatism, it may not be when measuring peripheral curvature.

4. Keratometers assume alignment of the corneal apex, line of sight, and instrument axis. However, this rarely occurs during actual measurement.

5. The formula used to calculate the radius (*r*) approximates the distance to the convex focal point, which in the case of the Reichert keratometer, may introduce up to 0.12 D of error. This error may increase if the instrument is not correctly focused or the operator accommodates during measurement.

6. Since the indexes may differ between manufacturers, one must be careful when comparing the readings in diopters between different instruments.

7. Reichert and similar keratometers are "one position" instruments, able to measure two meridians 90 degrees apart without moving the instrument position. While this allows for quick measurement, it decreases the clinician's ability to measure irregular astigmatism. The Haag-Streit ophthalmometer must be rotated to measure each meridian, allowing the clinician to better detect irregular astigmatism at the expense of efficiency.

Modern corneal topographers calculate a simulated keratometry reading that incorporates the same paraxial assumptions of traditional keratometry. These "simulated

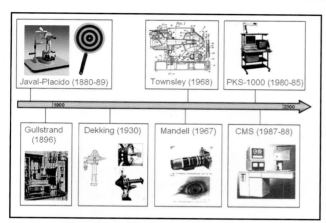

Figure 1-2. Topography timeline.

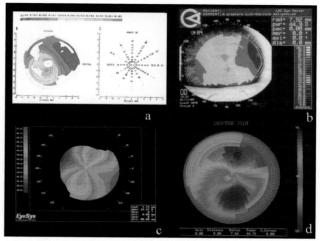

Figure 1-3. Early topographic maps.

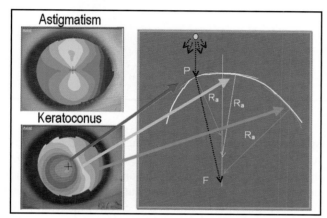

Figure 1-4. The colors of each point in an axial map represent the power associated with a sphere centered on the VK axis.

K" readings have been enriched by reporting curvature along "semi-meridians" of the steepest and flattest meridians at different zones (usually 3, 5, and 7 mm) to evaluate irregular astigmatism in the peripheral cornea.

KERATOSCOPY, CORNEAL TOPOGRAPHY, AND ITS COLOR MAPS

In 1880, A. Placido devised his keratoscopy target, a flat disk with alternating black and white rings. Soon after, in 1889, Javal attempted to give a quantitative measure of the corneal shape by placing Placido disks into his ophthalmometer, behind the arc that carried the ophthalmometric mires.[2] Although the actual inventor of the first photokeratoscope is still a matter of discussion,[3] it was Allvar Gullstrand who developed the algorithms for the first description of corneal topography based on quantitative measurements. In a paper published in 1896, part of

the work that earned him a Nobel prize in 1911, Gullstrand[4] followed Javal's suggestion to develop a method of using a measuring microscope described as a "dividing engine" to determine the distance between two points on a keratoscopic photograph. Instantaneous radius of curvature was deduced from Gullstrand's measurement through an arc-step algorithm, and the corneal meridian profiles that he was able to plot are surprisingly similar to those from modern computerized CT.

It took about 90 years for photokeratoscopy to enter the computer age. A timeline is shown in Figure 1-2. During those 90 years, several people contributed to the development of modern corneal topography. These include Dekking,[5] who in 1930 devised the first "cone," and Bonnet,[6] who in 1964 edited a book on corneal topography reporting elevation maps obtained by stereo-photographic measurement of eyes sprayed with talcum, a technique more recently replaced by fluorescein.[7] Mandell published several works on corneal shape models and contact lens fitting in the 1960s.[8–10] In 1979, Kuyama[11] made 3D isometric computerized maps, which were subsequently adopted by Sun/Nidek PKS-1000.

A major step in the clinical utility of corneal topography was the introduction of color-coded power maps. Several early maps are shown in Figure 1-3. The first two-dimensional, color-coded map was published by Maguire et al,[12] and this is shown in Figure 1-3A. Following the introduction of Maguire's map, fully integrated commercial computer assisted videokeratoscopes such as the CMS (Figure 1-3B) and TMS-1 (Computed Anatomy, New York, NY), the EyeSys CTS (Figure 1-3C) (EyeSys Technologies, Houston, TX), and the VISIO (Figure 1-3D) (Visioptic, Inc., Houston, TX) introduced maps in which each point in the cornea was assigned a color according to its power (Figure 1-4).

Figure 1-5. Classical "bow tie" image associated with astigmatism.

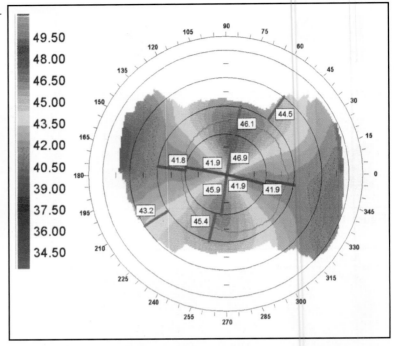

As corneal topography moved from a scientific curiosity to a clinical tool, disputes arose over what quantities were scientifically logical, most valuable for applications, most easily understood by clinicians, and ultimately most useful. A parallel set of disputes concerned the terminology for types of instruments, measurements, maps, and algorithms. It is not surprising that eye professionals confused types of maps with the algorithms that created them. False theoretical limits on some methodologies were assumed because of the limited computing power of earlier PCs. Much of the confusion could have been avoided by an earlier understanding of the relationship between measuring corneal shape and measuring corneal optics, and by recognizing the clinical potential of keratoscopy.

The Axial Map

For many keratoscopes designed in the mid-1980s, axial power was the primary quantity extracted from the raw data. As seen in Figure 1-4, the values and colors of each point P in an axial map represent the power associated to a sphere, Ra, having the same slant as the cornea and therefore refracting a ray of light in the same way at each point P. The assumption regarding the index used (1.3375) is similar to that of keratometry. The axial map is more a descriptor of corneal optics than shape.

The axial map is a traditional but poor descriptor of corneal refraction because it does not take into account spherical aberration.[13,14] Nor is the axial map a descriptor of shape. At each point P in Figure 1-4, the curvature and height of the centered sphere are not the same as the curvature and height of the cornea, and the discrepancy increases toward the periphery. Therefore, the axial map distorts shape. For example, in Figure 1-4, the map at the bottom left shows a wide red area that indicates a keratoconic cone. However, the size of the cone is exaggerated, and increasing the resolution of the depiction would not increase the map detail.

The axial map has some utility as a simple descriptor of corneal astigmatism, including cylinder, axis, and irregularity. The example at the top-left in Figure 1-4 and Figure 1-5 shows the classical "bow-tie" or "hourglass." The vertical "yellow-orange" axis of symmetry of the hourglass is the steeper meridian.

Despite its limitations, the axial map became known as "the corneal topography map" because of two factors. First, keratoscopes were thought of as merely Javal ophthalmometers or keratometers newly capable of measuring a larger corneal area with greater precision. In other words, they were used to assess the need for simple optical correction of optics. They were not intended to measure more sophisticated optical aberrations, much less the physical shape of the cornea. Second, the calculation of axial power from reflective data required only simple algorithms.[15–17]

THE "REVOLUTION" AROUND YEARS 1993–1996: NEW ALGORITHMS AND MAPS

The calculus required for data analysis was the limiting factor for several years following introduction of computer-assisted corneal topography. Since axial power was computed by algorithms[17,18] that did not reconstruct the physical surface of the cornea, it was thought impossible to extract accurate corneal height and instantaneous curvature from Placido disk images.[19] There were authors who proposed alternative algorithms. El Hage used a differential equation whose coefficients were fitted by polynomials.[20] Doss et al proposed an algorithm that attempted to overcome some of the spherical bias.[21] Wang et al proposed the first arc-step method,[22] van Saarloos proposed an alternative arc-step,[23] and Klein's more sophisticated algorithm[24] used parabolas instead of arcs. The three arc-step algorithms demonstrated that long-forgotten Gullstrand methods could not only approximate axial power, but also measure corneal shape. Unfortunately these approaches could not be practically implemented without further technical developments. The major challenge to implementing an arc-step algorithm was to calculate "local" quantities with high resolution while (1) controlling the "noise" that made maps inaccurate and non-reproducible, and (2) confining the calculus complexity to stay within the limits of available computer power.[23]

In the early to mid-1990s, the explosion of excimer laser refractive surgery necessitated more accurate instruments and more detailed representation of the corneal surface. The previous evaluation of keratoscopes on spheres[17,25–27] did not reflect their suitability for use in surgical design. The first evaluations made on aspheric test surfaces by Roberts,[28] Cohen, Tripoli et al,[29–32] and Carones et al[33] in 1993–1995 revealed the inadequacy of spherically biased methods for measuring height and curvature, especially in the periphery. It also became evident that the use of an appropriate arc-step algorithm on Placido disk images, rather than being impossible, was quite accurate (less or around 1 micron) for measuring corneal height and curvature.

Once released from the over-simplicity of axial power, instrument makers quickly developed new, useful quantities. An instantaneous curvature map, calculated by an arc-step algorithm, was introduced[34–36] by the Keratron (Optikon 2000, Rome, Italy). An example is shown in Figure 1-6. Curvature maps were soon adopted by most keratoscopes under different names (eg, instantaneous, true, IROC, local, tangential, or meridional).[a]

After the curvature map was introduced in keratoscopes, it quickly revealed its role as an accurate descriptor of corneal shape.[38] Along a meridional section of the cornea (Figure 1-7, right side), each zone has a center of curvature that is not on the corneal axis, except at the vertex. Without axial constraints, the curvature map can track and display all transitions between flat and steep zones and reveal any local distortions, from the center to the extreme periphery.[b]

The maps in Figure 1-7 illustrate the clinical value of the curvature map's depiction of detail. In both maps, the green-blue transition (circle a, about 7 to 8 mm in size) reveals an abrupt change of curvature delimiting the "apical zone"[38] or "optical cap." Bier's primitive cornea model described this zone in 1955[39] and defined the periphery around it as a "negative zone" in curvature. Actually this annular region may be very flat, but never goes to concavity. Information about corneal shape that cannot be seen in the axial map is revealed: (a) indicates the size of the "corneal cap," (b) the size of the keratoconus apex, (c) the surrounding flat zone, and (d) a mild warpage induced by normal lid pressure.

Curvature maps in Figure 1-8 show the degeneration of the cap with increasing keratoconus.

A power, or refractive map, where power is calculated according to ray tracing (Figure 1-9) was proposed at the same time by Roberts, and first introduced by EyeSys in the Holladay diagnostic summary.[40] In 1996 Barsky and others proposed a Gaussian curvature map[41–42], similar to that shown in Figure 1-10. Its purpose was to overcome a limit of both axial and instantaneous curvature maps. Since axial and instantaneous maps were based on a center, they did not retain the same appearance on eccentric corneas if the patient changed fixation. Unfortunately, the Gaussian map hides astigmatism, a clinically important feature. For this reason Barsky proposed overlaid arrows to represent the amount and direction of astigmatism at each point (as seen in the bottom left map in Figure 1-9). Though the Gaussian map is not common on commercial keratoscopes, it might yet find a useful application, such as in intraoperative situations when the patient cannot fixate.

---

a In their proposed standards, the ANSI committee has recently qualified the curvature map as "meridional curvature" to distinguish it from Gaussian and other non-directional measures. Unfortunately "meridional," besides being an uncommon term, neglects a more important distinction between curvature and axial power, both of which are measured along meridians. Therefore, while waiting for an eventual acceptance by CT manufacturers and by ISO, we will refer only to "curvature" in this text.

b Although the precise boundaries and terminology of the "zones" are controversial among authors in the clinical literature, they are usually referred to as a change in the corneal curvature.

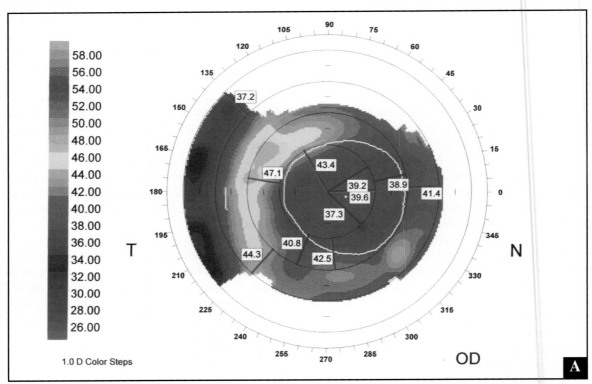

Figure 1-6A. An instantaneous curvature map showing a patient S/P myopic LASIK.

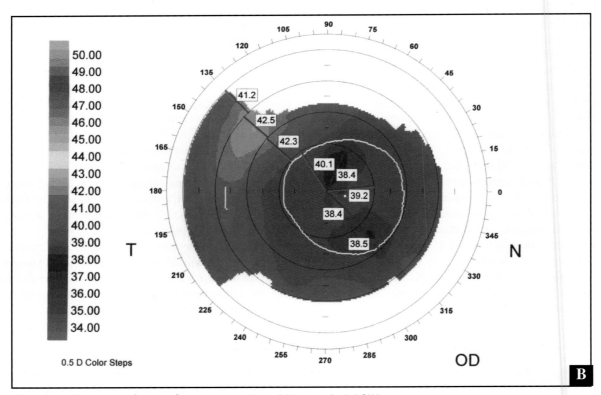

Figure 1-6B. An axial map showing a patient S/P myopic LASIK.

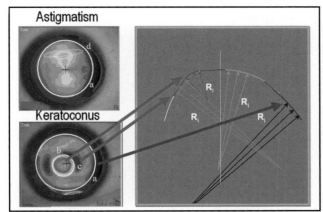

Figure 1-7. Instantaneous map's attention to corneal shape detail.

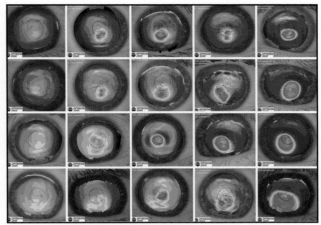

Figure 1-8. Progression of keratoconus shape in a number of different patients.

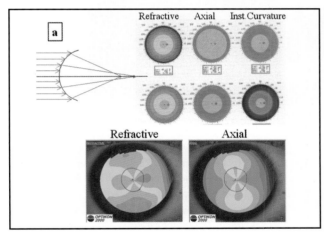

Figure 1-9. The refractive map: power is calculated according to ray tracing. (Courtesy of Dr. Cynthia Roberts.)

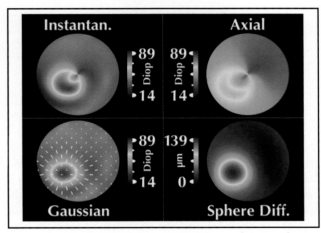

Figure 1-10. Gaussian map. (Courtesy of B. Barsky.)

Corneal surface reconstruction algorithms also made accurate measurement of corneal height feasible. Since a representation of absolute height from a plane would have little meaning, the quantity is generally shown in "spherical offset" maps. Construction is illustrated in Figure 1-11. The colors represent the height of the cornea with respect to a reference sphere, measured in a direction parallel to the axis. The points that are above the sphere appear in orange-red and those below the sphere are green-blue. This universally accepted color convention in corneal topography was inspired by geographic topography, in which warm colors represent hills and mountains and blue shades are sea depth. An alternative format of height representation is the *fluorescein map*, available in contact lens software modules of most corneal topographers, which can simulate fitting of spherical, aspherical, or toric contact lenses. An example of this can be seen in Figure 1-12.

Although description of this map is beyond the scope of this chapter, it can be a valuable tool for the clinical interpretation of corneal shape.

SUMMARY

Corneal topography has become an invaluable tool in ophthalmology due to advancements in technology and its application to refractive surgery. Newest advances include indexes for diagnosis of corneal diseases such as keratoconus, evaluation of the posterior cornea and other anterior segment structures, pachymetry measurement, and calculations for intraocular lens (IOL) measurements. Interpretation of maps such as those reviewed briefly in this chapter is a learned skill, and it is the goal of this book

Figure 1-11. Construction of an elevation map.

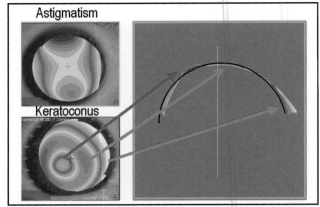

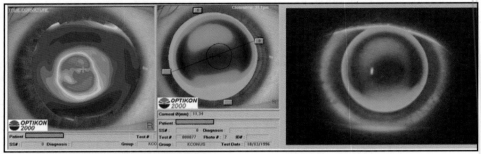

Figure 1-12. RGP simulation of fluorescein pattern

to educate the reader to better understand topography and its value in clinical decision-making. What follows is a review of corneal anatomy and optical properties, a technical review of the technology, map presentation and scaling, and in-depth information on system specific parameters, including using topography in refractive surgery.

REFERENCES

1. Horner DG, Salmon TO, Soni PS. Corneal topography. In: Benjamin WJ, Ed. *Borish's Clinical Refraction.* Philadelphia, PA: WB Saunders Company; 1998.

2. Reynolds A. Introduction: History of corneal measurement. In: Schanzlin D, Robin J, eds. *Corneal Topography Measuring and Modifying the Cornea.* New York: Springer-Verlag; 1991:vii–x.

3. Levene JR. The true inventors of the keratoscope and photo-keratoscope. *The British Journal for the History of Science Vol. 2.* 1965;8:324–342.

4. Gullstrand A. Photographic-ophthalmometric and clinical investigations of corneal refraction. *Am J Optom Arch Am Acad Optom.* 1966;43:143–214.

5. Dekking H. *Fotografie der cornea opperwlatke Assen.* Groninque th.med 1930 No. 2, Van Gorcum, im Bcm, 91, 360 (1930) no. 271; 1930.

6. Bonnet R, Le Grand Y, Rapilly C. *La Topographie Corneenne.* Paris, France: N. Desroches; 1964.

7. Warnicki JW, Rehkopf PG, Arrfa RC, Stuart JC. Corneal topography using a projected grid. In: Schanzlin D, Robin J, eds. *Corneal Topography Measuring and Modifying the Cornea.* New York: Springer-Verlag; 1991:25–32.

8. Mandell RB. Keratometry and contact lens practice. *The Optometric Weekly.* 1965;May 6:69–75.

9. Mandell RB. Corneal contour of the human infant. *Arch Ophthalmol.* 1967;77:345–348.

10. Mandell RB. Mathematical model of the corneal contour. *Brit J Physiol Opt.* 1971;26(3):183-197.

11. Kuyama H, Sasamoto K, Maruyama S, Itoi M. A new photokeratometer for contact lens in clinic. *J Jpn C L Soc.* 1979;21(3):80–84.

12. Maguire LJ, Singer DE, Kylce SD. Graphic presentation of computer-analyzed keratoscope photographs. *Arch Ophthalmol.* 1987;105:223–230.

13. Klein SA. A corneal topography algorithm that produces continuous curvature. *Optom Vis Sci.* 1992;69:829–834.

14. Roberts C. The accuracy of "power" maps to display curvature data in corneal topography systems. *Invest Ophthalmol Vis Sci.* 1994;35:3524–3532.

15. Gersten M, Mammone RJ, Brunswick NJ, Larchmont NY. *System for Topographical Modeling of Anatomical Surfaces.* US patent Nr. 4,863,260. Sep. 5, 1989.

16. Olsen T. On the calculation of power from curvature of the cornea. *Br Journ Ophthalmol.* 1986;70:152–154.

17. Koch DD, Foulks GN, Moran CT, Wakil JS. The corneal EyeSys system: accuracy analysis and reproducibility of first-generation prototype. *J Refract Corneal Surg.* 1989;6:423–429.

18. Gersten M, Mammone RJ, Brunswick NJ, Larchmont NY. System for topographical modeling of anatomical surfaces. US patent Nr. 4,863,260 Sep. 5, 1989. A radially aspheric surface. *J Refract Corneal Surg.* 1994;10:103-116.

19. Wilson SE, Wang JY, Klyce SD. Quantification and mathematical analysis of photokeratoscopic images. In: Shanzlin DJ, Robin JB, eds. *Corneal Topography: Measuring and Modifying the Cornea.* New York: Springer-Verlag; 1991:1–9.

20. El Hage SG. The computerized corneal topographer EH-270. In: Shanzlin DJ, Robin JB, eds. *Corneal Topography: Measuring and Modifying the Cornea.* New York: Springer-Verlag; 1991:11–24.

21. Doss JD, Hutson RL, Rowsey JJ, Brown R. Method for calculation of corneal profile and power distribution. *Arch Ophthalmol.* 1981;99:1261–1265.

22. Wang J, Rice DA, Klyce SD. A new reconstruction algorithm for improvement of corneal topographical analysis. *J Corn Refract Surg.* 1989;5:379–387.

23. van Saarloos PP, Constable IJ. Improved method for calculation of corneal topography for any photokeratoscopic geometry. *Optom and Vis Sci.* 1991;68:957–965.

24. Klein SA. A corneal topography algorithm that produces continuous curvature. *Optom Vis Sci.* 1002;69:829–834.

25. Wang J, Rice DA, Klyce SD. A new reconstruction algorithm for improvement of corneal topographical analysis. *J Corn Refract Surg.* 1989;5:379–387.

26. Hannush SB, Crawford SL, Waring GO III, Gemmill MC, Lynn MJ, Nizam A. Accuracy and precision of keratometry, photokeratoscopy and corneal modeling on calibrated steel balls. *Arch Ophthalmol.* 1989;107:1235–1239.

27. Maguire LJ, Wilson SE, Camp JJ, Verity S. Evaluating the reproducibility of topography systems on spherical surfaces. *Arch Ophthalmol.* 1993;111:259–262.

28. Wilson SE, Verity SM, Conger DL. Accuracy and precision of the corneal analysis system and the topographic modeling system. *Cornea.* 1992;11:28–35.

29. Roberts C. Characterization of the inherent error in a spherically-biased corneal topography system in mapping a radially aspheric surface. *J Refract Corneal Surg.* 1994;10:103–116.

30. Cohen KL, Tripoli NK, Holmgren DE, Coggins JM. Assessment of the power and height of radial aspheres reported by a computer-assisted keratoscope. *Am J Ophthalmol.* 1995;119:723–732.

31. Cohen KL, Tripoli NK, Holmgren DE, Coggins JM. Assessment of the height of radial aspheres reported by a computer-assisted keratoscope. *Invest Ophthalmol Vis Sci* (suppl). 1993;34:1217.

32. Tripoli NK, Cohen KL, Holmgren DE, Coggins JM. Assessment of radial aspheres by the Keratron keratoscope using an arc-step algorithm. *Am J Ophthalmol.* 1995;120:658–664.

33. Tripoli NK, Cohen KL, Obla P, Coggins JM, Holmgren DE. Height measurement of astigmatic test surfaces by a keratoscope that uses plane geometry reconstruction. *Am J Ophthalmol.* 1996;121:668–676.

34. Carones F, Gobbi PG, Brancato R, Venturi E. Comparison between two computer-assisted keratoscopes in measuring aspheric surfaces. *Invest Ophthalmol Vis Sci* (suppl) 1994:3748.

35. Brancato R, Carones F. *Topografia corneale computerizzata.* Milan, Italy: Fogliazza; 1994.

36. Mattioli R, Carones F, Cantera E. New algorithms to improve the reconstruction of corneal geometry on the Keratrontm videokeratographer. *Invest Ophthalmol Vis Sci.* 1995;36(suppl):1400.

37. Mattioli R, Tripoli, N. Corneal geometry reconstruction with the Keratron videokeratographer. *Optom Vis Sci.* 1997;74:881–894.

38. Brancato R, Carones F. *Topografia corneale computerizzata.* Milan, Italy: Fogliazza; 1994.

39. Kraff CR, Robin JB. Normal corneal topography. In: Shanzlin DJ, Robin JB, eds. *Corneal Topography: Measuring and Modifying the Cornea.* New York: Springer-Verlag; 1991:33-38.

40. Bier N. A study of the cornea in relation to contact lens practice. *Am J Optom.* 1956;33(6):291-304.

41. Holladay JT. Corneal topography using the Holladay diagnostic summary. *J Cataract Refract Surg.* 1997;23:209–221.

42. Barsky BA; Klein SA; Garcia DD. Gaussian power, mean sphere, and cylinder representations for corneal maps with applications to the diagnosis of keratoconus. *Invest Ophthalmol Vis Sci.* 1996;37(suppl):558.

43. Barsky B, Klein S, Garcia D. Gaussian power with cylinder vector field topography maps. *Optom Vis Sci.* 1997;74:917–925.

Anatomy and Physiology of the Cornea

Keming Yu, MD, PhD; Tracy Swartz, OD, MS; Helen Boerman, OD; and Ming Wang, MD, PhD

The cornea serves as the window of external images to the eye. Its characteristics of clarity and curvature are the most important principal requirements for its physiologic functions. The avascular cornea, together with the sclera, forms the outer shell of the eyeball, provides strong mechanical protection for the inner contents, and maintains the ocular contour.

The cornea is responsible for two-thirds of the total refractive power of the eye. Any slight change in the cornea contour changes the refractive error. Small focal changes of corneal smoothness or corneal tissue may produce visual distortion.

Maintenance of corneal transparency depends on the architecture of the stroma and a functional endothelium and epithelium. The cornea is a transparent, avascular tissue exposed to the external environment. The anterior corneal surface is covered by the tear film, and the posterior surface is directly bathed by the aqueous humor. The cornea is continuous with the opaque sclera and semitransparent conjunctiva. The transitional zone between cornea and sclera is the richly vascularized limbus, which contains a reservoir of pluripotential stem cells.

The shape of the anterior corneal surface is convex and aspheric. The adult cornea measures approximately 12 mm horizontally and 11 mm vertically. It is approximately 0.55 mm thick at the center, and increases gradually toward the periphery of the cornea where it is about 0.7 mm thick.

The radius of curvature of the corneal surface is not constant over the entire surface. It is steepest at the center of the cornea, and becomes flatter in the periphery. The average radius of curvature of the anterior corneal surface is about 7.8 mm (6.7 to 9.4 mm). The posterior surface is about 6.5 mm, and the central 3 mm optical zone of the cornea (where the surface is almost spherical) is about 7.5–8.0 mm.[1,2] The refractive power of anterior corneal surface and posterior surface is about +48.8 D and –5.8 D, respectively, and its absolute refractive power is about +43.0 D. The cornea thus contributes 74%, or 43.25 D, of the total 58.60 D of power of the normal human eye. The cornea is also responsible for most of the refractive astigmatism in the optical system.

OPTICAL PROPERTIES

The optical properties of the cornea are determined by the following factors: transparency, surface smoothness, contour, and refractive index. The arrangement of the collagen fibers in the cornea result in its clarity. Both the mean diameter of each collagen fiber and the mean distance between collagen fibers are quite homogenous and measure less than half of the wavelength of visible light (400 to 700 nm). The arrangement of collagen fibers is such that the incident ray scattered by each collagen fiber is cancelled by interference of other scattered rays,[3] which allows light to pass through the cornea.

The healthy and intact corneal epithelium and tear film play a crucial role in the maintenance of the cornea's smooth surface. Patients with dry eye syndrome suffer from the loss of proper lubrication, which may lead to superficial punctate keratopathy and a roughened corneal surface. If the corneal contour is altered due to pathological conditions, such as scarring, thinning, or keratoconus, irregular astigmatism results.

The total refractive index of cornea is 1.376. Light is most significantly refracted as it passes through the anterior surface. A refractive index of 1.3375 is used in calibrating the keratometer to account for the combined optical power of the anterior and posterior surfaces of the cornea.

CORNEAL VASCULAR SYSTEM

The cornea is one of the few avascular tissues in the body. This characteristic is the most important factor, as it is the way that the cornea maintains its transparency. The anterior ciliary artery, derived from the ophthalmic artery, forms a vascular arcade at the limbus. This arcade anastomoses with derivatives of the facial branch of the external carotid artery. Therefore, blood components in the cornea are supplied from both internal and external carotid arteries. Some corneal diseases cause vascularization of the cornea and induce loss of vision. Although a normal healthy cornea does not contain blood vessels, factors from the blood play various important roles in corneal metabolism and wound healing.

The cornea depends on glucose diffusing from the aqueous humor for nutrition. Oxygen is supplied primarily by diffusion from tear fluid. The direct exposure of the tear fluid to the atmosphere is essential for the supply of oxygen to the cornea. A small portion of the oxygen requirement is diffused from the aqueous humor and limbal circulation. The reduction of oxygen, as in long-term contact lens wear, may cause corneal hypoxia and stromal edema. Therefore, to avoid interference with corneal oxygenation, contact lens technology has been aimed at maximizing gas permeability. Eyelid exposure during sleep also decreases the amount of oxygen supplied to the cornea under normal physiologic conditions.

CORNEAL INNERVATON

The cornea is one of the most heavily innervated and most sensitive tissues in the body. The density of nerve endings in the cornea is the highest in the body, yielding a sensitivity of the cornea 100 times that of the conjunctiva. The cornea has two major nerve supplies: sensory innervation via fibers from the ophthalmic division of the trigeminal nerve (CN 5), whose cell bodies lie in the trigeminal ganglion, and sympathetic innervation via fibers whose cell bodies lie in the superior cervical ganglion. In terms of the quantity, the number of corneal sensory axons is greater than the number of sympathetic axons.

The nasociliary nerve, which arises from the ophthalmic division of the trigeminal ganglion, leaves the medial superior border of the trigeminal ganglion and enters the orbit through the superior orbital fissure. There it runs inferiorly and somewhat temporally to the superior rectus muscle, and just over the top of the optic nerve. The nasociliary nerve branches before it penetrates the sclera, so that one to three long ciliary nerves may pierce the sclera several millimeters from the optic nerve. In their intraocular course, the nerves travel in the suprachoroidal space, where they branch several times to form a loose network. Within the suprachoroidal space, there is branching and possible exchange between the axons of the long ciliary nerves and those from the short ciliary nerves. Thus, as those intraocular branches reach the corneoscleral limbus, there are as many as 12 to 16 circumferentially arranged branches containing a mixed population of fibers of sympathetic, as well as sensory, origin. Recurrent branches around the circumference innervate the conjunctiva bordering the limbus, as well as the limbal corneal epithelium. After entering the cornea, nerve trunks run in a quasiradial direction through the middle third of the stroma. They then branch anteriorly, forming a dense subepithelial plexus, and the nerves penetrate Bowman's layer and to innervate the corneal epithelium. Neurotransmitters in the cornea include acetylcholine, catecholamines, substance P, and calcitonin gene-related peptide.

MICROSCOPIC ANATOMY AND PHYSIOLOGY

The cornea can be divided into five layers: the epithelium, Bowman's layer, stroma, Descemet's membrane, and the endothelium. A microscopic section is seen in Figure 2-1. Although the tear film is not part of the cornea, it is intimately associated with the cornea anatomically and functionally.

The anterior surface of the cornea is covered by a layer of tear film. The most important function of the tear film is to protect the corneal epithelium. The tear film consists of three layers: a superficial lipid layer, an aqueous layer, and a mucin layer. The lipid layer is derived from meibomian gland secretions that retard water evaporation. The mucin layer is secreted by conjunctival goblet cells. The aqueous layer is produced primarily by the lacrimal glands located in the superior temporal orbit.[3] If the function of the lacrimal glands is affected due to an autoimmune disease—such as Sjögren's syndrome—severe dry eye will occur.[4] The total thickness of the tear film is about 7 μm. The respective thicknesses of the lipid layer, aqueous layer, and mucin layer are about 0.1 μm, 7 μm, and 0.05 μm.[5]

The volume of tear fluid is about 6.5 ± 0.3 μl.[6] The tear fluid contains various biologically important factors such as electrolytes, glucose, immunoglobulins, lactoferrin, lysosome, albumin, and oxygen. It also contains various kinds of biologically active substances such as prostaglandins, histamine, growth factors, and interleukins.[7,8] Therefore, the tear film serves not only as a

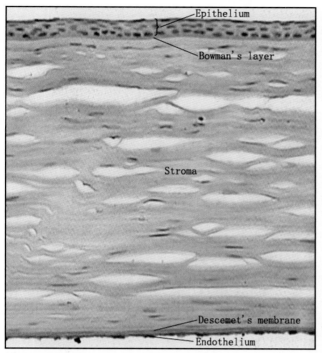

Figure 2-1. Microscopic section of the cornea.

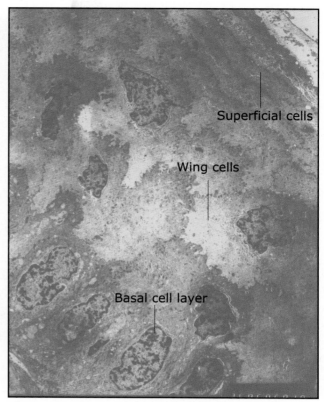

Figure 2-2. Layers of the corneal epithelium.

lubricant and nutritional source for the corneal epithelium, but also as the source of the regulatory factors for the maintenance and repair of the corneal epithelium.[9–11]

The cornea is covered by a multilayered nonkeratinized squamous epithelium that develops from the embryonic surface ectoderm. The epithelium is continuous at the limbus with that of bulbar conjunctiva. The more superficial layers of the five- to six-layered epithelium are flattened, whereas the basal layer consists of cuboidal-cylindric cells. Between the overlying squamous epithelial cells and the basal layer are cells that show elongated cytoplasmic processes, which in sagittal sections resemble wings; hence, it is called the *wing-cell layer*. This is illustrated in Figure 2-2. The epithelial cells are connected to one another by intercellular bridges.

The corneal epithelium is composed of stratified squamous epithelial cells and makes up about 5% (0.05 mm) of the total corneal thickness. The epithelium and tear film form an optically smooth surface. Tight junctions between superficial epithelial cells prevent penetration of tear fluid into the stroma. Continuous proliferation of perilimbal basal epithelial cells gives rise to the other layers that subsequently differentiate into superficial cells. With maturation, these cells become coated with microvilli on their outermost surface and then desquamate into the tears. This process of differentiation takes about 7 to 14 days. Basal

epithelial cells secrete a continuous, 50 nm thick, basement membrane composed of type IV collagen, laminin, and other proteins. Beneath the superficial cells are two to three layers of wing cells.

The columnar, cuboidal, single layer of basal cells is 18 to 20 μm high and 8 to 10 μm in diameter. Basal cells adhere to the basement membrane via hemidesmosomes that are linked to anchoring fibrils of type VII collagen.[12] They represent the germinative layer of the epithelium. Basal cells are a source of wing cells and superficial cells.

The basement membrane is secreted and derived from basal cells of corneal epithelium. It is about 40 to 60 nm thick. It has two important functions: it forms the scaffold for the organization of the epithelium, and it is a boundary that separates the epithelium from the stromal layer.[13]

Bowman's membrane is a layer of randomly arrayed collagen fibrils that merge into the more organized anterior stroma. Bowman's layer is not a membrane, but a simple condensation of collagen fibers and proteoglycans. It is an acellular membrane-like zone that is observed by light microscopy at the interface between the corneal epithelium and the corneal stroma. It is prominent in primates.

While other mammals have a similar zone, it is very thin (about 12 μm thick). Bowman's membrane plays an important role in the maintenance of the epithelial structure. It does not regenerate after injury.

The stroma is the main portion of the cornea. It occupies more than 90% of the total thickness of the cornea. The characteristics of the cornea, such as its transparency, constancy, shape, and physical strength are principally based on the anatomic and biochemical characteristics of the corneal stroma. Beneath the acellular Bowman's layer, the corneal stroma is composed of an extracellular matrix composed of collagen, proteoglycans, keratocytes, and nerve fibers. The cellular components occupy only 2% to 3% of the total volume of the stroma.[14] Type I and Type V fibrillar collagens are intertwined by filaments of Type VI collagen, as shown in Figure 2-3. The major corneal proteoglycan is decorin and the concentrations and ratios of proteoglycans vary from anterior to posterior surfaces.

Optimal corneal optics requires a smooth surface with a healthy tear film and epithelium. Clarity of the cornea depends on tight packing of epithelial cells to produce a layer with a nearly uniform refractive index and minimal light scatter. The regular arrangement of stromal cells and macromolecules is also necessary for a clear cornea. Keratocytes vary in density and size throughout the stroma. These corneal fibroblasts continually digest and manufacture stromal molecules. Stromal cells do not regenerate after injury.

Descemet's membrane serves as the basement membrane of the endothelium, and is secreted by the endothelium. It gradually increases in thickness from birth (3 μm) to adulthood (8 to 10 μm). Descemet's membrane is composed primarily of collagen type IV, and is resistant to enzymatic degradation. In certain corneal ulcerations, such as bacterial keratitis, Descemet's membrane remains intact and protrudes under the action of intraocular pressure. When Descemet's membrane is ruptured by an injury, aqueous humor penetrates into the corneal stroma and results in stromal edema. It does not regenerate.

The corneal endothelium is a single layer of hexagonal cells that covers the posterior surface of Descemet's membrane in a well-arranged mosaic pattern, as shown in Figure 2-4. Endothelial cells are about 5 μm thick and 20 μm wide. In a normal cornea, the dimensions of the endothelium are quite uniform. The density of the endothelium is about 3,500 cells/mm^2 in a young adult. Endothelial cells have a large nucleus and contain abundant cytoplasmic organelles. It does not proliferate in humans and many other animals, such as monkeys and cats, but it does proliferate in rabbits. The most important physiologic function of the corneal endothelium is to regulate the water content of the corneal stroma by ion transport systems.

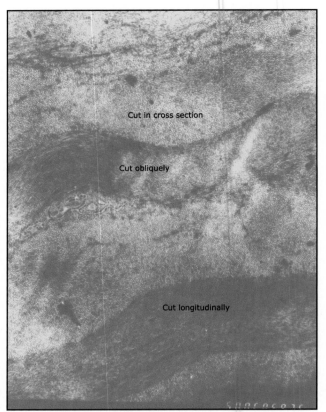

Figure 2-3. Collagen fibrils intertwined within the stroma.

The limbus is the transitional zone of the eye position between the transparent cornea and nontransparent sclera, which is about 1 mm wide. Stem cells located in the limbus are the important reservoir of corneal epithelial cells and respond to loss of corneal epithelium.

The highly specialized structure of the cornea is necessary for optical performance. Alteration of this structure by disease, trauma, age, or surgery will affect visual performance. Physical examination by slit lamp biomicroscopy and topographic evaluation may identify corneal abnormalities. The following chapters detail topographic examination of the cornea as it relates to healthy eyes, common corneal diseases, and refractive surgery.

REFERENCES

1. Polack FM. Morphology of cornea. *Am J Ophthalmol.* 1961;51:1051.

2. Hogan MJ, Alvarado JA, Weddell JE. *Histology of the Human Eye.* Philadelphia, PA: WB Saunders; 1971.

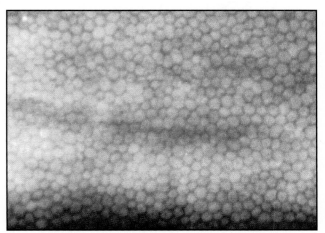

Figure 2-4. Hexagonal cell pattern of the corneal epithelium.

3. Records RE. Tear film. In: Records RE, ed. *Physiology of the Human Eye and Visual System.* New York, NY: Harper & Row; 1979:47.

4. Sjögren H, Block KK. Keratoconjunctivitis sicca and the Sjögren syndrome. *Surv Ophthalmol.* 1971;16:145.

5. Holly FJ, Lemp MA. Tear physiology and dry eyes. *Surv Ophthalmol.* 1977;22:69–87.

6. Scherz W, Doane MG, Dohlman CH. Tear volume in normal eyes and keratoconjunctivitis sicca. *Graefe's Arch Clin Exp Ophthalmol.* 1974;141–150.

7. Ohashi Y, et al. Presence of epidermal growth factor in human tears. *Invest Ophthalmol Vis Sci.* 1989; 30:1879–1882.

8. Van Setten G, Schultz G. Transforming growth factor-alpha is a constant component of human tear fluid. *Graefe's Arch Clin Exp Ophthalmol.* 1994;232:523–526.

9. Tsutsumi O, Tsutsumi A, Oka T. Epidermal growth factor-like, corneal wound healing substance in mouse tears. *J Clin Invest.* 1988;81:1067–1071.

10. Nishida T, Nakamura M, Mishma H, Otori T. Interleukin 6 promotes epithelial migration by a fibronectin-dependent mechanism. *J Cell Physiol.* 1992;153:1–5.

11. Nishida T. Extracellular matrix and growth factors in corneal wound healing.*Curr Opin Ophthalmol.* 1993; 4:4–13.

12. Gipson IK, Suprr-Michaud SJ, Tisdale AS. Anchoring fibrils from a complex network in human and rabbit cornea. *Invest Ophthalmol Vis Sci.* 1987;28:212–220.

13. Vracko R, Benditt EP. Basal lamina: the scaffold for orderly cell replacement. Observations on regeneration of injured skeletal muscle fibers and capillaries. *J Cell Biol.* 1972;55:406.

14. Otori T. Electrolyte content of rabbit cornea; straoma. *Exp Eye Res.* 1967;6:356–367.

The Optics of the Cornea

David Coward, OD; Tracy Swartz, OD, MS; and Ming Wang, MD, PhD

The cornea is the first structure that interacts with light as it is being transferred into the eye and contributes the greatest amount of refractive power. The cornea can be treated like an ophthalmic lens created from three different interfaces: tears, corneal tissue, and the aqueous humor. To calculate the power of the cornea, a thin lens formula can be used three times, once for each interface. The thin lens formula is:

$$F = (n - n^1)/r$$

where F is the total refractive power at the surface of the cornea, n is the refractive index of the first surface, and n^1 is the refractive index of the second surface. The radius, r, is the radius of curvature of the cornea in meters. For the average human cornea, the central anterior corneal radius of curvature is 7.8 mm and the posterior corneal radius of curvature is 6.5 mm. The indices of refraction are listed in Table 3-1.

When using the above thin lens equation, the tear–air interface power is 43.00. This first interface accounts for the majority of corneal power because the change in density from air to tears has the greatest differential. Using the thin lens equation for the tear–cornea interface and the cornea–aqueous humor interface, the resulting refractive powers are +5.10 D, and –6.20 D respectively. The total cornea power, calculated by combining these dioptric powers, is approximately +42.00 D for the average human cornea.[1]

PHYSICAL CONSIDERATIONS THAT REDUCE VISUAL ABERRATIONS

The majority of a patient's visual complaints arise from lower order aberrations, commonly known as refractive errors. Defocus is considered absent when the punctum remotum of the eye is at infinity in a situation where the eye is not accommodating and a congruent image is perfectly focused on the retina.[2] A hyperopic patient can use accommodation to focus the image on the retina, while a myope has to move the object closer than infinity to focus the image.

Even when lower order refractive errors are corrected with spectacles or contact lenses, uncorrected higher order aberrations may decrease visual quality.[3] Aberrations relevant to the cornea are spherical aberration, coma, and oblique astigmatism.

Spherical aberration is an expression of the difference in refracting power for peripheral rays relative to central rays. This occurs when a point source of light is refracted by a large-aperture optical system. Different zones of the aperture have different focal lengths and therefore do not focus the point source of light to the same location. Normally, spherical aberration is not important in the human eye because the pupil is sufficiently small. Figure 3-1 shows the effect of spherical aberration on the point spread function (PSF).

Coma occurs when an object is located off axis, or if the apex of the cornea is not properly aligned with the other optical elements of the eye. Similar to spherical aberration, it has little effect due to the pupil being relatively small. Coma can be thought of as a type of off-axis spherical aberration. It creates a series of images superimposed upon on each other, with the brightest image being the smallest one. Figure 3-2 shows the effect of coma on the the the PSF and Snellen E.

Oblique astigmatism is independent of pupil size and cornea. It is induced when rays pass through the cornea and obliquely induce astigmatism. This phenomenon explains how a spherical cornea may register astigmatism when measured obliquely.

| TABLE 3-1 |
| INDICES OF REFRACTION |

	Air	Tears	Cornea	Aqueous Humor
Index of refraction	1.00	1.336	1.376	1.336

Figure 3-1. A point of light has this appearance to a patient with significant spherical aberration.

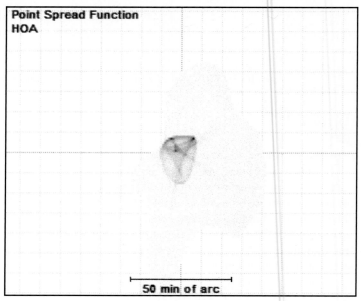

Figure 3-2. Coma results in a distortion of a point of light (left) and the Snellen E (right).

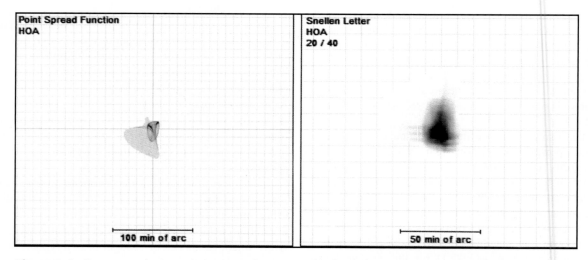

Corneal structure is such that aberrations are minimized. This is accomplished by the prolate shape and small angle Kappa. The cornea is not spherical, but rather aspheric. The curve flattens toward the periphery as you move away from the center, and the shape is described as prolate. Natural asphericity decreases the power of the peripheral parts of the cornea, resulting in decreased spherical aberration and coma.[4] The asphericity of the human cornea is described by factor Q, which represents the difference in curvature from the center to the periphery of the cornea. The average value for a human's cornea is –0.26. A perfect value for Q would be –0.50, but the junction of the cornea and sclera at the limbus prohibit this in nature.

Aberrations are further minimized by the location of the corneal apex. If the apex of the cornea aligns with the pupil center, it would naturally intercept the visual axis. When this does not occur, light rays get redirected and meet with the retina at oblique angles. These redirected rays result in a lessened retinal response, producing what is known as the *Stiles Crawford Effect.* The pupil normally reduces aberrant rays, which decreases the effect of oblique rays. Essentially, the same problem occurs if the pupil is not centered.[1]

Pupil size is uniquely suited to limited aberrations such as spherical aberration and diffraction. The pupil size that is best for limiting higher order aberrations and to minimize diffraction is 2.5 mm. The average pupil size is 5 mm, with younger patients naturally having larger pupils.[5]

CORNEAL OPTICS S/P KERATOREFRACTIVE SURGERY

Keratorefractive surgery changes the natural shape of the cornea, typically decreasing the natural safeguards against aberrations. Keratorefractive surgeries are successful because the optical properties of the eye can be manipulated by changing the shape of the cornea. The prolate structure of the cornea is changed by the removal of a convex positive meniscus for myopic ablations, a concave positive meniscus for hyperopic corrections, and a toric positive meniscus in astigmatic corrections.

The size of angle Kappa in reference to the ablation zone becomes important when this angle is large. If the visual axis is far from the geometric center of the cornea, the ablation will be effectively decentered. This is most often problematic with a hyperopic treatment when the central cornea is steeped around the visual axis.[6] In refractive surgery, pupil size related to the treatment zone remains important. Patients with pupil size greater than 8 mm should be identified and appropriately educated about visual side effects before undergoing keratorefractive sur-

gical correction.

Physiologically, the response of the cornea is complex following ablative procedures. The amount of tissue removed can be predicted by Munnerlyn's formula.

$$T = S^2 D / 3$$

where S is the diameter of the treatment optical zone, D is the refractive correction, and T is the maximum amount of corneal tissue removed in microns. Clinically, for every diopter of correction, approximately 12 microns of tissue are removed when using a 6 mm ablation.

Ablative, incisional, and INTACS procedures all change keratometric readings. A 0.8 D change is K is associated with a 1 D change in refraction.[4] This is important for surgical planning, because creating a cornea that is too flat (less than 35 D) or too steep (more than 52 D) can result in a disabling loss of visual quality.[7]

Note that the ratio of refractive change to keratometric change is not 1:1. The mismatch is thought to result from the change in posterior corneal curvature following keratorefractive surgery. In myopic ablative procedures, the posterior corneal surface is thought to become more negative; at the same time, the anterior corneal surface becomes less positive. The natural power ratio between the two surfaces is altered, and the assumptions used in keratometry create significant errors in power measurements.

IOL CALCULATIONS S/P REFRACTIVE SURGERY

A considerable amount of research has been done to improve the ability to calculate IOL powers after a refractive procedure. Several methods are available to cataract surgeons to aid them in IOL power calculation. The clinical history method, sometimes referred to as the refraction derived method, involves subtracting the change in refractive error induced by refractive surgery from the average corneal power measured prior to surgery. The equation to determine the change in the corneal power from the known pre- and postoperative refractive and keratometry values is: $RE\Delta_{sp} = MR_{preop} - MR_{postop}$. A sample calculation is shown in Table 3-2.

To determine the change in corneal power based on the refraction in the corneal plane, the change in refraction must be converted using the following equation:

$$RE\Delta_{cp} = RE\Delta_{sp} / 1 + (0.014 * RE\Delta_{sp})$$

This value can then be subtracted from the preoperative keratometry value to determine the keratometry value for the corneal plane (K_{cp}).

TABLE 3-2

AN EXAMPLE OF THE CLINICAL HISTORY METHOD

	OD	OS
Ks preop	45.00 (Average)	45.50 (Average)
MR preop	−6.00	−4.50
MR postop	−0.25	−0.50
Ks postop	40.75	41.25

	OD	OS
$RE\Delta_{sp} = MR_{postop} - MR_{preop}$	$RE\Delta_{sp} = -6.00 - (-0.25) = -5.75D$	$RE\Delta_{sp} = -4.50 - (-0.50) = -4.00$
$K_{sp} = K_{preop} + RE\Delta_{sp}$	$45.00 - 5.75 = 39.25$ D	$45.50 - 4.00 = 41.50$ D

TABLE 3-3

AN EXAMPLE OF THE CONTACT LENS METHOD

	OD	OS
OR_{sp} = MR with CL + CL power	$ORsp = -3.00 + (-3.00) = -6.00$	$ORsp = -1.50 + (-1.50) = -3.00$
BC of CL = 337.5/BC(mm)	$337.5/7.4 = 45.61$	$337.5/7.5 = 45.00$
$OR_{cp} = OR_{sp} /1 + (0.014 * OR_{sp})$	$-6.00/1 + (0.014 * -6.00) = -5.55$	$-3.00/1 + (0.014 * -3) = -2.13$
K_{CL} = BC of CL + OR_{cp}	$45.61 + (-5.55) = 40.06$ D	$45.00 + (-2.13) = 42.87$ D

The contact lens method utilizes the known values of lens power and base curve combined with over-refraction to determine the power of the cornea (Table 3-3).[8]

Videokeratography measures the central corneal power inside the 3-mm zone measured by keratometry, and may give a more accurate power to use in IOL calculation formulas. For eyes that have had refractive surgery, the corneal power derived from clinical history, contact lens refraction, or videokeratography should be used in a third-generation theoretic formula, such as the Hoffer Q, Holladay, or SRK/T, to calculate the intraocular lens power used during cataract surgery.[9]

Cheng and Lam[10] investigated the K-value obtained from the Gaussian optics formula (CalK) based on post-operative corneal topography by Orbscan II (Bausch & Lomb, Rochester, NY) and ultrasound pachymetry, comparing them to those obtained from the clinical history method (estK). A high correlation was noted between K-values obtained by the clinical history method and the Gaussian optics formula (R = 0.97, P < .001). The mean difference between the two methods was 0.13 D. However, Preussner et al found ray tracing superior to Gaussian optics in calculating corneal power, which is essential in IOL lens calculation.[11]

Aramberri recommends adjusting the SRK/T formula using the double K method. He found using the preoperative K value from keratometry or topography for the effective lens position calculation, and using the clinical history method with the vergence formula, improved the accuracy of IOL calculation S/P keratorefractive surgery.[12] Gimbel and Sun[13] evaluated target refractions based on measured and refraction-derived keratometric values by comparing them with postoperative achieved refractions. Differences between target refractions were calculated using five IOL formulas and two A-constants. Refraction derived keratometry values led to more accurate IOL power calculations, along with using Holladay 2 or Binkhorst 2 formulas.

Chen et al[14] suggested using the flattest keratometry value by calculation, and aiming for a −1.50 D rather than plano in lens calculation to reduce the likelihood of hyperopia after cataract surgery following keratorefractive surgery. Gimbel et al[15] also recommended using the smaller of the actual or refraction derived keratometric values for calculating IOL power. As increasing numbers of baby-boomers who are S/P keratorefractive surgery qualify for cataract surgery, it is likely specific parameters will develop to avoid hyperopic postoperative results.

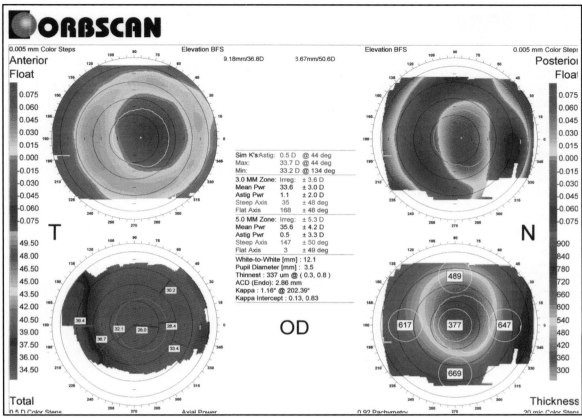

Figure 3-3A. Postoperative topography showing severe oblation OD.

CASE REPORT:
KERATOREFRACTIVE SURGERY FOR HIGH MYOPIA RESULTS IN FLAT CORNEA

A 24-year-old male interested in LASIK presented with an unremarkable medical and ocular history. Manifest refractions of −10.75 DS OD, −10.50 DS OS yielded acuity of 20/20. Preoperative keratometric readings were 41.12/41.87 @100 OD and 40.87/41.37 @090 OS. Ultrasound pachymetry was 550 OD and 555 OS. Anterior and posterior segment were healthy. The patient underwent LASIK for full correction of his myopia.

Postoperative day 1 the patient saw 20/40 OD and 20/50 OS. He returned to clinic one month later seeing 20/40 unaided in each eye, and reporting poor night vision and starbursts around lights. His refraction was −0.75 +2.00 x 020, 20/30 OD and −1.25 +1.75 x 157, 20/25 OS.

Over the next four months the patient complained of dryness and poor driving vision, especially at night. Refraction of −1.50 +1.50 x 045 corrected the right eye to 20/40, and pl +0.50 corrected the left to 20/30. As demonstrated in Figures 3-3A and B, postoperative keratometry

readings are less than 35 D. The severely oblate shape was causing his night vision issues. The Orbscan maps demonstrate that the inferior cornea is bowing forward. The instability of the posterior cornea also causes a loss of asphericity; however, it is difficult to estimate how much this is changing the BCVA. The situation is compounded by evidence of decentration of the ablation zone, shown in Figures 3-4A and 3-4B. Coma predominates the higher order aberrations, due to misalignment of the optic axis and the corneal center of curvature.

CASE REPORT:
HYPEROPIC KERATOREFRACTIVE SURGERY RESULTS IN STEEP CORNEA

A 19-year-old female presented for a LASIK evaluation. Manifest refraction was +1.75 +0.50 x 25, 20/40 OD and +0.75, 20/25 OS. Cycloplegic refraction found more hyperopia: +4.25 (20/50) OD and +1.50 (20/40) OS. Her preoperative topography was normal. After considerable discussion, she elected to undergo LASIK in both eyes.

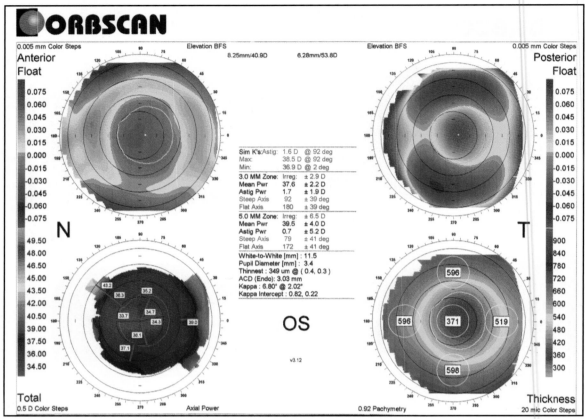

Figure 3-3B. Postoperative topography showing severe oblation OS.

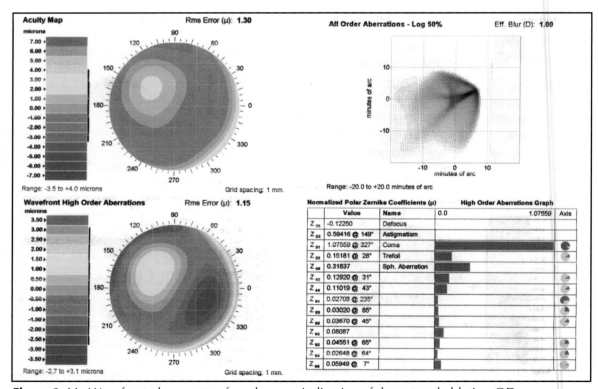

Figure 3-4A. Wavefront aberrometry found coma, indicative of decentered ablation OD.

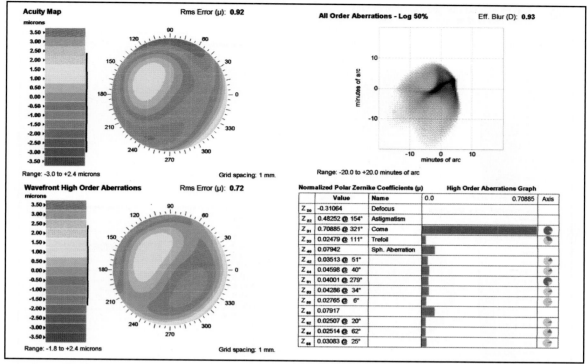

Figure 3-4B. Wavefront aberrometry found coma, indicative of decentered ablation OS.

The latent hyperopia OD was partially addressed, and the goal was a correction of +2.75 OD, +1.00 OS. She underwent bilateral femtosecond laser-assisted keratomileusis using a VISX Star 4 laser (VISX USA, Inc., Santa Clara, CA).

At one month, the patient was seeing 20/30 and 20/25 uncorrected and was extremely happy with her results. However, at 18 months S/P LASIK, the patient presented complaining of the vision OD. UCVA dropped to 20/50 OD. Manifest refraction found +1.50 +1.25 x 180 while the cycloplegic again revealed more hyperopia: +3.00 +1.25 x 180, yielding a VA of 20/30. Her visual complaint was relieved with simple hyperopic correction, and the patient underwent an enhancement of +1.50 +1.25 x 180.

At one month, she presented complaining of decreased vision OD, multiple images, and "an unbalanced feeling." Manifest refraction found –1.50 +0.75 x 75, and corrected her to only 20/50. Her wavefront aberrometry measurements revealed coma OD, shown in Figures 3-5A and 3-5B. Interestingly, the Wavescan and I-Trace both found hyperopic refractions, as shown in Table 3-4. The coma suggested a decentered apex, and topography revealed a significant steepening just above the geographical center. Her elevation map is shown in Figure 3-6.

Neither correction of the manifest refraction with a soft lens nor Alphagan-P to change the pupil size corrected the patient's complaint. While a gas permeable contact lens did restore functional vision, the patient is not able to tolerate the lens. It appears that the patient only uses the apex of the cornea for vision, resulting in the preferred myopic refraction. As time progresses and the natural smoothing of the cornea occurs, her symptoms are lessening and a custom treatment may or may not be necessary in the future.

CONCLUSION

Understanding of natural corneal optics, and how they are changed with keratorefractive surgery, is required for all corneal surgeons. Surgical planning must incorporate the knowledge to safeguard the patient from visual quality issues arising from drastic changes in corneal architecture. While night vision issues, glare, and distortion are minimized by increased ablation zones and improved ablation profiles, significant treatments in less-than-ideal patients may result in undesirable topographical abnormalities.

REFERENCES

1. Robin JB, Rich LF, Elander RE. *Principles and Practice of Refractive Surgery.* Philadelphia, PA: WB Saunders; 1997: Chapters 3–4.

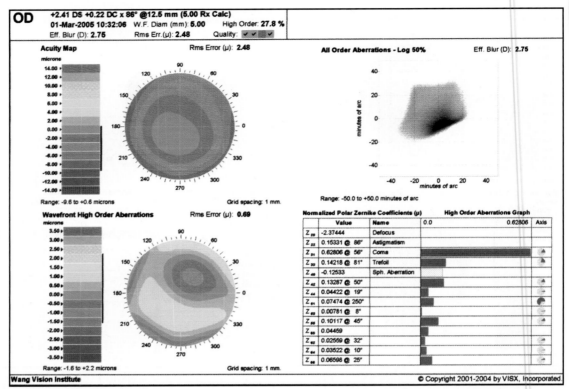

Figure 3-5A. Wavefront aberrometry showing hyperopia with coma aberration, WaveScan.

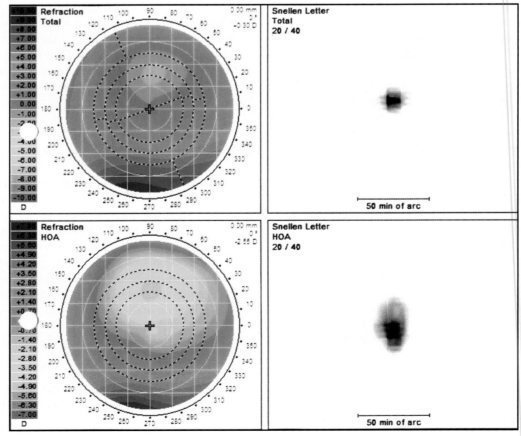

Figure 3-5B. Wavefront aberrometry showing hyperopia with coma aberration, iTrace.

TABLE 3-4 VARIABLE REFRACTION S/P HYPEROPIC LASIK (CASE 11)	
METHOD	**Refraction**
WaveScan	+1.74 +0.85 x 75 (5.0 mm)
I-Trace	+2..07 +.045 x 118 (5.0 mm)
Autorefractor	+1.75
Manifest	-1.50+0.75 x 75

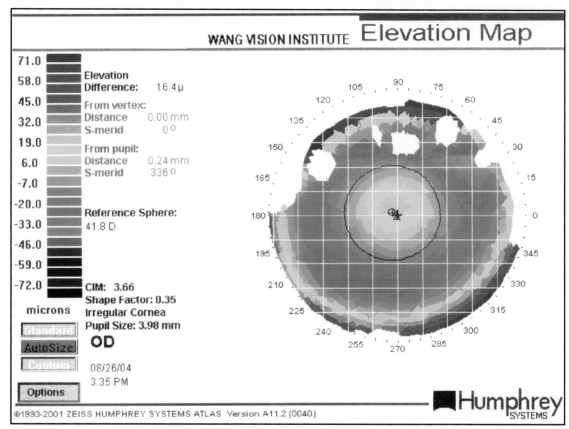

Figure 3-6. Elevation topography S/P repeated hyperopic ablation with mild decentration superiorly.

2. Fannin TE, Grosvenor T. *Clinical Optics.* 2nd ed. Boston, MA: Butterworth-Heinemann; 1996: Chapters 6, 12.

3. Klyce S. Night vision after LASIK. *Ophthalmol.* 2004; 111:1–2.

4. Munnerlyn C, Koons S, Marshall J. Photorefractive keratectomy: a technique for laser refractive surgery. *J Cat Refract Surg.* 1988;14:46.

5. Baikoff G, Lutun E, Ferraz C, Wei J. Analysis of the eye's anterior segment with optical coherence tomography: static and dynamic study. *J Fr Ophthalmol.* 2005; 28(4):343–352.

6. Freedman KA, Brown SM, Mathews SM, Young RS. Pupil size and the ablation zone in laser refractive surgery: considerations based on geometric optics. *J Cat Refract Surg.* 2003;29(10):1924–1931.

7. Klyce S. Night vision after LASIK. *Ophthalmol.* 2004; 111:1-2.

8. Haigis W. Corneal power after refractive surgery for myopia: contact lens method. *J Cat Refract Surg.* 2003;29; 1397–1411.

9. Hoffer KJ. Intraocular lens power calculation for eyes after refractive keratotomy. *J Refract Surg.* 2004;20(6): 783–789.

10. Cheng CK, Lam DS. Keratometry for intraocular lens power calculation using Orbscan II in eyes with laser in situ keratomileusis. *J Refract Surg.* 2005:21;365–368.

11. Preussner PR, Wahl J, Lahdo H, Dick B, Findl O. Ray tracing for intraocular lens calculation. *J Cat Refract Surg.* 2002;28:1412–1419.

12. Aramberri J. Intraocular lens power calculation after corneal refractive surgery: double-K method. *J Cat Refract Surg.* 2003;29:2063–2068.

13. Gimbel HV, Sun R. Accuracy and predictability of intraocular lens power calculation after laser in situ keratomileusis. *J Cat Refract Surg.* 2001;27:571–576.

14. Chen L, Mannis MJ, Salz JJ, Garcia-Ferrer FJ, GE J. Analysis of intraocular lens power calculation in post-radial keratotomy eyes. *J Cat Refract Surg.* 2003;29:65–70.

15. Gimbel HV, Sun R, Furlong MT, van Westenbrugge JA, Kassab J. Accuracy and predictability of intraocular lens power calculation after photorefractive keratectomy. *J Cat Refract Surg.* 2000;26:1147–1151.

Chapter 4

Topographic Technologies

Tracy Swartz, OD, MS; Zuguo Liu, MD, PhD; Xiao Yang, MD;
Mei Zhang, MD, PhD; and Ming Wang, MD, PhD

The principles of topography are based on the reflections of a concentric ring of light upon the cornea. Variations in curvature and astigmatism are represented as an asymmetry of the keratographic patterns. Modern keratoscopes incorporate complex images in the analysis of topographic anomalies. Topographic evolution has been driven by the propagation of refractive surgery and the demand for increasing precision.

This chapter will explore the evolution of keratoscopes. New technologies have met the demand for increased precision in evaluation of complex corneal shapes. These include Placido disk imaging, three-dimensional topography, PAR, slit-scanning topography, Scheimpflug imaging, ultrasound, and interferometric systems. This chapter contains a brief overview of each system.

PLACIDO DISK IMAGING

Placido disk imaging is based on the overlay of concentric mires on the cornea. Keratoscopes permitting the direct observation of illuminated mires upon the cornea demonstrate the placido ring. The closer the mires, the steeper the axis. The wider the rings, the flatter the axis. It was the first technology to be used to evaluate the shape of the cornea in conjunction with computer analysis. While systems may differ somewhat, all contain a transilluminated Placido target in the shape of a cone or disk, an imaging system containing an objective lens and camera, a video frame grabber, and a computer for image analysis. The number, position, color, and thickness of the rings varies between systems.

Placido systems are typically divided into two types: near (also called small targets) or distance (called large targets). Near target systems typically allow for imaging with lower illumination and enjoy greater corneal coverage. However, they are sensitive to focusing adjustments, and facial anatomy may hinder measurement. Large target systems require more illumination and are less sensitive to focusing error, but cover less of the cornea.[1]

Most systems project images of illuminated keratoscope rings onto the corneal surface to produce a virtual image of the Placido disk about 4 mm behind the corneal vertex.[2] An example is shown in Figure 4-1. They directly measure the curvature of the cornea, and calculate the elevation map using a coordinate system from the curvature data. However, this requires assumptions about the corneal geometry. Elevation is generated by fitting slope data to a predefined mathematical model that may be spheric, aspheric, or a conical section. While this practice is reasonable in normal corneas, it may result in serious error in diseased eyes or eyes having undergone keratorefractive surgery.[3]

Studies regarding the accuracy of early Placido disk systems found acceptable levels of accuracy and reproducibility. However, most test objects were spheres.[4] Systems tend to be more accurate centrally than peripherally, and defocus increases errors. Clear surfaces are required for clear mires. Reported accuracy of dioptric power varies from 0.1 D to 0.25 D, and from approximately 0.018 mm to 0.045 mm in the radius of curvature.[5]

ASTRAMAX THREE-DIMENSIONAL TOPOGRAPHY

The AstraMax (LaserSight Technologies, Inc., Winter Park, FL) uses a three-dimensional grid system, shown in

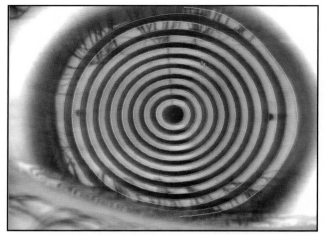

Figure 4-1. A Placido image. (Courtesy of Joe Wakil, MD.)

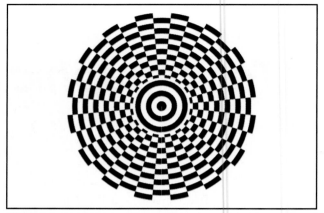

Figure 4-2. AstraMax system's polar grid. (Courtesy of Aleksandar Stojanovic, MD.)

Figure 4-2. Rather than using a Placido disk, a polar grid provides both radial and concentric data points, enabling measurement of radial distance and rotational concentric changes in the cornea. The AstraMax uses three cameras to obtain multi-angled shots, generating 35,000 data points in 0.2 seconds. The three-dimensional system measures each data point independently, free from any memory data of an adjacent point. The device discards data of poor quality from any monocular angle. A raw image is shown in Figure 4-3.

The AstraMax also offers limbus-to-limbus measurements (12 mm), scotopic and photopic pupil size, anterior and posterior corneal evaluation, and orbital pachymetry. The AstraMax target is projected onto the eye, and the three-camera system detects the leading and trailing edge of the light as it travels through the eye. This method yields thousands of pachymetry readings, as opposed to the traditional ultrasound method that gives only one reading at each application.[6] Unfortunately, no literature reports of the system's reliability or validity exist.

Two systems measure elevation directly: the PAR Corneal Topography System (PAR CTS) and the Orbscan. A triangulation method is used by both of these systems to measure the elevation of the corneal surface, and curvature data is calculated without the error of geometrical assumption.[7]

THE PAR CORNEAL TOPOGRAPHY SYSTEM AND RASTERPHOTOGRAMMETRY

Rasterstereography is a method of topographical evaluation of the cornea that creates an elevation map. Unlike Placido disk of systems, it does not depend on the reflec-

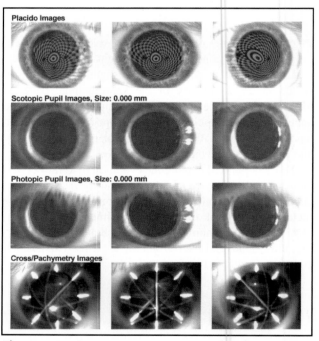

Figure 4-3. Raw AstraMax image of a keratoconic cornea.

tivity of the corneal surface, and can provide information about the entire corneal, limbal, and interpalpebral conjunctival surfaces.[8] Since a smooth reflective surface is not required, images can be obtained with epithelial irregularity or defects, sutures, or stromal ulceration.

The PAR CTS was the first topography system to produce an elevation map of the corneal surface using rasterstereography.[9] It projects a grid onto the corneal surface and computes elevation data based on the distortion of the grid. The PAR CTS requires that a small amount of fluorescein be placed in the tear film, and the images are collected using standard fluorescence-based photography.

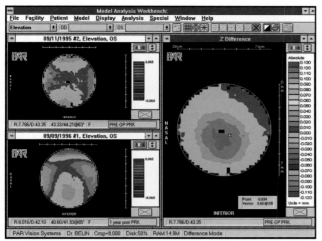

Figure 4-4A. PAR CTS displays for a cornea S/P myopic LASIK. (Courtesy of Michael W. Belin, MD.)

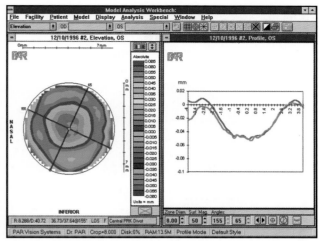

Figure 4-4B. PAR CTS displays the corresponding ablation profile for the same eye. (Courtesy of Michael W. Belin, MD.)

Image acquisition is rapid and relatively insensitive to focusing. From the known geometry of the grid projection and imaging system paths, rays can be intersected into three-dimensional space to compute the X, Y, and Z coordinates of the surface.[10]

PAR CTS can provide elevation, curvature, and keratometry maps. A topographical map of an eye S/P myopic LASIK and its ablation profile are shown in Figure 4-4. Unlike Placido disk-based videokeratoscopes, the PAR CTS produces a true elevation map and requires neither a smooth reflective surface nor precise spatial alignment for accurate imaging.[11] Based on the fact that the cornea is an asymmetric refractive surface, the PAR corneal elevation map can be obtained by comparing corneal height with a spherical reference surface. The actual corneal surface is either above or below this reference surface measured at individual points.

Unlike Placido disk-based videokeratoscopes, which require a smooth reflective surface,[12] the system demonstrates the ability to image irregular, de-epithelialized, and keratinized corneas. PAR CTS can be installed on slit lamp microscopes, surgical microscopes, or automatic optometry instruments, allowing topographical examination intraoperatively.

Currently, there is limited information on normal corneal topography with the PAR CTS, and it is rarely used in clinical practice. Naufal et al[13] investigated corneal elevation maps in 100 normal eyes of 50 subjects using the PAR CTS. Five categories were identified in their study: unclassified, regular ridge, irregular ridge, incomplete ridge, and island. They found that the surface of the normal cornea was not smooth and spherical, and surface irregularities ranged from small central islands of

elevation to complete, elevated bands crossing the cornea. Priest et al investigated the accuracy and precision of the elevation topography from Tomey Topographic Modeling System (TMS-1) (Nagoya, Japan) and PAR CTS. Based on quantitative analysis of elevation measurements, they concluded that the PAR CTS represented surface topography more accurately than the TMS-1.[13]

SLIT-SCANNING TOPOGRAPHY

While the PAR CTS failed to gain popularity among ophthalmic surgeons, the Orbscan (Bausch & Lomb, New York, NY) slit-scanning system is well-known. Slit-scanning technology is currently utilized by a single system, the Orbscan. The Orbscan uses a slit-scanning beam similar to the parallel piped one used in biomicroscopy and direct stereotriangulation to measure the anterior corneal surface. During the 1.5-second examination, two slit-scanning lamps project a series of 40 slit beams angled at 45 degrees to the right and left of the video axis. Twenty slits are projected from the left and 20 from the right. Proprietary software image registration attempts to minimize the influence of involuntary eye movements during data acquisition.

The typical display used for the Orbscan incorporates four images: the anterior and posterior elevation maps, the curvature (axial) map, and the pachymetry map. An example is shown in Figure 4-5. When used for screening, Tanabe et al recommend using 10 or 20 μm scales for elevation maps, which best identify abnormal corneas.[14]

Modis et al[15] investigated the anterior and posterior corneal shape, curvature, and thickness of normal human

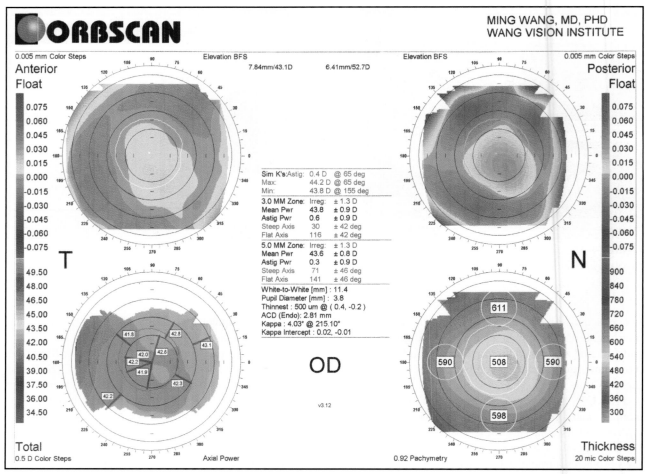

Figure 4-5. Typical Orbscan quad map of an eye with mild irregular astigmatism.

corneas using the Orbscan. Slit-scanning topography seems to be a reliable technique for evaluating normal corneas not only for anterior shape and curvature, but also for a real pachymetry gradient recording.[15]

In addition to curvature and elevation mapping of the cornea, the technology also yields pachymetry data. However, the accuracy of these measurements remains controversial. It is generally accepted that Orbscan measurements of central corneal thickness were greater than ultrasonic pachymeter measurements in virgin eyes.[16] The role of Orbscan pachymetry is limited by lack of repeatability for peripheral measurements, however, and is recommended for central CT measurements only.[17]

Kawana et al[18] compared central corneal thickness measurements of three pachymetry devices in eyes after LASIK. They found in post-LASIK eyes, Orbscan II slit-scanning topography significantly underestimated corneal thickness. Noncontact specular microscopy gave smaller thickness readings than ultrasonic pachymetry, but these two units showed an excellent linear correlation.[18]

SCHEIMPFLUG IMAGING

The Pentacam (Oculus, Inc., Lynnwood, Wash., USA) utilizes Scheimpflug imaging. It is a rotating Scheimpflug camera that provides 50 Scheimpflug images during one scan in less than 2 seconds with 500 true elevation points per image. The Pentacam has two integrated cameras. One is located in the center for the purposes of detection of the size and orientation of the pupil, and to control fixation. The second is mounted on the rotating wheel to capture images of the anterior segment. The Scheimpflug image is a complete picture from the anterior surface of the cornea to the posterior surface of the lens, as shown in Figure 4-6. The slit images are photographed on an angle from 0 to 180 degrees to avoid shadows from the nose. It generates 25,000 true elevation points for each surface, including the center of the cornea. Possible eye movements are captured and corrected internally.[19]

The Pentacam provides a complete analysis of the anterior and posterior surface topography of the cornea, including

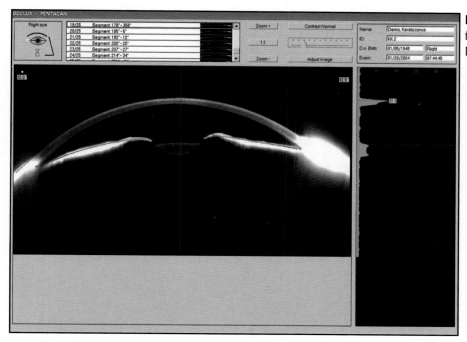

Figure 4-6. Pentacam Scheimpflug image (Courtesy of Oculus, Inc.)

curvature, tangential, and sagittal (axial) maps. The topography of the anterior and posterior surfaces of the cornea is generated from a true elevation measurement, and is illustrated in Figure 4-7. The Scheimpflug principle allows data capture in patients with significant keratoconus and other severe irregularities, which may prevent successful Placido imaging. The anterior and posterior corneal elevation maps can be shown with various reference bodies, which can be fitted in "float" or on the corneal apex.

The Pentacam calculates the pachymetry of the cornea from limbus to limbus and displays corneal thickness in a colored map. An example is shown in Figure 4-8. The Pentacam offers the correction of intraocular pressure (IOP), which is affected by corneal thickness. This is useful for glaucoma screening and management.

The True Net Power map reflects the true power of the cornea in its entirety, and facilitates improved IOL calculation for postkeratorefractive patients.[20] The Pentacam also provides a corneal wavefront analysis for both surfaces using Zernike indices to detect high-order aberrations attributable to the corneal surfaces.

ARTEMIS ULTRASOUND DIGITAL TOPOGRAPHY

This system uses high-frequency ultrasound scanning enhanced by digital signal processing. Ultrasonic echo data from consecutive parallel B-scans of the cornea spaced at 250-micron intervals are digitized and stored. Using the I-scan obtained by computing the analytic signal magnitude of the deconvolved ultrasound signal, layer thickness measurements are made with a precision of 2 microns standard deviation at 120-micron intervals along each scan plane. The data are stored as an array, $z(x,y)$, mapping thickness (z) onto horizontal and vertical (x,y) spatial coordinates. Pachymetric maps are then constructed by plotting local thickness against measurement point position. This technique provides the corneal surgeon with a new tool for the topographic evaluation of the thickness of anterior corneal layers in normal and pathologic corneas with high precision. The resolution of the Artemis is sufficient to distinguish individual corneal layers such as the epithelium, stromal component of the flap, and residual stromal bed. In addition, the technique is not limited to optically transparent tissue.[21] An example of the images obtained with this technology is shown in Figure 4-9. The common display used is the C12 array, illustrated in Figure 4-10. This array was created from scans of the right cornea of a patient scanned prior to LASIK and then six months postoperatively.

Reinstein et al[22] investigated precision, imaging resolution, three-dimensional thickness mapping, and clinical utility of a new prototype three-dimension very high frequency (VHF) (50 MHz) digital ultrasound scanning system for corneal epithelium, flap, and residual stromal thickness after LASIK. They found that VHF digital ultrasound arc-B scanning provides high-resolution imaging and high-precision three-dimensional thickness mapping

Figure 4-7A. Pentacam anterior elevation map. (Courtesy of Oculus, Inc.)

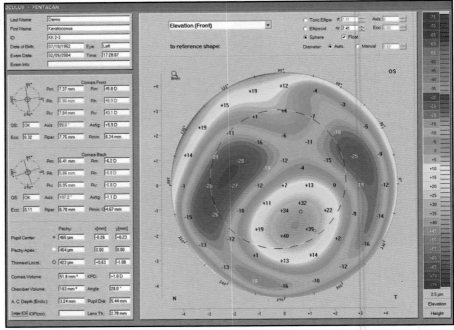

Figure 4-7B. Pentacam posterior elevation map. (Courtesy of Oculus, Inc.)

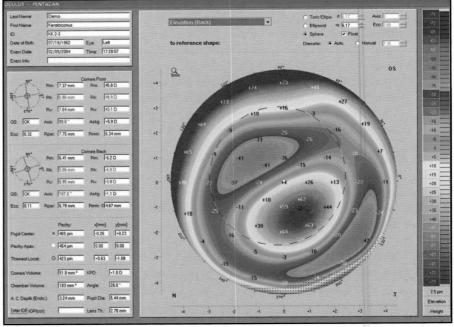

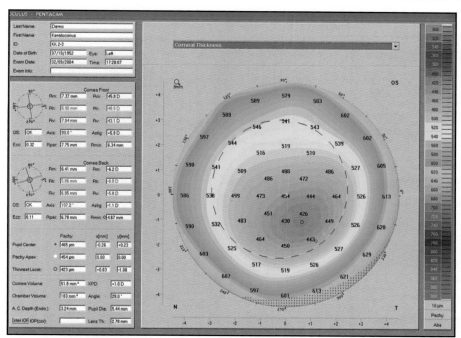

Figure 4-8. An ultrasound image of a cornea S/P LASIK. (Courtesy of Oculus, Inc.)

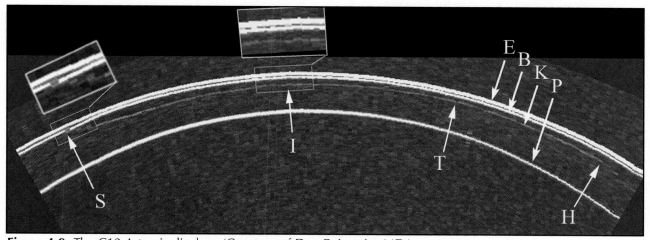

Figure 4-9. The C12 Artemis display. (Courtesy of Dan Reinstein, MD.)

of corneal layers, enabling accurate anatomical evaluation of the changes induced in the cornea by LASIK.[22]

INTERFEROMETRIC SYSTEM

This technique utilizes laser holographic interferometry fringe patterns to depict deviations of the corneal surface. Interferometry is based on the principles of light wave interference. It records the interference pattern generated on the corneal surface by two coherent wavefronts. High accuracy is theoretically possible.[23] Fringe patterns can be interpreted as contour maps of surface elevations where the difference between the two consecutive fringes is equal to an elevation difference of half the light wavelength (about 0.5 μm). The shape of the cornea can be calculated by adding this amount to the reference sphere elevation. Unfortunately, interferometric methods are sensitive to eye movements, and a system is required to maintain head position. Despite reported sensitivity of less than 0.1 D of curvature within the 5 mm vertex,[5] the system is too complicated to gain a foothold in the field.

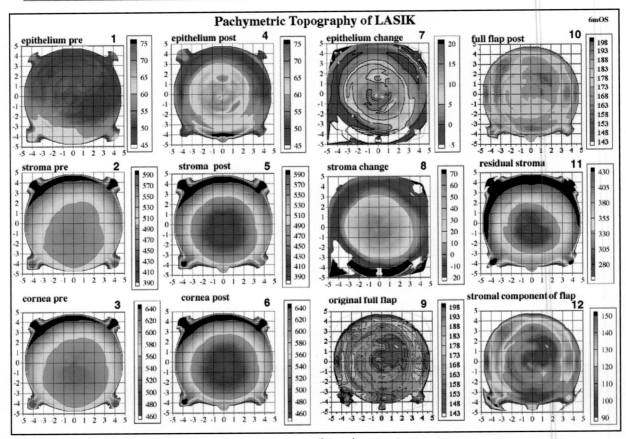

Figure 4-10. Pentacam pachymetry maps. (Courtesy of Oculus, Inc.)

CONCLUSION

Understanding of the type of topographic technology, and how each system derives the maps, is important for clinical interpretation. Placido disk and slit-scanning systems are the most widely used and understood by clinicians. The use of Scheimpflug images to create corneal topographic maps is the most recent addition to the field, and its evaluation of the structures posterior to the anterior surface may enable us to verify the slit-scanning technology's information and continue to help us to increase our understanding of pachymetry and the posterior surface changes that occur in some patients.

REFERENCES

1. Corneal topography. *Ophthalmology.* 1999;106(8):1628–1638.

2. Binder PS. Videokeratography. *CLAO J.* 1995;21(2):133-44.

3. Mandell RB. The enigma of the corneal contour. *CLAO J.* 1992;18:267–273.

4. Koch DD, Foulks GN, Moran CT, Wakil JS. The corneal EyeSys system: accuracy analysis and reproducibility of the first generation prototype. *Refract Corneal Surg* 1989;5:24–29.

5. Mejia-Barbosa Y, Malacara-Hernandez D. A review of methods for measuring corneal topography. *Opt Vis Sci.* 2001;78:240–253.

6. Surgicals Division Custom Ablation: A Myth or Reality. Website. Available at: http://www.medicalsintl.com/2001issue11.html. Viewed on July 26, 2005.

7. Litoff D, Belin MW, Winn SS, Smith RS. PAR technology corneal topography system. *Invest Ophthalmol Vis Sci.* 1991;32(suppl 4):922S.

8. Arffa RC, Warnicki JW, Rehkopf PG. Corneal topography using rasterstereography. *Refract Corneal Surg.* 1989;5(6):414–417.

9. Nemeth J, Erdelyi B, Csakany B. Corneal topography changes after a 15 second pause in blinking. *J Cataract Refract Surg* 2001;27:589–592.

10. Belin MW, Litoff D, Strods SJ, Winn SS, Smith RS. The PAR technology corneal topography system. *Refract Corneal Surg.* 1992;8(1):88–96.

11. Belin MW, Cambier JL, Nabors JR, Ratliff CD. PAR corneal topography system (PAR CTS): the clinical application of close-range photogrammetry. *Optom Vis Sci.* 1995;72(11):828–837.

12. Belin MW, Zloty P. Accuracy of the PAR corneal topography system with spatial misalignment. *CLAO J.* 1993;19(1):64–68.

13. Naufal SC, Hess JS, Friedlander MH, Granet NS. Rasterstereography-based classification of normal corneas. *J Cataract Refract Surg.* 1997;23:222–230.

14. Tanabe T, Oshika T, Yomidokor A, et al. Standardized color-coded scales for anterior and posterior elevation mapping of scanning slit corneal topography. *Ophthalmology.* 2002;107(7):1298–1302.

15. Modis L Jr, Langenbucher A, Seitz B. Evaluation of normal corneas using the scanning-slit topography/pachymetry system. *Cornea.* 2004;23(7):689–694.

16. Giraldez Fernandez MJ, Diaz Rey A, Cervino A, Yebra-Pimentel E. A comparison of two pachymetric systems: slit-scanning and ultrasonic. *CLAO J.* 2002;28(4):221–223.

17. Cho P, Cheung SW. Repeatability of corneal thickness measurements made by a scanning slit topography system. *Ophthalmic Physiol Opt.* 2002;22(6):505–510.

18. Kawana K, Tokunaga T, Miyata K, Okamoto F, Kiuchi T, Oshika T. Comparison of corneal thickness measurements using Orbscan II, non-contact specular microscopy, and ultrasonic pachymetry in eyes after laser in situ keratomileusis. *Br J Ophthalmol.* 2004;88(4):466–468.

19. Gerste RD. Five in one: an innovation that combines several diagnostic strategies. *Ophthalmo-Chirurgie* (Special Edition). 2004:1–4.

20. Holladay JT, Belin MW, Maus M, Chayet AS, Vinciguerra P. Next generation technology for the cataract & refractive surgeon. *Cataract and Refractive Surgery Today.* 2005; January(suppl):1–2.

21. Reinstein DZ, Silverman RH, Trokel SL, Coleman DJ. Corneal pachymetric topography. *Ophthalmology.* 1994; 101(3):432–438.

22. Reinstein DZ, Silverman RH, Raevsky T, et al. Arc-scanning very high-frequency digital ultrasound for 3D pachymetric mapping of the corneal epithelium and stroma in laser in situ keratomileusis. *J Refract Surg.* 2000;16(4): 414–430.

23. American Academy of Ophthalmology. Corneal topography. *Ophthalmology.* 1999;106(8):1628–1638.

Axial, Elevation, and Pachymetric Mapping

Ilan Cohen, MD; Tracy Swartz, OD, MS; Ray-Ann Lin, MD; and Ming Wang, MD, PhD

The cornea is a convex structure responsible for the refraction of light. Corneal topography depicts the variations on the surface of the cornea. Because the cornea is not perfectly spherical, nor does it perfectly coincide with any other geometrical abstraction, we need to consider the characteristics on each point along its surface in order to understand its properties.

The cornea has two surfaces responsible for the refraction of light: the anterior and the posterior surfaces. The anterior surface is more important because approximately 90% of refraction occurs there. The posterior surface contributes roughly 10% of the total corneal power in a virgin eye. This assumption could lead to significant errors in eyes with keratoconus or post-keratorefractive surgery.

Numerous topographers enable measurement of the surface characteristics of the cornea. Each one uses slightly different formulas or techniques to derive the topographical map. To complicate matters, each topographer offers a wide range of plots to display the information obtained, based on user preferences. This chapter will discuss some of the most popular aspects of topography and the principal concepts in the anatomy of the map.

Topographers capture data from points on the corneal surface using various technologies. Placido imaging or slit scanning are the most commonly used systems. From these primary data points, a wide range of maps can be displayed by the computer. The maps are usually color coded for easier interpretation by the clinician.

CURVATURE MAPS

The most commonly used curvature map is the axial map. This map depicts the anterior curvature of the cornea at each point along its surface, usually up to a diameter of 7 mm. In order to know the curvature of a point on a spherical surface, we need to find the circle that best fits the plane curve at the surface point of interest, and determine the local radius of curvature (K), where $K = 1/R$. The radius of curvature (R) is measured in millimeters. Curvature is the inverse of the radius, measured in diopters. The optical power of the cornea at any given point is a function of the curvature at that point, but is not the same as the curvature. The smaller the radius of curvature, the more curved the surface. Curvature may be displayed using several types of maps: axial, tangential, and meridional.

Axial curvature maps are obtained by measuring the curvature of the cornea at each point relative to a specified axis, usually the visual axis. The local radius for a corneal surface point can be measured as the distance from the point to the optic axis along the normal. Unfortunately, this requires the assumption that the center of curvature for the specific surface point is located along the optic axis. This radius is then called the axial radius of curvature. The center for all surface points is on the optic axis for spherical surfaces only, and the cornea is an aspheric surface. While this assumption was acceptable for keratometry, it introduces significant error in the corneal periphery. This effectively smooths small variations on the surface of the cornea, and provides a less irregular map that is easier to read and understand.[1] The axial map gives a global view of the corneal curvature as a whole. However, axial maps tend to ignore minor variations in the local curvature. A comparison between an axial map and a tangential map for the same eye are shown in Figure 5-1. Figure 5-1A is an axial map,which is less irregular than Figure 5-1B, which is a tangential map.

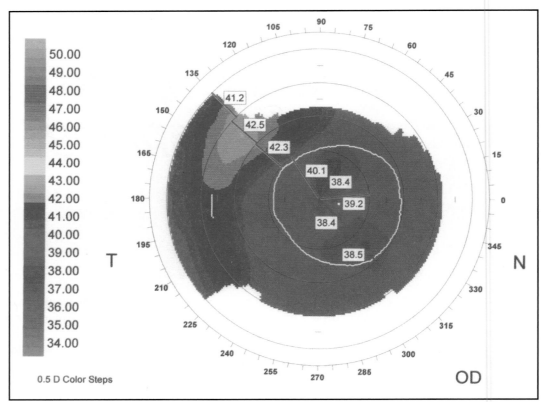

Figure 5-1A. An axial curvature map.

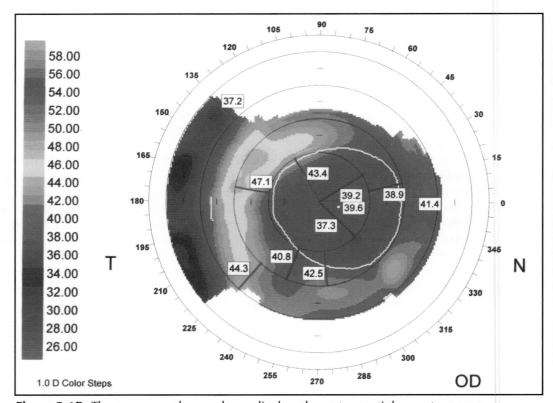

Figure 5-1B. The same eye shown above displayed as a tangential curvature map.

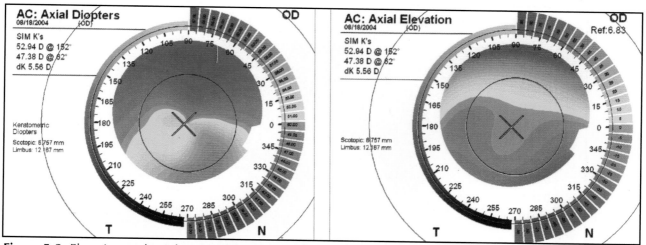

Figure 5-2. Elevation and axial maps of the same eye show that the inferior portion is not actually elevated, but rather depressed below that of the reference sphere due to the sharp curve of the cornea inferiorly.

The tangential map uses calculations based on a different mathematical approach to more accurately determine the peripheral corneal configuration. Tangential maps represent the local curvature of the cornea at each point. Tangential maps are sometimes referred to as "local curvature" or "instantaneous curvature" for this reason. Since the axis of reference is different for each point, there is a higher degree of variability from point to point.[2] There is also a smaller number of mathematical assumptions (ie, the sphericity of the cornea) used in this formula. The tangential map can recognize sharp power transitions more readily than the axial map, and eliminates the "smoothing" appearance that appears on the axial map for most topographers. Because tangential maps are more likely to illustrate focal irregularities, they are useful in contact lens fitting.

When reading a curvature map, it is important not to confuse "steepness" (typically pictured by hotter colors) with height. Curvature simply means that the shape of the cornea is changing, but it does not tell the direction of the change. For example, a curvature map of a keratoconic cornea characteristically shows red inferiorly, corresponding to the inferior distortion of the cornea inherent to the disease. The elevation map of the same eye in Figure 5-2 shows that the inferior portion is not actually elevated, but rather is depressed below that of the reference sphere, due to the sharp curve of the cornea inferiorly.

ELEVATION MAPS

A topographical map of a landscape depicts each point on the map in relationship to sea level. In corneal topography, an elevation map needs to be depicted with relation to a reference plane. This plane is often a sphere with a diameter that most closely resembles the overall diameter of that specific cornea. Each point on the cornea that coincides with the reference sphere is represented by the color green. Warmer colors represent points that are higher than the reference plane, and cooler colors represent points lower than the reference plane. Remember that the refractive power of the cornea is not represented by the elevation itself, but by changes in elevation.

In refractive surgery, elevation maps are extremely important. Since removing tissue most directly affects the elevation of the cornea, we have to understand elevation topography in order to grasp the effects that we are imparting on the cornea. The cornea is usually prolate, not perfectly spherical. Therefore, in order for a topographical map to have a quantitative and qualitative meaning, we need to know how the reference sphere correlates to the corneal surface. This attribute may be fixed in some topographers and can be chosen by the user in others.

Changing the size, shape, or alignment of the reference sphere will have an impact on the topography map just as changing the sea level would impact the heights of structures on the land surface. For practical applications, the reference plane is usually set to a sphere. The size of the sphere is chosen such that it best fits the cornea in question.

Choices for alignment include: float, centered, pinned, or apex. In Figures 5-3A through 5-3D, the same eye has been mapped using the four choices. When using float alignment, there are no constraints assigned to the reference sphere. The diameter and the location of the sphere are chosen to maximize the area of contact between the reference sphere and the cornea. This is the default alignment for most topographers. When using centered alignment, the center of the sphere is constrained to the viewing axis with

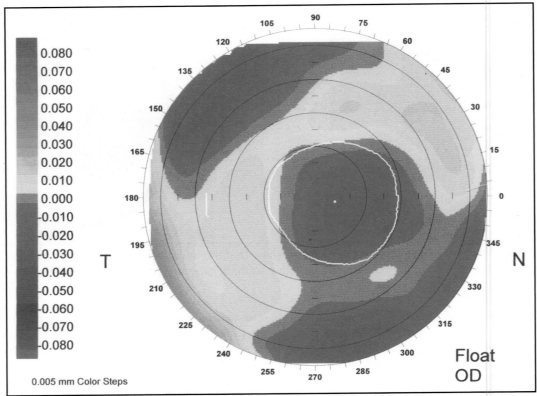

Figure 5-3A. Operator choices for alignment of anterior elevation map displays include float alignment, where there are no constraints assigned to the reference sphere.

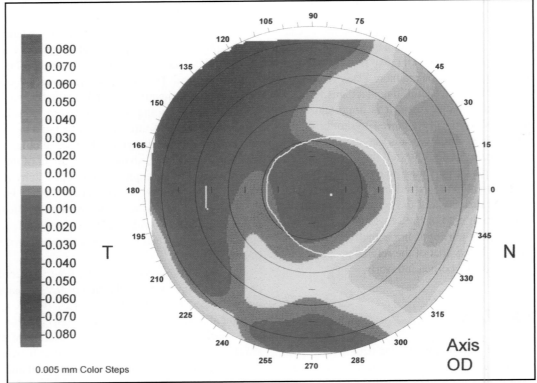

Figure 5-3B. Operator choices for alignment of anterior elevation map displays include centered alignment, where the center of the sphere is constrained to the viewing axis.

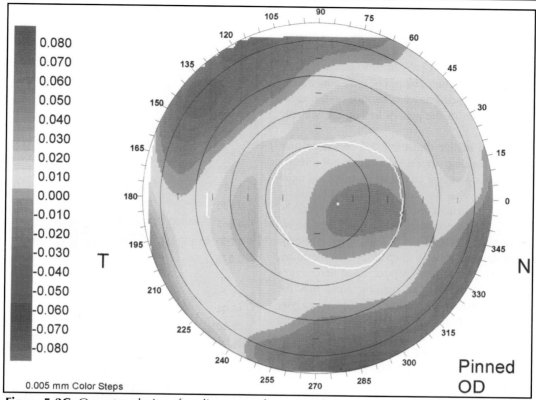

Figure 5-3C. Operator choices for alignment of anterior elevation map displays include pinned alignment, which forces the reference sphere and the data surface to intersect on the viewing axis.

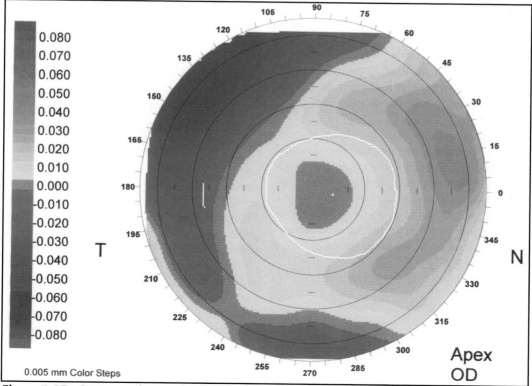

Figure 5-3D. Operator choices for alignment of anterior elevation map displays include apex alignment, which imposes both the center and pinned constraints.

the ability to move along that axis. Pinned alignment imposes the pin (P) constraint, which forces the reference sphere and the data surface to intersect on the viewing axis. The sphere center may be off axis in this scenario. Apex alignment imposes both center and pin (C + P) constraints. The sphere surface intersects the data surface on the viewing axis, and the center of the sphere lies on the viewing axis.

It is important to realize that the axial curvature map and anterior elevation map are related, but do not directly correspond. Figure 5-4 shows an elevation map and axial power map in an eye that has with-the-rule astigmatism. When we follow the vertical axis from a point superiorly toward the center, we see that elevation increases as we approach the center and decreases as we move inferiorly. This means that the curvature is steep along this meridian, as shown in the axial map. The steep meridian here is represented by the vertical bow-tie pattern. Note that the warm and cold colors are somewhat reversed when you compare an elevation map to a curvature map because a change in elevation causes a change in curvature.

In refractive surgery, we often need to compare pre- and postoperative topographical maps. The goal is to determine where tissue was removed and how much tissue was removed. We can then correlate this to the refractive effect that was achieved with the keratorefractive surgery. Elevation mapping directly illustrates tissue removal. Some programs perform a pre- and postoperative analysis based on the anterior elevation and pachymetry maps to calculate the exact amount of tissue that was removed at each point. This is useful in detecting postsurgical irregularities such as decentered ablation or central islands. Curvature maps should not be used to identify decentered ablations as they may exaggerate the decentration, exemplified in Figure 5-5.

General understanding of the anterior elevation topographical map can be applied to the posterior elevation topography. The posterior elevation map is created much like the anterior elevation map in design, with the exception that it represents the posterior surface of the cornea. The choices for alignment of the posterior surface elevation maps are the same as those for the anterior surface: float, centered, pinned, or apex. These are shown in Figure 5-6.

PACHYMETRY MAPS

Slit scanning and Scheimpflug imaging technology yield pachymetry data. Using slit-scanning technology, the pachymetry map is defined as the distance from the anterior to posterior surface, in the direction perpendicular to the anterior surface.[3] It gives us information not only

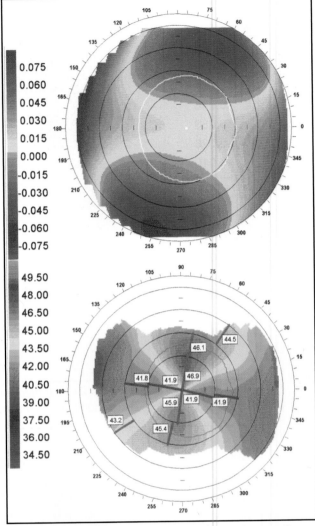

Figure 5-4. An elevation and axial power map in an eye showing with-the-rule astigmatism.

about the central or paracentral points of the cornea customarily obtained by ultrasound pachymetry, but also about the distribution of the thickness along the surface. Figure 5-7 shows a pachymetric map from a healthy patient (Figure 5-7A) and a patient with keratoconus (Figure 5-7B).

Pachymetry information is useful in glaucoma assessment, as well as in screening refractive surgery candidates and estimating residual corneal bed thickness postoperatively. This data is invaluable when combined with the other maps to arrive at conclusions where keratoconus or forme fruste keratoconus is suspected. Figure 5-8 illustrates the subtle differences between the two diagnoses.

Pachymetry maps are also valuable in the differential diagnosis of keratoconus and pellucid marginal degeneration (PMD). As can be seen in Figure 5-9, corneal thinning

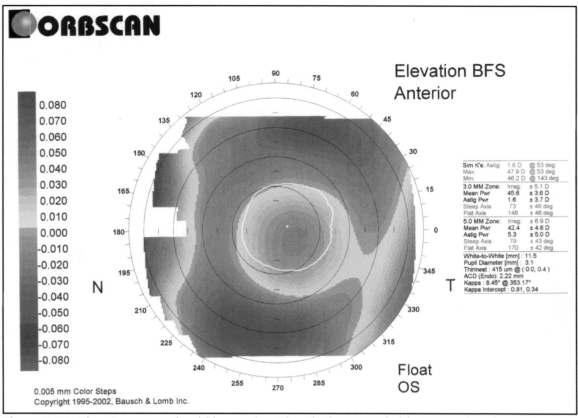

Figure 5-5A. Elevation maps should be used to identify decentered ablations, rather than using curvature maps.

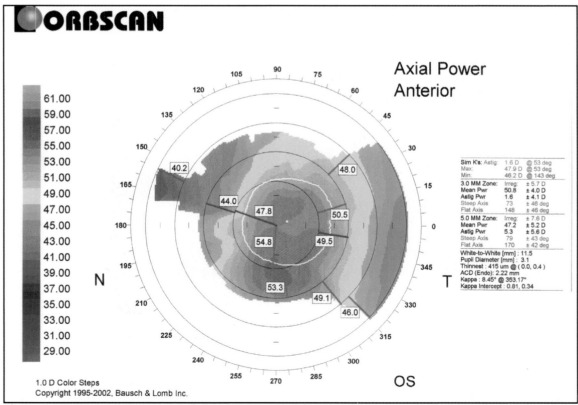

Figure 5-5B. Curvature maps tend to exaggerate the decentered area, and should not be used to identify decentered ablations.

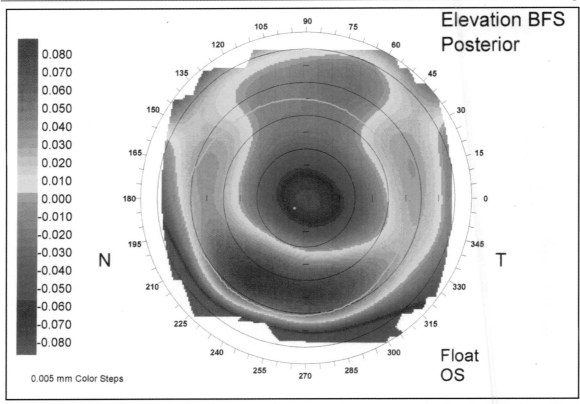

Figure 5-6A. Operator choices for alignment of posterior elevation map displays include float alignment. where there are no constraints assigned to the reference sphere.

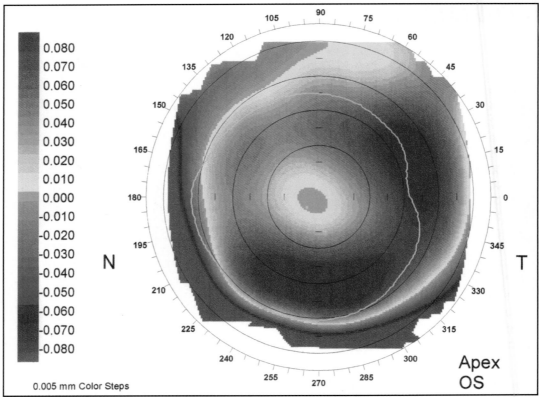

Figure 5-6B. Operator choices for alignment of posterior elevation map displays include centered alignment, where the center of the sphere is constrained to the viewing axis.

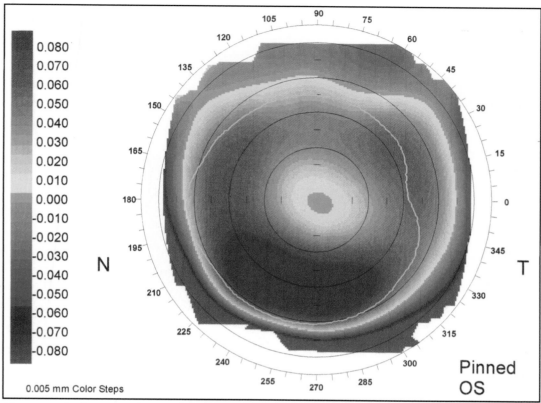

Figure 5-6C. Operator choices for alignment of posterior elevation map displays include pinned alignment, which forces the reference sphere and the data surface to intersect on the viewing axis.

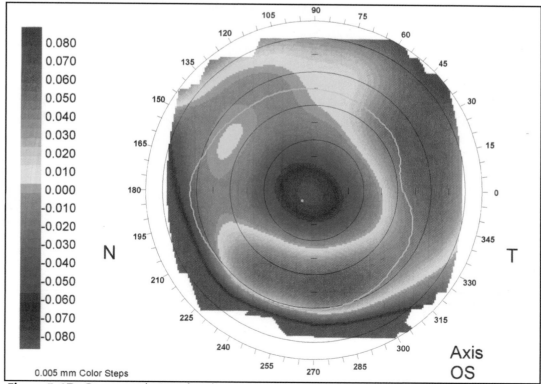

Figure 5-6D. Operator choices for alignment of posterior elevation map displays include apex alignment, which imposes both the center and pinned constraints.

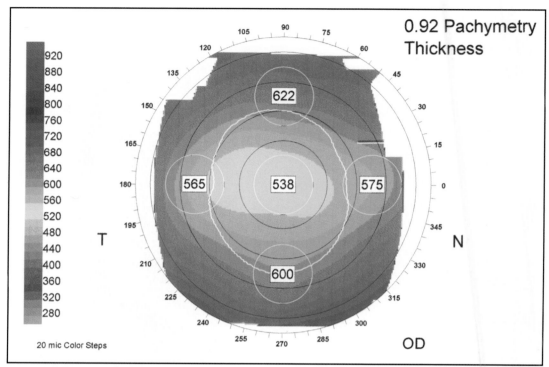

Figure 5-7A. Pachymetry maps from a healthy patient.

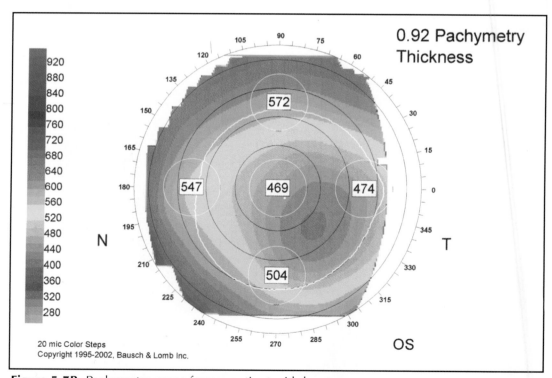

Figure 5-7B. Pachymetry maps from a patient with keratoconus.

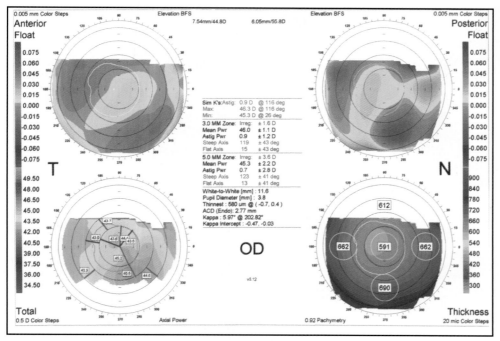

Figure 5-8. Subtle topographic abnormalities in forme fruste keratoconus.

corresponds to the apex of the cone in keratoconus (Figure 5-9A), and inferior to it in cases of PMD (Figure 5-9B). Early topographical signs may only be found on the posterior surface using slit-scanning topography in forme fruste keratoconus.

Topographic Map Interpretation

When looking at a topography map, you need to consider the clinical picture and interpret the map in that perspective. Correct identification of the type of map is crucial: Is it a curvature map or elevation map? When comparing maps over time, it is necessary to note the scale used. Some clinical entities that commonly interfere with the accuracy of topographic maps include corneal opacities, dry eye and insufficient tear film, eye movements, and contact lens wear.

A corneal scar can interfere with the data acquisition by a slit-scan topographer. The slit-scanning unit may misinterpret the opacity as a corneal surface, resulting in errors in both pachymetry and posterior elevation maps. A disrupted tear film can interfere with the reflection of light from the cornea, create artificially steepened areas, or lead to miscalculations based on missing data points. Irregularities resulting from a dry eye can be seen in Figure 5-10. INTACS segments can also result in loss of data in certain systems, as seen in Figure 5-11.

Minimal eye movements are required for data collection, especially for the slit-scanning systems where data

capture requires more time. Some topographers may accomplish this process faster than others and this may be helpful in patients who have difficulty opening their eyes or that cannot maintain fixation for long.

Contact lens wear may distort the shape of the cornea. An example of contact lens warpage in a gas permeable lens wearer is shown with a tangential map in Figure 5-12. This is not uncommon in hard contact lens wearers and prolonged soft contact lens wear. These eyes may resemble early keratoconus on topography. For this reason, it is recommended that contact lens wear be discontinued for a sufficient duration to allow the cornea return to its natural shape.

Epithelial surface irregularities such as superficial punctate keratitis, recurrent corneal erosions, and abrasions can also interfere with topography. They typically cause focal irregularities or loss of data (seen as white spots on maps). It is important to let such irregularities heal before important topography-based decisions are made.

Conclusion

In conclusion, topography has become an indispensable tool for the ophthalmologist in assessing the qualities of the corneal surface. The ability to interpret and understand various topographical maps can be complex given the

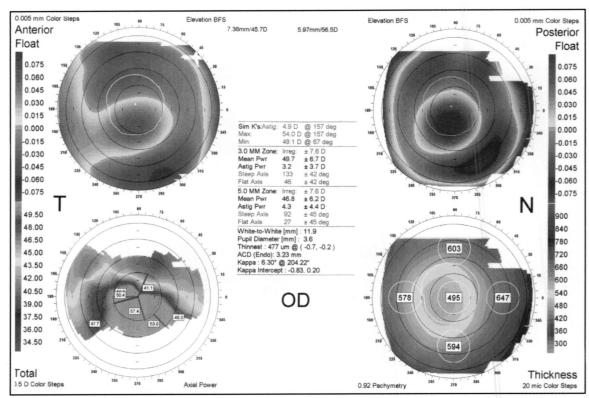

Figure 5-9A. The ectasia in keratoconus tends to be central.

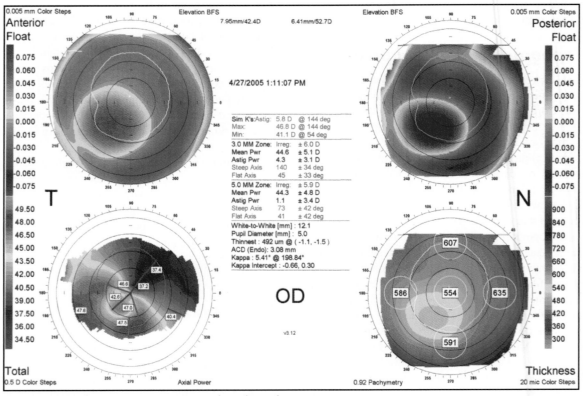

Figure 5-9B. The ectasia in PMD tends to be inferior.

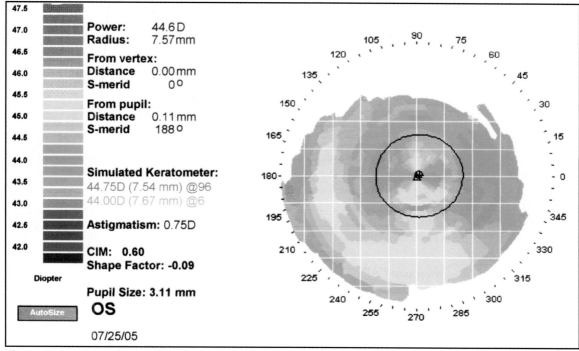

Figure 5-10. Central irregularities commonly found in dry eye patients.

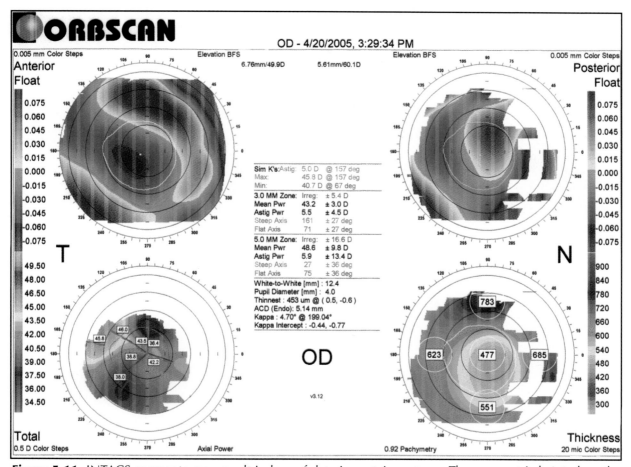

Figure 5-11. INTACS segments may result in loss of data in certain systems. The segment is located on the right side of each map.

variety of technology available. It is especially important for the refractive surgeon who assesses the eligibility of a candidate for elective surgery to understand the characteristics of the different types of maps for proper interpretation and clinical utility.

REFERENCES

1. Applegate RA. Comment on characterization of the inherent error in a spherically-biased corneal topography system in mapping a radially aspheric surface. *Refract Corneal Surg.* 1994;10:113–114.

2. Roberts C. Characterization of the inherent error in a spherically-biased corneal topography system in mapping a radially aspheric surface. *Refract Corneal Surg.* 1994; 10:103–116.

3. Marsich MW, Bullimore MA. The repeatability of corneal thickness measures. *Cornea.* 2000;19(6):792–795.

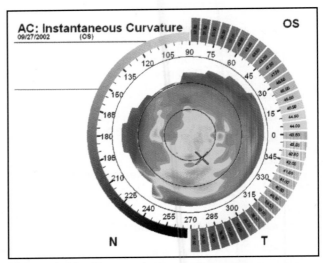

Figure 5-12. Contact lens warpage as seen on an instantaneous curvature map.

Topographical Scales

Ralph Chu, MD and Megan Buliano, OD

In order to view a topographical map correctly, it is important to understand the general shape of the curvature patterns and how it relates to scaling. The same map can appear differently, depending on the scale used to display the curvature. Thus, determining which scale to use in a particular situation is key to success.[1]

Initially, a standardized absolute scale was proposed,[2] ranging from 9.0 D to 101.5 D. The central portion of the range was measured with 1.5 D step intervals and the extreme limits of the range in 5.0 D step intervals. Although this range covered the entire power spectrum seen in corneal practice, salient topographic features were occasionally lost within the 5.0 D intervals, particularly at the low end of the scale. Hence, this was modified by the Klyce/Wilson Scale,[3] which ranged from 28.0 D to 65.5 D in equal 1.5 D step intervals. It has still been argued that the 1.5 D interval is so wide that irregularities in corneal topography may be masked. An example of changes in topographic patterns associated with increased step size is shown in Figure 6-1. Figure 6-1A shows more detailed irregularity compared to its counterpart (Figure 6-1B), due to smaller step size.

However, it has been demonstrated that the 1.5 D scale can detect all the topographic characteristics identified by a more sensitive 1.0 D scale in a consecutive series of patients that included contact lens-wearing corneas, early to moderate and advanced keratoconus, penetrating keratoplasties, extracapsular cataract extraction, excimer laser photorefractive keratotomy, radial keratotomy, aphakic epikeratophakia, and myopic epikeratophakia.[4]

In 1999, the American National Standards Institute (ANSI) issued a report entitled *Corneal Topography Systems—Standard Terminology, Requirements* (ANSI Z-80.23–1999).[5,6] This standard was anticipated to encompass the presentation of information, the standardized scale, scale interval, and the representative color palette used for curvature and elevation maps. It would allow users of corneal topographers to directly compare the topography maps produced by different manufacturers. However, Annex B of the ANSI standard, which defines scale intervals, the scale center, and a color convention, does not specify a single, well-defined color palette but rather suggests a variety of numeric and color scale combinations.[5]

In an effort to overcome this potential point of confusion, an alternative color scale was proposed—the Universal Standard Scale (USS). The USS was able to overcome the problems encountered with the ANSI standard by associating a single, well-defined numerical scale with a single, well-defined color palette. Table 6-1 highlights the differences between the ANSI and USS scales. This method has been shown to produce maps that were consistent and could be rapidly and correctly interpreted. The USS displays a range of powers that encompasses 99.9% of both naturally occurring and surgically induced corneal shapes. The USS scale is based on 1.5 D intervals and a well-defined color scale that would be most relevant for average clinical uses.[7] The 1.5 D interval gives the best sensitivity, specificity, and range.[7]

Table 6-1 describes the ability of topography scales to display corneal powers by relating interval size to dioptric range. There is no standardization of topographic scales between commercial companies. This makes it more difficult to compare examinations performed using different systems. For example, in the absolute/standardized scale default mode, the Humphrey Atlas (Carl Zeiss Meditec, Dublin, CA) ranges from 38.5 to 50.0 D in 0.50 D intervals, while the out-of-the-box absolute default scale for the Tomey TMS IV (Tomey Corporation, Nagoya, Japan) ranges from 9 D to 101.5 D.

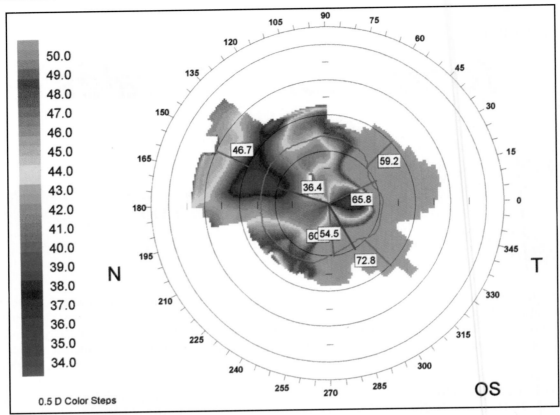

Figure 6-1A. Axial map shown at a 0.5 D step size.

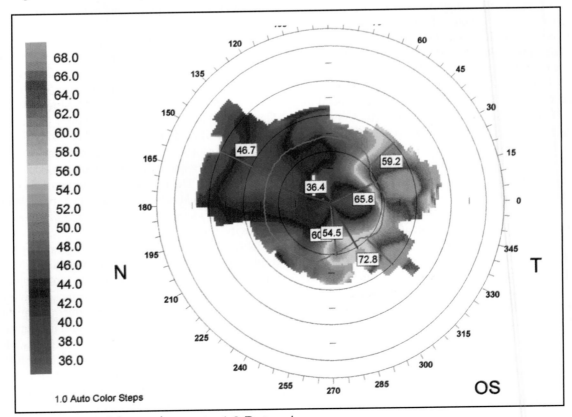

Figure 6-1B. Axial map shown at a 1.0 D step size.

TABLE 6-1

THE ABILITY OF TOPOGRAPHY SCALED TO DISPLAY CORNEAL POWERS BY RELATING INTERVAL SIZE TO DIOPTRIC RANGE

Scale Name	Interval Size	Range of Powers (D)	Displayed Powers (% of 388 topographic maps of 12 corneal conditions)
ANSI	1.5	29–59	99.2
ANSI	1.0	34–54	96.6
ANSI	0.5	39–49	86.2
USS	1.5	30–67.5	99.9

TABLE 6-2

ASSOCIATIONS TYPICALLY USED BY COLOR SCALES

COLOR	POWER (D)	
Red	48.0	Steep
Orange/Yellow	45.0	
Yellow/Green	43.5	Average
Green/Light blue	42.0	
Blue	39.0	Flat

When evaluating a topographic display, either a printed report or on the instrument's screen, one should study maps in a structured way to avoid mistakes in interpretation. The guidelines below will aid in successful interpretation of the maps.[8]

- Check name of patient, date of exam, and examined eye.
- Check the type of scale.
- Type of measurement (height in microns, curvature in mm, power in diopters).
- Step interval.
- Study the map (type of map, form of abnormality).
- Evaluate statistical information.
- Compare with map of contralateral eye.
- Compare with previous maps (verify they are the same scale).
- Apply statistical analysis or other needed software application.
- Explain the exam results to the patient.

Once a topographic image has been captured, it is scaled and graphically represented in a color-coded contour map. Depending on the scale used for color conversion, identical maps may, in fact, appear to be different.

Scale ranges and color representation vary among topographers, which makes direct comparisons between topographers open to interpretation.

COLOR SCALE

The color-coded contour map of corneal surface power has been adopted as a standard presentation scheme in corneal topography. The color-coded contour map markedly facilitates the viewer's interpretation through the association of power with color and recognition of pathologic features with the patterns formed by the map contours. Warm colors, red and orange, are used to represent relatively higher powers (steeper curvatures); green and yellow are used for powers associated with normal corneas; and cool color hues of blue are used to denote relatively lower powers (flatter curvatures). Table 6-2 describes the colors used. This concept, along with standard scale, provides an intuitive basis for the interpretation of corneal topography.[4]

Color-coded contour maps were initially developed for videokeratoscopy. With the introduction of projection-based topography systems, a similar color-coded system was applied to elevation maps. For these, the high areas were depicted by the warm colors and low areas were depicted by the cool colors. As a result it is extremely important to verify both the type of scale and the type of map being studied. For example, in a case of keratoconus, the red area on a height map corresponds to the highest point, which is the apex of the cone. In the same case, the red area on a curvature or power map is the steepest area, which is usually located adjacent to the cone inferiorly.

As you can see in Figure 6-2, the absolute/standardized scale significantly expands the dioptric range used. Clinically significant irregularities may be masked when comparing eyes with widely disparate curvature readings. When the range is standardized, the steepest curvatures

Figure 6-2A. Illustrates an auto scale.

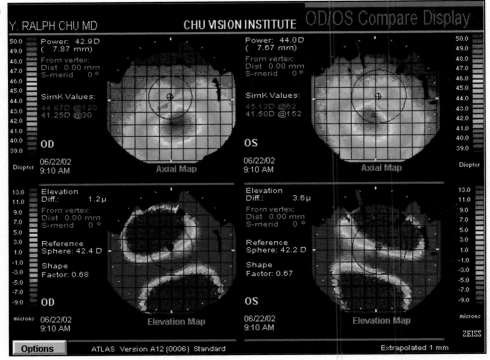

Figure 6-2B. Illustrates a standard scale of the same eye.

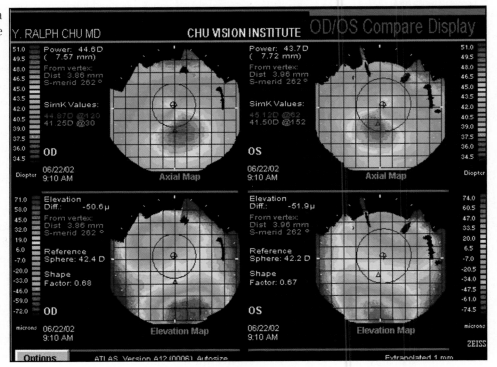

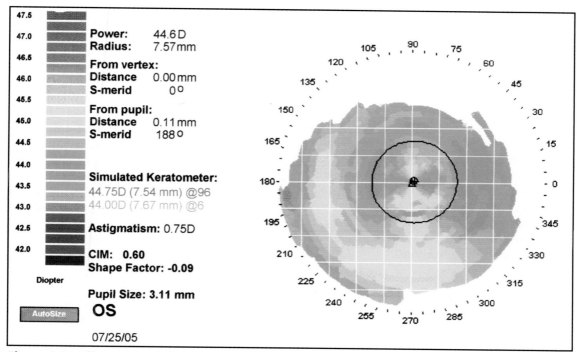

Figure 6-3A. Illustrates a defect on auto scale.

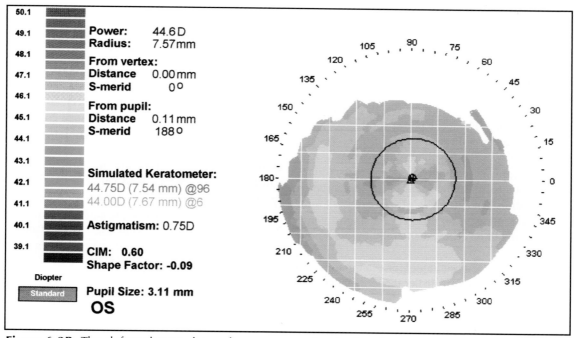

Figure 6-3B. The defect shown above disappears on standard scale.

appear red, while the flattest curvatures appear blue. General patterns remain the same, but intricate curvature changes disappear because the interval of measurement also increases from 0.25 D to 0.50 D.[1]

The use of a standardized and fixed color scale for routine clinical examination is important for consistent and correct evaluation of corneal topography. Scales that adapt themselves, like the autosize/normalized scale, to the range of powers on an individual cornea can lead to confusion. A physiologic asymmetry or astigmatism may by amplified by an adaptable scale like the autosize/normalized scale and may lead to misdiagnosis as pathologic. An example of this is shown in Figure 6-3. This patient has a mild dry eye. The irregular astigmatism is more evident using the auto scale. Alternatively, a cornea with substantial irregular astigmatism can be made to look less abnormal with an adjustable scale.[4]

The allocation of colors on an absolute/standardized scale is related to the distribution of corneal powers in the normal population. Central corneal power has an approximate Gaussian distribution (represented by a bell shaped curve). The mean central corneal power is 43.50 D, which is depicted by a color from the middle of the spectrum. Approximately 66% of the population has a central corneal power within one standard deviation of the mean (42 to 45 D) and this is represented by the adjacent colors on the scale. Less than 3% of the population has a central corneal power beyond ± 3 S.D., represented by red and dark blue. If these colors are present on an absolute scale map, the cornea is unlikely to be normal.[7]

AUTOSIZE/NORMALIZED SCALE

The normalized scale (relative, adaptive) or autoscale automatically adjusts and subdivides a specific cornea into several dioptric intervals based on the actual dioptric range of the cornea measured. Based on color representation, maps may appear to represent similar dioptric curvatures when using this scale, but depending on a patient's specific corneal curvature, these intervals may vary in range and dioptric value. This may falsely give the appearance that all maps represent equal curvatures.

A normalized scale uses a set number of colors, which are automatically adjusted to fill the range of dioptric values for that single map. The mean power for that cornea is positioned in the center of the scale. The normalized scale has the advantage over the absolute scale by fusing narrower steps between the contours, which provides more detail. Some systems limit how small the steps can be so that the information generated is still clinically relevant. However, as the scale may be different for almost every examination, it should be checked carefully before studying the map.

The automatic scale is a useful tool for examining a single eye in greater detail, as the smaller range will highlight variation and subtle changes with the caveat that normal variations may seem accentuated to the point of being questionable surgical candidates. For example, the use of a normalized scale can produce a pair of maps of similar appearance for a patient with advanced keratoconus in one eye (using a large step interval) and a subclinical cone in the other eye (using a small step interval).[7]

The automatic scale may also be beneficial in patients S/P LASIK with visual complaints. Figure 6-4 shows a patient S/P Hyperopic LASIK with decentered apex. The extent of the decentration appears larger using the automatic scale.

STANDARD/ABSOLUTE SCALE

The standard or absolute scale assigns the same color to a specific dioptric interval of curvature and forces that cornea's parameters to fit within that range. Although the range varies by instrument, each individual instrument's range is consistent. Therefore, for each map viewed a direct comparison of images from different eyes or from curvature changes of one eye (preoperative and postoperative refractive surgery patients) can be made quickly and accurately. Since, to date, there has so been no standardization of scales between commercial companies, this makes it more difficult to directly compare examinations performed using different systems.

A potential limitation of the standard scale is its inability to highlight subtle corneal changes that are important to evaluate when considering refractive surgery. Misinterpretation can exist due to the large range in intervals and loss of detail. Since the ranges and parameters are standard, two different maps can be compared—unlike with the autosize scale. This scale is most useful when comparing maps over time and with varying interpreters. It gives the best results for gross evaluations of the cornea.

CONCLUSION

It has long been recognized that corneal topography displays should be constructed in a standardized fashion that is consistent with the user's expectations and needs. Improperly designed and loosely defined color scales can easily introduce confusion and errors of interpretation. For example, too small a step size for the contour interval will tend to emphasize clinically insignificant detail. Insufficient color contrast between adjacent contours may mask clinically significant findings by making contours difficult to distinguish from one another. For routine clinical exams, it may be best to use the standard scale for mapping. It will be the most consistent when monitoring corneal maps over time. Table 6-3 reviews the differences between the scales.

When evaluating topographic maps, the way you view a map will depend on the information you want to gain from the map. If your goal is to compare two different eyes, you may want to consider viewing in standardized scale. This will allow a direct comparison of colors and aid in a quicker evaluation. When evaluating an eye for refractive surgery, the autosize/normalized scale may be a more useful tool. Smaller variations will be observed, allowing examination in greater detail. In some instances, one scale may not be preferred over another and comparison of the same eye in different scales is necessary. This will allow for enhanced evaluation of subtle corneal

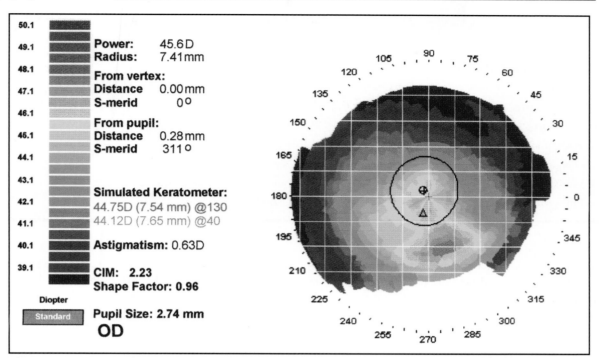

Figure 6-4A. Manipulating the scale can minimize the appearance of advanced keratoconus in this eye using a large step interval.

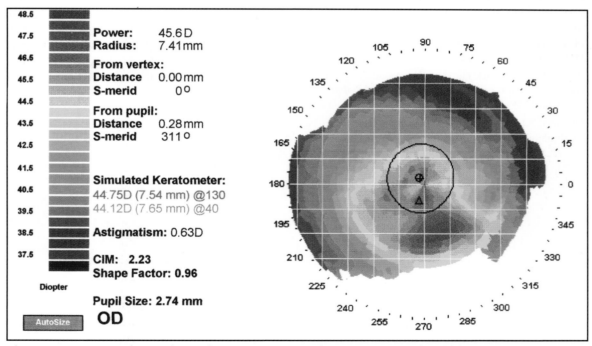

Figure 6-4B. Manipulating the scale can exaggerate the appearance of mild keratoconus in a sub-clinical cone using a small step interval.

TABLE 6-3

COMPARISON OF TOPOGRAPHICAL SCALES

Color Standardized/Absolute Scales	Normalized/Relative/Autosize
Standardized	Non-standardized
Good for comparison	Comparison of maps is more difficult
Large step sizes	Small steps
Low resolution	High resolution
Wide range of powers	Narrow range of powers
Good for screening	Subtle features can be detected
Good for gross pathology	Good for detail

nuances (autosize), with a broader corneal view (standard scale), helping you avoid possible over-analysis of clinically insignificant findings or a misdiagnosis of early corneal changes.

REFERENCES

1. Lebow KA. Making scaling work for you. *Contact Lens Spectrum.* 1999:50.

2. Maguire LJ, Singer DE, Klyce SD. Graphic presentation of computer-analyzed keratoscope photographs. *Arch Ophthalmol.* 1987;105:223–230.

3. Wilson SE, Klyce SD, Husseini ZM. Standardized color-coded maps for corneal topography. *Ophthalmology.* 1993;100:1723–1727.

4. Oshike T, Klyce SD. Corneal topography: basic concepts. In: Brightbill FS, ed. *Corneal Surgery—Theory, Technique, and Tissue.* 3rd ed. St. Louis, MO: CV Mosby; 1999.

5. Smolek M, et al. The universal standard scale: proposed improvements to the American National Standards Institute (ANSI) scale for corneal topography. *Ophthalmology.* 2002;109:361–369.

6. Secretariat, Optical Laboratories Association. *American National Standard for Ophthalmics—Corneal Topography Systems: Standard Terminology, Requirements.* Merrifield, VA: Optical Laboratories Association. American National Standards Institute; 1999:ANSI Z80.23-1000.

7. Corbett MC, Rosen ES, O'Brart DPS. Presentation of topographic information. In: *Corneal Topography: Principles and Applications.* London: BMJ; 1999:31–59.

8. Simón GL, Simón S, Simón JM, Simón C. Fundamentals on corneal topography. In: Boyd BF, ed. *LASIK and Beyond LASIK.* Panama: Highlights of Ophthalmology; 2001:9–59.

SECTION II

TOPOGRAPHIC APPLICATIONS

Topography of the Normal Cornea

Zuguo Liu, MD, PhD; Xiao Yang, MD; and Mei Zhang, MD, PhD

The cornea is a transparent structure that comprises the anterior one-sixth of the outer wall of the eye. It is a critical structure that not only keeps the eyeball intact, but also contributes three-quarters of the refractive power of the whole eye. Accordingly, even subtle changes to the corneal shape may greatly impact the refractive power of the entire eye. In recent years, great progress has been achieved in corneal topography, which allowed clinicians to obtain detailed information about the shape of the entire cornea. Much evidence has shown that corneal contour often undergoes obvious changes during the processes of many corneal diseases. Such changes not only provide evidence for their early diagnosis, but also enable clinicians to follow disease progression and predict the outcome of certain corneal disorders.

Recently, tremendous development has been made in keratorefractive surgery, which requires more detailed information about corneal topography than ever before. Though keratoscopy has been widely used in the clinic, it can only reveal some qualitative changes of the corneal surface. Corneal keratometry also provides quantitative information of the corneal surface, but it can only detect the refractive power of the central cornea within 3 mm in diameter. In the last decade, the introduction and development of computer-assisted corneal topography enabled clinicians to acquire detailed information about the entire corneal surface, providing both qualitative and quantitative information. Furthermore, the newly developed Orbscan corneal topographer can provide a refractive map of the anterior corneal surface, elevation maps of the anterior and posterior corneal surfaces, and a pachymetry map of the entire cornea in a single screen examination. The intensive studies on corneal topography and the application of newly developed instruments not only promote the development of refractive corneal surgery, but also benefit traditional corneal surgeries, such as corneal graft and postoperative evaluation of corneal surgeries. They also provide valuable explanations to previously misunderstood visual problems.

THE GENERAL STRUCTURE AND FUNCTION OF THE CORNEA

Although the cornea comprises only one-sixth of the outer wall of the eyeball, its structure and function are very complicated. In addition to keeping the eyeball intact, the cornea must maintain its normal shape and transparency to allow for normal vision. Several factors may affect the normal shape of the anterior corneal surface, such as corneal thickness, curvature, and regularity of the anterior and posterior surface.

The corneal thickness is uneven in different regions of the cornea, with the thinnest part located in the central cornea. The thickness of the cornea increases gradually from 0.50 mm in the central cornea to the limbus, which is about 1.2 mm thick. Because of this difference, the curvature of the anterior corneal surface differs from that of the posterior surface. The radius of curvature averages 7.8 mm on the central anterior surface and 6.7 mm posteriorly.[1]

The surface of the cornea is covered by tear film to maintain lubrication. When evaluating corneal topography, the images obtained reflect the tear film contour in front of the cornea. Since the tear film profile is determined by the anterior corneal surface, the curvature of the tear film reflects that of the underlying anterior corneal surface. Most of the refractive power of the whole eye is attributed to the anterior corneal surface. Therefore, a healthy anterior corneal surface is required for 20/20 visual acuity.

Figure 7-1. Three-zone category of the corneal surface.

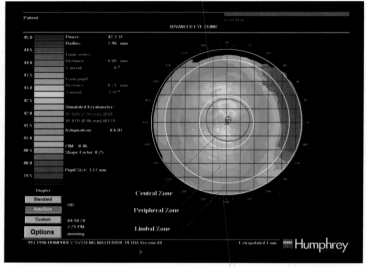

Histologically, the cornea consists of five layers: epithelium, Bowman's layer, stroma, Descemet's layer, and endothelium. The corneal epithelium is the superficial layer of the cornea, which consists of five to eight layers of cells with a thickness of 50 to 100 μm. The cells in the outermost layer are polygonal cells with a flat cell body and nucleus, which do not undergo keratinization under normal circumstances. This makes it possible to form a very smooth anterior corneal surface. If the corneal thickness, curvature, or smoothness and regularity of the anterior surface are altered, visual function will be jeopardized.

SURFACE ZONES OF THE CORNEA

The cornea is a continuous transparent structure, with no visible borders. To facilitate topographic analysis, the cornea may be divided into zones. For optical and anatomical purposes, we can simply divide the corneal surface into two major regions: the central optical zone and the peripheral zone.[2] Central vision occurs through the central cornea's optical zone. Its shape, size, and curvature vary from person to person. Peripheral vision occurs through the peripheral cornea when the pupil is widely dilated.

There are two methods to categorize corneal surface zones topographically. Using the three-zone method, the cornea is divided into the central, peripheral, and limbal zones. Using the four-zone method, the cornea is divided into the central, paracentral, peripheral, and limbal zones.[3] In our experience, the three-zone category is simpler to apply and more practical clinically. We will discuss the three-zone category (Figure 7-1) in this chapter.

The central zone, also called the apical zone or corneal cap, is approximately 4 mm in diameter. Basically, the apical zone is the area around the corneal apex, where the refractive power variation is little. There are several definitions used to determine the apical zone. Mandell[4] defined the corneal cap as being the "central corneal area of maximum and constant meridional curvature." He considered the refractive power variation in this zone to be less than 0.25 D. Ericksen defined the apical zone to be the area surrounding the corneal apex where the power varies by no more than 1 D.[4] Others have defined it as the area around the apex where the curvature differs by less than 0.05 mm.[3,5] Dingeldein and Klyce[6] did not confirm the existence of a definable apical zone. They suggested that it was arbitrary and anatomically incorrect to divide the cornea into zones. But it is useful for fitting contact lenses and corneal refractive surgery.

Although each author holds a different opinion, all share a common understanding that the central zone should be the area with little variation of corneal refractive power and a relatively regular shape, resembling a sphere. It should be kept in mind that neither the central nor the peripheral zone is discrete, and the size of the central zone differs among eyes.

The optical zone of the cornea plays an important role in the planning and the evaluation of corneal refractive surgery and is critical in the maintenance of normal visual function. For the normal cornea, the optical zone can be defined as the central spherical area that overlaps the entrance pupil. The aim of corneal refractive surgery is to reconstruct the optical zone of the cornea. The size of optical zone in corneal refractive surgery may vary from 3 to 7 mm in diameter.

In radial keratotomy and intracorneal implants, the surgery is performed in the peripheral cornea, leaving the central optical zone untouched. The amount of refractive correction can be controlled by adjusting the diameter of optical zone. Correcting different amounts of refractive error in myopia is accomplished by changing the size of the optical zone.

The geometric center of the cornea is defined as the intersection of the horizontal and vertical axis of the cornea. The distance between the geometric center and the visual axis varies among different individuals. In corneal refractive surgery, both the localization of ablation zone and the measurement of corneal topography are based on the visual axis.

The corneal peripheral zone is localized between the central and limbal zone. This area encompasses the paracentral and peripheral zone defined in the four-zone category, 4 to 11 mm in diameter. In this zone, the cornea flattens gradually toward the limbus, creating asphericity. The peripheral zone of the cornea plays an important role in the centration and fitting of contact lenses. Corneal keratometry can only measure the corneal curvature on the central cornea within 3 mm in diameter. Thus, this instrument cannot meet the requirement for contact lens design. The introduction of computerized corneal topography enables clinicians to obtain more detailed information about the peripheral cornea, which greatly promotes the progress of corneal contact lens manufacturing. Moreover, the peripheral zone of the cornea also has to be taken into account when performing corneal refractive surgery. An accurate evaluation of the corneal peripheral zone will help clinicians rule our irregularities in candidates.

The limbal zone can be defined as the area that connects the cornea and the sclera. This zone may suffer from corneal thinning disorders such as Terrien's marginal degeneration. The thinning of the limbus can change the refractive power of the limbal zone, which will indirectly result in the alteration of refractive power of the central cornea.

TOPOGRAPHY OF THE NORMAL CORNEA

When performing keratoscopy, the normal cornea reflects a series of regular concentric rings. An irregular and distorted reflection indicates an irregular corneal surface. The keratometer measures the refractive power of the anterior surface of the central 3 mm, using the reflected mires from four points along two meridians at right angles. The corneal curvature can be converted to diopters using an assumed refractive index, which gives a reading of the total corneal power. The meridian with the greatest refractive power is perpendicular to that with the least refractive power. Under normal circumstances, due to the upper eyelid pressure, the greater power is usually on the vertical meridian, producing with-the-rule astigmatism. Because corneal keratometry determines the curvature by measuring the central 3 mm, it cannot detect the changes outside the central cornea.

Placido-based videokeratoscopes comprise the vast majority of the units used in clinical practice today. The normal cornea examined by computerized corneal topography shows a higher refractive power in the central cornea and a gradual reduction of refractive power (1 to 3 D) when moving toward the limbus, corresponding to a gradual color change on the absolute scale map. On the color-coded dioptric map, normal corneas show several kinds of distinctive topographic patterns.

There are several studies regarding a classification system for normal corneal topography. Knoll defined four normal corneal topographic patterns by using the amount of central asymmetry and peripheral flattening along the horizontal meridian: (1) central symmetry with less than 2 mm of peripheral flattening; (2) central symmetry with greater than 2 mm of peripheral flattening; (3) central asymmetry with less than 2 mm of peripheral flattening; and (4) central asymmetry with greater than 2 mm of peripheral flattening.[7] Since measurements were obtained along the horizontal meridian, it was difficult to get information about radial asymmetry and from other areas of the cornea.

In 1990, Bogan et al[8] presented a new category system, which was widely accepted. Anterior refractive power was classified into five patterns according to the shape of the hottest color on the map: round, oval, symmetric bowtie, asymmetric bowtie, and irregular pattern (Figure 7-2). Each pattern contributes to a different proportion. They found that asymmetric bowtie was the most common topographic pattern, with a proportion of 32.1%.

In 1997, Kanpolat et al[9] evaluated corneas of emmetropic eyes with keratometric astigmatism of 0.50 D or less. They used the same classification of corneal topographies and the proportion of topography patterns as described in Table 7-1. Liu et al evaluated the normal cornea in a Chinese population sample using TMS-1 and found most were consistent with Bogan's, but with fewer irregular patterns in Chinese eyes.[10] Most changes in irregular patterns are due to eccentric fixation, dryness, or a depressed surface on the cornea. It has been suggested that the asymmetric bowtie pattern and the irregular pattern may represent an early stage of keratoconus in some cases. In addition, wearing contact lenses will also affect corneal topography, and this should be taken into account when analyzing the corneal topography of a contact lens wearer.

Most studies report average central corneal power between 43.50 ± 1.50 D and average corneal astigmatism between 0.50 ± 1.50 D.[6,8,10,11] Alvi et al[12] reported that for 95% of normal corneas, corneal contours will be steeper than 38.50 D, flatter than 47.50 D, and have a contour range less than 4.25 D when using the EyeSys CAS. Most studies found that peripheral flattening is asymmetric in the majority of normal eyes, and flattening is closer to the

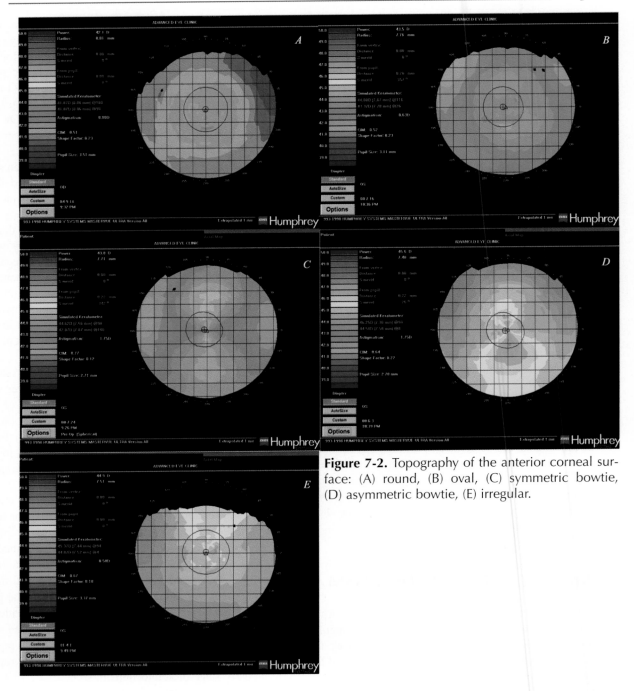

Figure 7-2. Topography of the anterior corneal surface: (A) round, (B) oval, (C) symmetric bowtie, (D) asymmetric bowtie, (E) irregular.

visual axis on the nasal side.[6,8–11] Using the TMS-1 Corneal Topography System, Liu et al[10] found that the average corneal powers were 43.45 ± 1.47 D, 43.45 ± 1.37 D, 43.16 ± 1.42 D, and 42.84 ± 1.45 D on the visual axis, 3-mm zone, 5-mm zone, and 7-mm zone, respectively. The difference of the average power was 0.65 ± 0.47 D between ring 1 and ring 15, and 1.78 ± 0.89 D between ring 1 and ring 25. The average corneal astigmatism was 0.93 ± 0.34 D on the 7, 8, 9 rings.[10]

Bafna et al[13] found that the average refractive power of the central cornea was 42.86 D, the average powers for the axial map were 43.09 D, 43.10 D, 42.75 D, and 42.21 D at the 1-mm zone, 3-mm zone, 5-mm zone, and 7-mm zone, respectively. Edmund[14] found the average corneal area within which the power varied by less than 0.5 D around the visual axis was 2.03 mm² in right eyes and 1.88 mm² in left eyes.

Normal corneal shape is aspheric, steeper centrally, and flatter progressively toward the limbus.[6] There are several

Topographic pattern	Bogan (1990) %	Kanpolat (1997) %
Round	22.6	14.0
Oval	20.8	11.4
Symmetric bowtie	17.5	29.0
Asymmetric bowtie	32.1	33.3
Irregular	7.1	12.3

TABLE 7-1
THE TOPOGRAPHIC PATTERNS AND PROPORTIONS IN THE NORMAL CORNEA

TABLE 7-2
DIFFERENT TYPES OF CONIC SECTIONS AND THE CORRESPONDING VALUES OF THE DIFFERENT MEASURES OF ASPHERICITY[15]

	e^2	$SF(=e^2)$	$p(=1-e^2)$	$Q(=-e^2)$
Hyperbola	>1	>1	<0	<−1
Parabola	1	1	0	−1
Prolate ellipse	$0 < e^2 < 1$	$0 < SF < 1$	$0 < p < 1$	$-1 < Q < 0$
Circle	0	0	1	0
Oblate ellipse	<0	<0	>1	>0

descriptors to describe corneal aspheric shape.[15] Vision scientists often assume the corneal profile in any meridian to be a conic section. A conic section can be fully described using two parameters: the apical radius and the eccentricity (e).[16] The eccentricity indicates the departure of the peripheral curvature from the apical radius and so defines the degree of asphericity. There are other descriptors such as shape factor (SF), Q, and p, used to describe a conic section, as shown in Table 7-2. It can be a circle, an ellipse, a parabola, or a hyperbola. A normal cornea is a prolate conic section. That means that the curvature flattens from the apex to the periphery and $0 < SF < 1$. This is called positive asphericity. In the corneas that underwent corneal refractive surgeries or orthokeratology, an oblate conic section may occur. The curvature steepens from the apex to the periphery and $SF < 0$. This is called negative asphericity (Figure 7-3). Table 7-3 summarizes the mean asphericity data for the anterior surface of the normal cornea.

Corneal apex location is important for the design and fitting of contact lenses, and its relation to the visual axis is important to centralizing the optic zone in keratorefractive surgery. The location of the corneal apex varies considerably in different individuals. Tomlinson and Schwartz[17] found that 63% of the corneal axes in normal corneas were temporal to the vertical meridian, 16.3% were paranasal to the vertical meridian, and 21% were on the vertical meridian. The corneal apex was located equally superiorly, inferiorly, and on the horizontal meridian. Sixty-two percent of the corneal apex was located within 0.5 mm of the visual apex. Edmund[14] found that the median position of the apex for the right eye was 0.54 mm temporal and 0.47 mm superior to the visual axis. For the left eye the position of the apex was 0.42 mm temporal and 0.60 mm superior to the visual axis. Rabinowitz et al[11]

measured the steepest point on the cornea and its location relative to the center of the videokeratography. They found that the median site of the corneal apex was superotemporal to the visual axis, which was located in any quadrant around this point and clustered in the vertical meridian. This is in agreement with the work of Edmund.[14] Dingeldein and Klyce[6] did not attempt to locate the corneal apex precisely, but they found the area of greatest power surrounded the visual axis in 52% of the eyes. The location varied considerably from subject to subject with respect to the visual axis. In the investigation on normal corneas in the Chinese population, Liu et al found no corneal apexes on the visual axis,[10] with 69% of corneal apexes inferior to the visual axis.

Dingeldein and Klyce[6] noticed a high degree of mirror image symmetry between the right and left eyes in most individuals. Rabinowitz et al[11] also found the enantiomorphism in the normal corneas. They found that the mirror image symmetry extended to the apex, as described by Edmund[14] and to the acute angle between the steepest radial axis above and below the horizontal meridian. There is also a high degree of symmetry within an individual eye above and below the horizontal meridian. An example can be seen in Figure 7-4.

There are several quantitative indices available from computer-assisted corneal topography. The analysis of quantitative indices allows detection of unusual videokeratography patterns, and description of variation commonly found in keratoconus. Rabinowitz et al[11] analyzed both eyes of 195 normal subjects with a TMS-1 videokeratoscope using quantitative indices. Results are reported in Table 7-4. We analyzed normal corneas of Chinese people using the same indices and obtained similar results, except a smaller SAI (0.247 ± 0.008) and a smaller SRI (0.194 ± 0.181).[10]

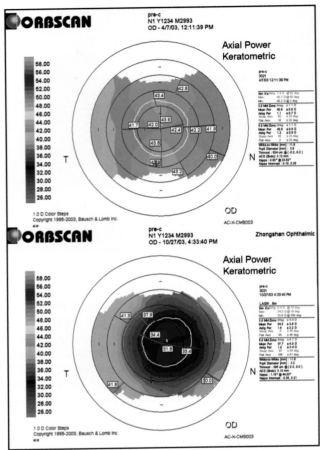

Figure 7-3. Asphericity of the corneal surface. The top image shows positive sphericity (preoperative); the bottom image shows negative sphericity (postoperative).

	e^2	SF$(=e^2)$	$p(=1-e^2)$	$Q(=-e^2)$
Townsley[54]	0.30	0.30	0.70	–0.30
Mandell and St Helen[55]	0.23	0.23	0.77	–0.23
Kiely et al[56]	0.26	0.26	0.74	–0.26
Guillon et al[57]	0.18	0.18	0.82	–0.18
Patel et al[58]	0.03	0.03	0.97	–0.03
Eghbali et al[59]	0.18	0.18	0.82	–0.18
Carney et al[60]	0.33	0.33	0.67	–0.33

TABLE 7-3

SUMMARY OF MEAN ASPHERICITY DATA FOR THE ANTERIOR SURFACE OF THE CORNEA[15]

While the majority of topographic systems utilize Placido imaging, other systems enable direct measurement of elevation. The Orbscan has such a capability. It calculates the elevation of the anterior and posterior surfaces of the cornea (relative to a best-fit-sphere) as well as the thickness of the entire cornea. Figure 7-5 shows a topographical elevation map of the anterior and posterior surfaces of the cornea. Liu et al classified elevation maps into five patterns according to the a classification scheme used by the PAR CTS: regular ridge, irregular ridge, incomplete ridge, island, and unclassified patterns.[18] Anterior and posterior elevation patterns are described in Table 7-5. It has been found that the most common anterior corneal elevation pattern is the island (71.74%), followed by the incomplete ridge, regular ridge, irregular ridge, and unclassified patterns. The island is also the most commonly observed posterior corneal elevation pattern (32.61%), followed by the regular ridge, incomplete ridge, and irregular ridge (Table 7-5). No unclassified pattern appears in posterior corneal elevation map patterns,[18] shown in Figure 7-6.

In addition to the elevation maps, Orbscan also measures the curvature of the anterior corneal surface.[18] Using the same classification scheme obtained by TMS-1 corneal topography system,[8] Liu et al found that the symmetric bowtie was the most commonly observed topographic pattern on the axial power maps of the anterior corneal surface (39.13%), followed by the oval, asymmetric bowtie, round, and irregular.[18] The axial power pattern of the anterior corneal surface is described in Table 7-6. The distribution differs slightly from the results obtained by the TMS-1 system (see Table 7-1). The mean simulated keratometry (Sim K) measurement was 44.24 ± 1.61 D/43.31 ± 1.66 D, which was not statistically different from the mean Sim K values in a study of normal corneal topography with the TMS-1 reported by Bogan et al.[8] The mean keratometric astigmatism was 0.90 ± 0.41 D, which was also not significantly different from that reported by Bogan et al[8] and another investigation of normal corneal topography with PAR CTS reported by Naufal et al.[19] Mean astigmatism in the 3-mm, 5-mm, and 7-mm diameter zones was 1.22 ± 1.08 D, 0.94 ± 0.44 D, and 1.51 ± 0.91 D, respectively. There was a decrease in the refractive power of the cornea and an increase in the irregularity from the center to the periphery of the cornea in both the anterior and posterior corneal surfaces.

Corneal thickness is an important factor in determining the eligibility of subjects for refractive surgery.[20,21] Pachymetry is also important in the diagnosis of corneal diseases, such as keratoconus[22,23] and the monitoring of corneal conditions after surgery.[24,25] Corneal thickness can be evaluated with a number of methods including ultrasonic pachymetry,[26-28] optical slit lamp pachymetry,[28] specular microscopy,[27] confocal microscopy,[29,30] and partial coherence interferometry.[31] The cornea thickens gradually

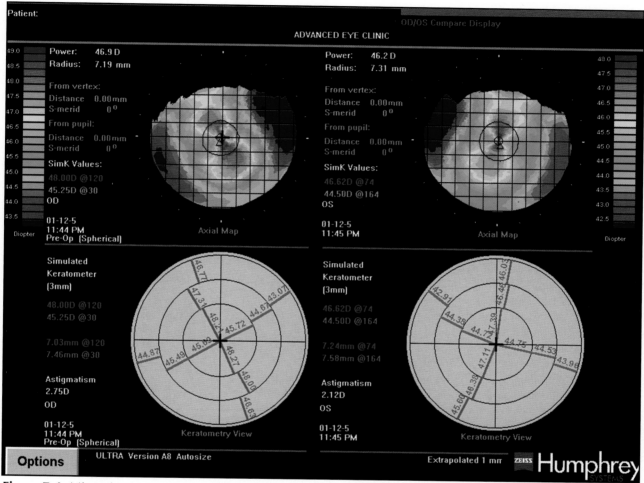

Figure 7-4. Mirror image symmetry of the corneal surface in both eyes of one subject.

TABLE 7-4		
QUANTITATIVE INDICES IN NORMAL CORNEAS[11]		
	Right Eye	**Left Eye**
Sim K (D)	43.7 ± 1.5	43.8 ± 1.5
Min K (D)	43.2 ± 1.5	4.3 ± 1.6
Central K (D)	43.7 ± 1.4	43.8 ± 1.4
SRI	0.54 ± 0.17	0.54 ± 0.17
SAI	0.33 ± 0.13	0.30 ± 0.11
I-S values	0.20 ± 0.53	0.28 ± 0.54
CA		
Power (D)	44.5 ± 1.5	44.6 ± 1.5
Distance (mm)	0.70 ± 0.25	0.68 ± 0.29
Degree	157.8 ± 50.3	165 ± 102.2

TABLE 7-5		
ELEVATION PATTERN OF THE ANTERIOR AND POSTERIOR CORNEAL SURFACES		
Identified pattern	**Anterior (%)**	**Posterior (%)**
Regular ridge	4.34	30.43
Irregular ridge	2.17	13.04
Incomplete ridge	19.57	23.91
Island	71.74	32.61
Unclassified	2.17	0
Total	100	100

from the center to the periphery. Our study found the thinnest site on the entire cornea was an average of 0.55 ± 0.03 mm in thickness and was located at an average of 0.90 ± 0.51 mm from the visual axis. This site was most commonly located in the inferotemporal quadrant (69.57%), followed by the superotemporal, inferonasal, and superonasal quadrants.[18] The location of the thinnest site on the cornea is illustrated in Figure 7-7.

Lam and Chan[32] reported that the thinnest region of the cornea was found in the inferiortemporal quadrant for the right eye and inferior for the left eye. We evaluated average pachymetry in nine circles of 2-mm diameter that are located in the center of the cornea and at eight locations in the mid-peripheral cornea (superior, superotemporal, temporal, inferotemporal, inferior, inferonasal, nasal, and superonasal), each located 3 mm from the visual axis. Among the nine regions evaluated, the central cornea was found to be the thinnest (0.56 ± 0.03 mm). The superior cornea was the thickest (0.64 ± 0.03 mm), followed in order of decreasing thickness by the superonasal, inferonasal, inferior, superotemporal, nasal, inferotemporal, and temporal zones.

The classification system for corneal pachymetry pattern was first presented by Liu et al[18] and is described in Table 7-7 and illustrated in Figure 7-8. The warmest color in the pachymetry map, which identifies the thinnest area of the cornea, is used to designate one of four different patterns: round, oval, decentered round, and decentered oval. The majority of eyes have either oval (47.83%) or round (41.30%) patterns. There is no statistical difference in corneal thickness of the thinnest site or the central and mid-peripheral measured sites between eyes.

Normal Variation of Corneal Topography

Under normal conditions, the physiological functions of our body vary periodically. Accordingly, corneal topography undergoes a periodical variation with the body's changes in physiological function. Several factors cause variation of corneal topography, including eyelid pressure, time of day, blinking, tear film stability and tonicity, and hormone levels. Age and gender can affect hormone levels, which also impact the corneal topography.

Early in 1869, Snellen suspected eyelid pressure resulted in changes of corneal shape. In 1965, Masci[33] noticed that there was a shift toward against-the-rule astigmatism when the eyelid was fully retracted. He concluded that eyelid pressure resulting from the eyelids in normal position could cause a with-the-rule astigmatism. When the lid fissure is fully opened, the cornea can form an against-the-

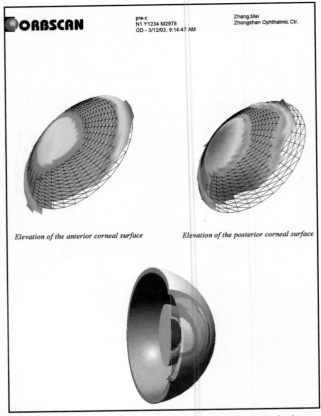

Figure 7-5. Three-dimensional image of corneal elevation in the same eye.

rule astigmatism. Wilson et al[34] noticed that the shift toward against-the-rule astigmatism when eyelids are retracted is caused by the steepening in the horizontal meridian without flattening in the vertical meridian. We believe both meridians contribute to against-the-rule astigmatism formation after the eyelid is fully retracted.

There have been several investigations recently that have evaluated the effects of eyelids on corneal shape (Figure 7-9). Lieberman and Grierson[35] used surface modeling to create central corneal elevation difference maps of four normal eyes with and without lid contact to the corneal surface. Surface modeling demonstrated that the lids influenced the corneal shape. A study conducted by Buehren et al[36] investigated the stability of the ocular surface in the inter-blink period, and found significant changes were apparent in the upper and lower regions of the maps, indicating that corneal shape is related to eyelid pressure. Some other authors also reported that bilateral monocular diplopia may appear after prolonged reading.[37,38] They theorized that reading for a long period of time will result in ptosis, and pressure from the upper lid can lead to alteration of the corneal shape.[38] Currently, the

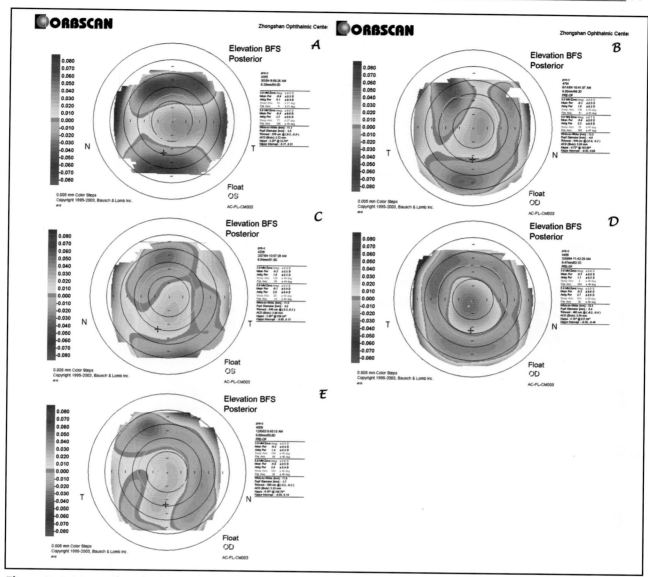

Figure 7-6. No unclassified pattern appears in the posterior corneal elevation map.

TABLE 7-6	
AXIAL POWER PATTERN OF THE ANTERIOR CORNEAL SURFACE	
Identified pattern	**Percent (%)**
Round	6.52
Oval	26.07
Symmetric bowtie	39.13
Asymmetric bowtie	23.91
Irregular	4.53
Total	100

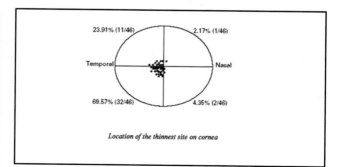

Figure 7-7. Location of the thickness site and average corneal thickness of a normal cornea measured by the Orbscan.

Identified pattern	Percent (%)
TABLE 7-7	
PACHYMETRIC PATTERNS	
Round	41.30
Oval	47.83
Decentered round	2.18
Decentered oval	70.0
Total	100

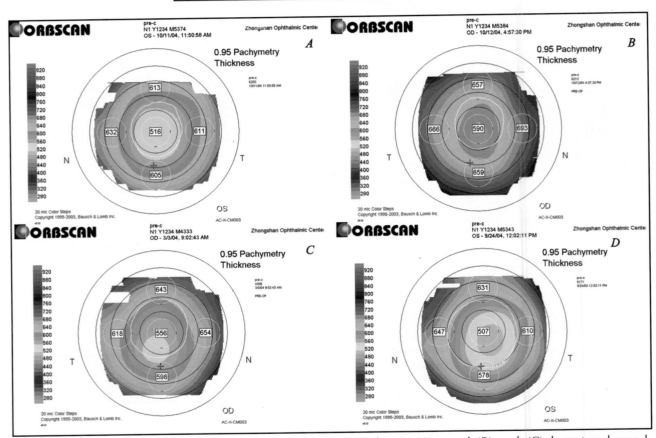

Figure 7-8. Pachymetric patterns on maps generated with the Orbscan: (A) round, (B) oval, (C) decentered round, (D) decentered oval.

effect of upper eyelid pressure on corneal shape is widely accepted.

Corneal topography varies at different times during one day. The corneal topography obtained during waking hours has subtle differences from that obtained during sleep. During sleep, the anterior cornea thickens by 3% to 8%, which will recover to baseline within 1 to 12 hours in the following waking hours. About 75% of the recovering occurs within the first 2 hours.[3] It has not been fully under-stood why corneal thickness increases during sleep. It is now believed to be related to the tear film tonicity. The eyes are closed during sleep, which will cause hypoxia in the tear film and the weakening of the corneal epithelial pump function, which will eventually result in the edema of anterior corneal stroma. Interestingly, the visual acuity of normal corneas does not change upon wakening, when the eyelids are opened. The reason is still unclear. In corneal endothelial dysfunction disorders, such as Fuchs'

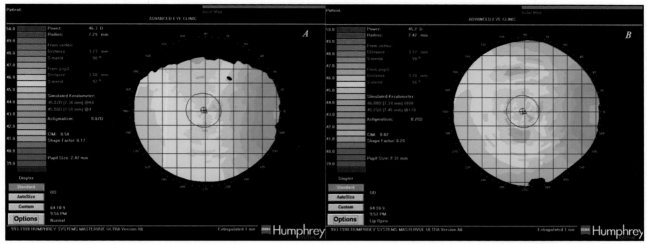

Figure 7-9. Effects of the eyelid on the corneal shape. (A) normal eyes with eyelid contact to the corneal surface; (B) normal eyes without eyelid contact to the corneal surface.

TABLE 7-8

ELEVATION PATTERN BY PAR SYSTEM[24]

Identified pattern	Percent (%)	Corneal astigmatism (Mean ± SD)
Unclassified	3	0.74 ± 0.69
Island	29	0.84 ± 0.64
Regular ridge	17	0.99 ± 0.71
Irregular ridge	28	1.176 ± 0.616
Incomplete ridge	23	0.77 ± 0.54
Total	100	

dystrophy and bullous keratopathy, the corneal edema is more severe during sleep, so some patients may feel an obvious visual acuity decrease in the morning that recovers in the afternoon. It may be because the corneal thickness undergoes very severe changes in these patients and the corneal edema is more significant during sleep. In addition, Ousley and Terry[39] measured the corneal topography of 12 eyebank eyes with videokeratoscopes at the four stages of hydration and dehydration to evaluate the effect of corneal thickness changes on the central and paracentral corneal topography. The results showed that dehydration produced average central and paracentral corneal steepening. It seems that daily dehydration of the normal cornea can partly explain the corneal power increase both in the horizontal and vertical meridian from morning to evening. Another factor that can affect corneal shape is the mechanical pressure coming from the eyelids

during sleep. The corneal curvature is relatively flatter in the morning due to the nightly eyelid pressure and steeper in the afternoon when the pressure is diminished.[40] When compared to the measurement in the morning, the corneal curvature increased by about 0.10 D in the afternoon. However, such physiological variation does not appear to be of any clinical significance.

Blinking and tear film stability can also affect corneal surface regularity. Nemeth et al[41] took measurements 5 and 15 seconds after a complete blink in 12 healthy subjects. They found that during the pause in blinking, both the mean SRI value and the SAI value increased, but there were no significant changes in the values for corneal refractive power or astigmatism. The stability of the tear film during pauses in blinking was considered the reason for this phenomenon. Because corneal topographers measure the shape of the tear film on the corneal surface, a steady tear film can provide a smooth, regular anterior surface. After a long pause time in blinking, the tear film will break and will affect the corneal surface. Another example for the effect of tear film on corneal topography comes from the corneal topography of dry eye patients. Liu and Pflugfelder[42] reported that the SRI and SAI were significantly elevated and that the potential visual acuity (PVA) was significantly reduced in dry eye patients as compared to normal subjects. After the instillation of artificial tears, the SRI, SAI, and mean astigmatism all decreased and the PVA improved in dry eyes. They suggested that the SRI and SAI could be used as objective diagnostic indices for dry eye as well as for evaluating the severity of this disease and the effect of artificial tears. The effect of the tear film can be noted in Figure 7-10.

Another physiological factor that affects corneal topography and curvature is the hormone level. The hormone levels in females vary with the menstrual cycle. Estrogens

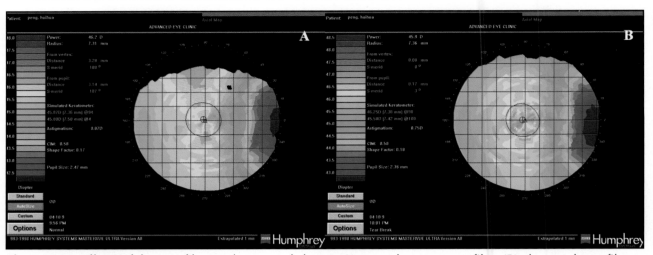

Figure 7-10. Effects of the tear film on the corneal shape. (A) normal cornea tear film; (B) abnormal tear film.

have a major effect on tissue hydration, with higher levels of hormone being associated with increased water retention.[43] It may also have an effect on corneal hydration and topography. The level of estrogen is low at the beginning of the menstrual cycle and then increases gradually. The peak concentration occurs at ovulation (in the middle of the menstrual cycle), and by the end of menstruation the level of estrogens is at its lowest. Several studies have attempted to demonstrate changes in corneal hydration and topography over the menstrual cycle and the results are different. Kiely et al[44] investigated corneal curvature and thickness in six women over one cycle. They found significant corneal steepening in both the horizontal and vertical meridians at the beginning of the cycle; the cornea then flattened gradually. This study also revealed cyclic variations in corneal thickness—thinning occurring toward the end of menstruation and thickening occurring at and shortly after ovulation. The changes of corneal thickness and topography during the menstrual cycle are consistent with the change of estrogen. More recently, Handa et al[45] found that diurnal variation of corneal curvature was significant, approximately 0.83 D in young females after menses, and corneal curvature became flatter during menses in young females. However, in 1996, Oliver et al[46] evaluated the effect of the menstrual cycle on corneal curvature. The results showed that no detectable temporal effect occurred within the menstrual cycle. One explanation is that the variability of measurement with the EyeSys CAS may be masking actual changes occurring during the menstrual cycle. Another reason may be that the sample size is too small in Oliver's study. A longitudinal study with a larger sample size is necessary to evaluate the effects of hormones on the corneal topography.

While aging, the structure and function of ocular surface, including tear film stability and eyelid tension,

undergo some physiological changes that may affect the corneal curvature and topography. Different hormone levels between genders will also affect corneal topography. Several researchers have attempted to evaluate age- and/or gender-related differences in corneal curvature and topography. Most of these studies have showed that the normal cornea shifts from with-the-rule to against-the-rule astigmatism while aging.[47–51] With respect to changes in the corneal meridians, the horizontal meridian may steepen with age.[49,50] The changes of corneal curvature with age may be attributed to the decrease of interfibrillar spacing of corneal collagen and the thickening of collagen bundles.[52] These structural changes may alter the rigidity and elasticity of the cornea. We conjecture that the decreased eyelid tension with age may be another reason for the shift of corneal astigmatism patterns and the change of the corneal meridians. Additionally, Goto et al noticed that corneal irregularity increased with age.[50] The reason for this finding may be decreased tear film stability that occurs as a result of aging.[53]

With respect to gender-related corneal topography changes, Hayashi et al[48] and Goto et al[50] found that with age, men tended to have more against-the-rule astigmatism. They noticed that the horizontal meridian of men steepened and, concurrently, the vertical meridian flattened. In contrast, both meridians of women became steeper with age. This may be because a woman's eyeball is shorter than a man's. Goto et al[50] speculated that the decrease in sex hormone levels may have a greater influence on the changes of corneal curvature in men than in women. However, Rabinowitz et al[11] reported that neither videokeratography patterns nor indices differed significantly with gender or with age. Further studies should be done to determine the effects of age and gender on corneal topography.

The cornea is a unique geometric and biomechanical structure. The comprehensive understanding of its shape will help in the diagnosis of corneal diseases, and the design and evaluation of corneal surgeries. These days, computerized corneal topography has enabled physicians to study a much more detailed corneal shape on every point of the entire cornea. It was also revealed that the shape of the normal cornea does not remain unchanged, but varies with physiological period, time of day, and sleep.

ACKNOWLEDGMENTS

Preparation of this chapter was supported by the National Natural Science Foundation of China (2003, 30371514) and the National Science Foundation for Distinguished Young Scholars of China (2002, 30225044) to Dr. Z. Liu.

NOTE

The authors have no commercial interest in any of the instruments mentioned in this chapter.

REFERENCES

1. Garner LF, Owens H, Yap MK, Frith MJ, Kinnear RF. Radius of curvature of the posterior surface of the cornea. *Optom Vis Sci.* 1997;74:496–498.

2. Miller D, Carter J. A proposed new division of corneal functions. In: *The Cornea. Transactions of the World Congress on the Cornea III.* New York: Raven Press; 1980.

3. Burris TE, Holmes-Higgin D. Topography—the fine art of corneal surface measurement. In: Bores LD, ed. *Refractive Eye Surgery.* Massachusetts, MA: Blackwell Science; 2001.

4. Mandell RB. *Contact Lens Practice: Corneal Topography.* Springfield, MO: Charles C Thomas; 1984.

5. Ludlam WM, Wittenberg S, Rosenthal J, Harris G. Photographic analysis of the ocular dioptric components. 3. The acquisition, storage, retrieval and utilization of primary data in photokeratoscopy. *Am J Optom Arch Am Acad Optom.* 1967;44:276–296.

6. Dingeldein SA, Klyce SD. The topography of normal corneas. *Arch Ophthalmol.* 1989;107:512–518.

7. Knoll HA. Corneal contours in the general population as revealed by the photokeratoscope. *Am J Ophthalmol.* 1961;38:389–397.

8. Bogan SJ, Waring GO III, Ibrahim O, Drews C, Curtis L. Classification of normal corneal topography based on computer-assisted videokeratography. *Arch Ophthalmol.* 1990;108:945–949.

9. Kanpolat A, Simsek T, Alp NM. The evaluation of normal corneal topography in emmetropic eyes with computer-assisted videokeratography. *CLAO J.* 1997;23:168-171.

10. Liu Z, Chen J, Li S, Me G, Ge J. The normal corneal topography in Chinese. *Chinese Journal of Practical Ophthalmology.* 1994;12:652–654.

11. Rabinowitz YS, Yang H, Brickman Y, et al. Videokeratography database of normal human corneas. *Br J Ophthalmol.* 1996;80:610–616.

12. Alvi NP, McMahon TT, Devulapally J, Chen TC, Vianna MA. Characteristics of normal corneal topography using the EyeSys corneal analysis system. *J Cataract Refract Surg.* 1997;23:849–855.

13. Bafna S, Kohnen T, Koch DD. Axial, instantaneous, and refractive formulas in computerized videokeratography of normal corneas. *J Cataract Refract Surg.* 1998;24:1184–1190.

14. Edmund C. Location of the corneal apex and its influence on the stability of the central corneal curvature: a photokeratoscopy study. *Am J Optom Physiol Opt.* 1987;64:846–852.

15. Lindsay R, Smith G, Atchison D. Descriptors of corneal shape. *Optom Vis Sci.* 1998;75:156–158.

16. Burek H. Coincs, cornea and keratometry. *Optician.* 1987;194:18–33.

17. Tomlinson A, Schwartz C. The position of the corneal apex in the normal eye. *Am J Optom Physiol Opt.* 1979;56:236–240.

18. Liu Z, Huang AJ, Pflugfelder SC. Evaluation of corneal thickness and topography in normal eyes using the Orbscan corneal topography system. *Br J Ophthalmol.* 1999;83:774–778.

19. Naufal SC, Hess JS, Friedlander MH, Granet NS. Rastersterreography-based classification of normal corneas. *J Cataract Refract Surg.* 1997;23:222–230.

20. Edmund C. Posterior corneal curvature and its influence on corneal dioptric power. *Acta Ophthalmol (Copenh).* 1994;72:715–720.

21. Consultation section. Refractive surgical problem: low corneal thickness to have LASIK. *J Cataract Refract Surg.* 2003;29:11–13.

22. Rao SN, Raviv T, Majmudar PA, Epstein RJ. Role of Orbscan II in screening keratoconus suspects before refractive corneal surgery. *Ophthalmology.* 2002;109:1642–1646.

23. Auffarth GU, Wang L, Volcker HE. Keratoconus evaluation using the Orbscan Topography System. *J Cataract Refract Surg.* 2000;26:222–228.

24. Kamiya K, Miyata K, Tokunaga T, Kiuchi T, Hiraoka T, Oshika T. Structural analysis of the cornea using scanning-slit corneal topography in eyes undergoing excimer laser refractive surgery. *Cornea.* 2004;23:S59–64.

25. Flanagan G, Binder PS. Estimating residual stromal thickness before and after laser in situ keratomileusis. *J Cataract Refract Surg.* 2003;29:1674–1683.

26. Remon L, Cristobal JA, Castillo J, Palomar T, Palomar A, Perez J. Central and peripheral corneal thickness in full-term newborns by ultrasonic pachymetry. *Invest Ophthalmol Vis Sci.* 1992;33:3080–3083.

27. Argus WA. Ocular hypertension and central corneal thickness. *Ophthalmology.* 1995;102:1810–1812.

28. Salz JJ, Azen SP, Berstein J, Caroline P, Villasenor RA, Schanzlin DJ. Evaluation and comparison of sources of variability in the measurement of corneal thickness with ultrasonic and optical pachymeters. *Ophthalmic Surg.* 1983;14:750–754.

29. Lemp MA, Dilly PN, Boyde A. Tandem-scanning (confocal) microscopy of the full-thickness cornea. *Cornea.* 1985;4:205–209.

30. Yaylali V, Kaufman SC, Thompson HW. Corneal thickness measurements with the Orbscan Topography System and ultrasonic pachymetry. *J Cataract Refract Surg.* 1997;23:1345–1350.

31. Rainer G, Findl O, Petternel V, et al. Central corneal thickness measurements with partial coherence interferometry, ultrasound, and the Orbscan system. *Ophthalmology.* 2004;111:875–879.

32. Lam AK, Chan JS. Corneal thickness at different reference points from Orbscan II system. *Clin Exp Optom.* 2003;86:230–234.

33. Masci E. On ophthalmometric astigmatism: modifications of the corneal curvature in relation to the palpebral activity and scleral rigidity. *Boll Ocul.* 1965;44:755–763.

34. Wilson G, Bell C, Chotai S. The effect of lifting the lids on corneal astigmatism. *Am J Optom Physiol Opt.* 1982;59:670–674.

35. Lieberman DM, Grierson JW. The lids influence on corneal shape. *Cornea.* 2000;19:336–342.

36. Buehren T, Collins MJ, Iskander DR, Davis B, Lingelbach B. The stability of corneal topography in the post-blink interval. *Cornea.* 2001;20:826–833.

37. Mandell RB. Bilateral monocular diplopia following near work. *Am J Optom Arch Am Acad Optom.* 1966;43:500–504.

38. Ford JG, Davis RM, Reed JW, Weaver RG, Craven TE, Tyler ME. Bilateral monocular diplopia associated with lid position during near work. *Cornea.* 1997;16:525–530.

39. Ousley PJ, Terry MA. Hydration effects on corneal topography. *Arch Ophthalmol.* 1996;114:181–185.

40. Kiely PM, Carney LG, Smith G. Diurnal variations of corneal topography and thickness. *Am J Optom Physiol Opt.* 1982;59:976–982.

41. Nemeth J, Erdelyi B, Csakany B. Corneal topography changes after a 15 second pause in blinking. *J Cataract Refract Surg.* 2001;27:589–592.

42. Liu Z, Pflugfelder SC. Corneal surface regularity and the effect of artificial tears in aqueous tear deficiency. *Ophthalmology.* 1999;106:939–943.

43. Fox SI. *Reproduction Human Physiology.* Dubuque, IA: William C Brown Pub; 1993:584–632.

44. Kiely PM, Carney LG, Smith G. Menstrual cycle variations of corneal topography and thickness. *Am J Optom Physiol Opt.* 1983;60:822–829.

45. Handa T, Mukuno K, Niida T, Uozato H, Tanaka S, Shimizu K. Diurnal variation of human corneal curvature in young adults. *J Refract Surg.* 2002;18:58–62.

46. Oliver KM, Walsh G, Tomlinson A, McFadyen A, Hemenger RP. Effect of the menstrual cycle on corneal curvature. *Ophthalmic Physiol Opt.* 1996;16:467–473.

47. Goh WS, Lam CS. Changes in refractive trends and optical components of Hong Kong Chinese aged 19-39 years. *Ophthalmic Physiol Opt.* 1994;14:378–382.

48. Hayashi K, Hayashi H, Hayashi F. Topographic analysis of the changes in corneal shape due to aging. *Cornea.* 1995;14:527–532.

49. Lam AK, Chan CC, Lee MH, Wong KM. The aging effect on corneal curvature and the validity of Javal's rule in Hong Kong Chinese. *Curr Eye Res.* 1999;18:83–90.

50. Goto T, Klyce SD, Zheng X, Maeda N, Kuroda T, Ide C. Gender- and age-related differences in corneal topography. *Cornea.* 2001;20:270–276.

51. Topuz H, Ozdemir M, Cinal A, Gumusalan Y. Age-related differences in normal corneal topography. *Ophthalmic Surg Lasers Imaging.* 2004;35:298–303.

52. Malik NS, Moss SJ, Ahmed N, Furth AJ, Wall RS, Meek KM. Aging of the human corneal stroma: structural and biochemical changes. *Biochim Biophys Acta.* 1992;1138:222–228.

53. Patel S, Farrell JC. Age-related changes in precorneal tear film stability. *Optom Vis Sci.* 1989;66:175–178.

54. Townsley MG. New knowledge of the corneal contour. *Contacto.* 1970;14:38–43.

55. Mandell RB, St Helen R. Mathematical model for the corneal contour. *Br J Physiol Opt.* 1971;26:183–197.

56. Kiely PM, Smith G, Carney LG. The mean shape of the human cornea. *Optica Acta.* 1982;29:1027–1040.

57. Guillon M, Lydon DP, Wilson C. Corneal topography: a clinical model. *Ophthal Physiol Opt.* 1986;6:47–56.

58. Patel S, Marshall J, Fitzke FW. Shape and radius of the posterior corneal surface. *Refract Corneal Surg.* 1993;9:173–181.

59. Eghbali F, Yeung KK, Maloney RK. Topography determination of corneal asphericity and its lack of effect on the refractive outcome of radial keratotomy. *Am J Ophthalmol.* 1995;119:275–280.

60. Carney LG, Mainstone JC, Henderson BA. Corneal topography and myopia. A cross-sectional study. *Invest Ophthalmol Vis Sci.* 1997;38:311–320.

Chapter 8

Topographic Presentation of Common Corneal Diseases

Zhenpin Zhang, MD, PhD

Corneal topography is instrumental in diagnosis of subtle diseases of the cornea when biomicroscopy and refraction fail to identify a problem. This is especially true for early keratoconus within the field of refractive surgery. Unpredictable results and dissatisfaction from patients may be attributed to the coexistence of undiagnosed early keratoconus in refractive surgery patients. Videokeratography screening allows the physician to rule out these early ectasias and other topographic abnormalities before embarking on refractive surgery. This chapter discusses the topographic characteristics, clinical manifestations, and possible physiology of noninflammatory corneal diseases, including keratoconus, pellucid marginal degeneration (PMD), dry eye, and pterygium.

KERATOCONUS AND PELLUCID MARGINAL DEGENERATION

Keratoconus is a bilateral noninflammatory corneal ectatic disease in which the cornea develops a conical shape due to thinning of the corneal stroma, with subsequent irregular astigmatism and myopia leading to marked impairment of vision. The key clinical features used to identify keratoconus have remained essentially the same since the introduction of the slit lamp biomicroscope. Only relatively recently has the development of computerized corneal topography revolutionized the diagnosis of early keratoconus.

The incidence of keratoconus in the general population varies, although it seems relatively high as new corneal topography techniques become more widespread. A long-term study in Minnesota found a prevalence of 54.5 per 100,000 in the general population.[1] Early forms of the disease may go undetected without anterior corneal topography. In a series of patients who sought refractive surgery for myopia, changes suggestive of keratoconus were found in 5.5% (5 of 91 patients) when computerized videokeratography was performed.[2] The variability in the reported incidence reflects the subjective criteria often used to establish the diagnosis. Keratoconus occurs in all ethnic groups with no male or female preponderance. It is most commonly an isolated condition, but may coexist with many other disorders, such as atopy, vernal keratoconjunctivitis, Down syndrome, Leber's congenital amaurosis, retinitis pigmentosa, and retinopathy of prematurity. The cause of keratoconus is unknown. Corneal thinning appears to result from loss of structural components in the cornea. But the underlying biochemical process and its etiologic basis remain poorly understood. Recent studies suggest that enzyme abnormalities in the corneal epithelium, such as increased expression of lysosomal enzymes and decreased levels of inhibitors of proteolyic enzymes, may play a role in corneal stromal degradation.[3,4] Gelatinolytic activity in the stroma may occur because of decreased function of enzyme inhibitors. Promoters of the genes involved in these enzyme activities may be abnormal as well. Regulatory proteins that may play a role in controlling the numerous enzymes involved are being studied. Abnormalities in corneal collagen and its cross-linking may be the cause of keratoconus. Eye rubbing and other factors such as contact lens wear may also play a role. The cytokine interleukin-1 has been suggested as a mediator of eye rubbing and stroma degradation.[5]

Keratoconus has its onset at puberty and is progressive until the third to fourth decade of life, when it usually arrests. It may commence later in life and progress or arrest at any age. The corneal thinning induces irregular astigmatism, myopia, and protrusion, leading to mild to

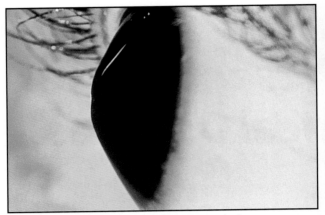

Figure 8-1. Steepening of the cornea in keratoconus.

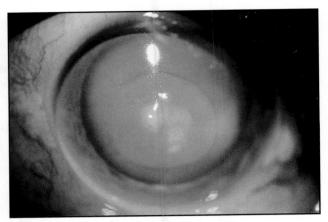

Figure 8-2. Fleischer ring.

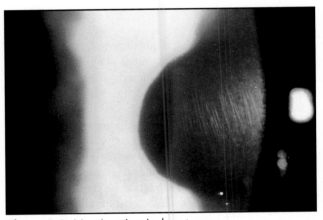

Figure 8-3. Vogt's striae in keratoconus.

marked impairment in the quality of vision, although patients never become totally blind from their disease. It is a progressive disorder ultimately affecting both eyes, although only one eye may be affected initially. In Amsler's study of 600 cases, 22% had clinically obvious keratoconus in both eyes, 26% had clinical keratoconus in one eye and latent keratoconus in the other, and 52% had latent keratoconus bilaterally.[6] Progression was highly variable and most often asymmetric. The cone could remain stationary, progress rapidly over 3–5 years, and arrest or progress intermittently over an extended period of time. When Amsler re-examined 286 eyes 3 to 8 years after the diagnosis, only 20% of his patients, including 66% of the latent cases, had progressed. Progression was most likely to occur in patients between 10 and 20 years of age, decreased slightly between ages 20 and 30, and was less likely to increase after age 30.[7]

Symptoms are highly variable and depend on the level of progression. Early in the disease there may be no symptoms. In advanced disease there is significant distortion of vision accompanied by profound visual loss. Clinical signs differ depending on the severity of the disease. In moderate to advanced disease, any one or combination of signs may be detectable by slit lamp examination of the cornea. These include steepening of the cornea (Figure 8-1), thinning of the corneal apex, clearing zones in the region of Bowman's layer, scarring at the level of Bowman's layer, and deep stromal stress lines that clear when the lids are pressed upon during slit lamp examination. A ring of iron deposition often accumulates within the epithelium at the base of the cone, and is called a Fleischer ring (Figure 8-2). The steepening of the cornea leads to various clinical signs. Protrusion of the lower eyelid on downgaze is termed "Munson's sign." Rizutti's sign can be found by focusing a light beam temporally across the cornea resulting in an arrowhead pattern at the nasal limbus. Charleau's sign is a dark reflex in the area of the cone when observed using a direct ophthalmoscope. Vogt's striae (Figure 8-3)

are vertical lines in the deep stroma and Descemet's membrane that parallel the axis of the cone, which transiently disappear on gentle digital pressure. Other accompanying signs might include epithelial nebulae, anterior stromal scars, an enlarged corneal endothelial reflex, and subepithelial fibrillary lines.

Patients with advanced disease may occasionally present with a sudden onset of visual loss accompanied by pain. Acute hydrops (Figure 8-4) is caused by rupture of Descemet's membrane with acute overhydration of the cornea and accumulation of lakes of fluid within the corneal stroma. The overlying corneal epithelium may become edematous, and fluid may leak through the corneal epithelium. The ruptured Descemet's membrane curls in on itself, and over time endothelial cells spread over the posterior stromal defect to lay down a new Descemet's membrane and recompensate the cornea. The corneal edema is ultimately replaced by scarring (Figure 8-5).

The cornea may appear normal on slit lamp biomicroscopy early in the disease. There may be slight distortion or steepening of keratometry mires centrally or inferiorly. In

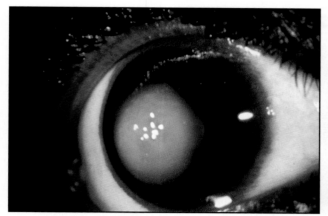

Figure 8-4. Acute hydrops.

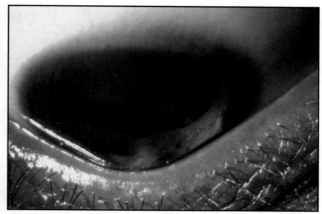

Figure 8-5. Central scarring.

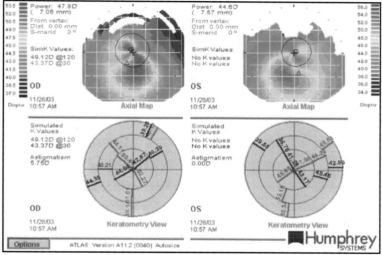

Figure 8-6. Skewing of the steepest radial axes above and below the horizontal meridian in keratoconus.

such instances, where the cornea appears normal but keratoconus is suspected, measuring the anterior topography of the central and paracentral cornea is extremely useful to confirm the diagnosis.[8]

Amsler[6] was the first to describe early corneal topographic changes in keratoconus using a photographic Placido disk before clinical or biomicroscopic signs could be detected in 1938. He classified keratoconus into clinically recognizable stages and an earlier latent stage recognizable only by Placido disk examination of corneal topography. The latter was subdivided into 2 categories: keratoconus fruste and early or mild keratoconus. Keratoconus fruste was characterized by a 1 to 4 degree deviation of the horizontal axis of the placido disk. Early or mild keratoconus showed a 4 to 8 degree deviation. Only slight degrees of asymmetric oblique astigmatism could be detected in these early forms. Similar findings were absent in patients with regular astigmatism.

The Placido disk is a simple tool for early diagnosis of keratoconus. Instrument tilt or poor alignment with respect to the corneal plane in hand-held keratoscopes may result in mis-interpretation of the deviation of the horizontal axis. Reproducibility thus poses a potential problem with this device. Early forms of keratoconus are best detected with videokeratography. Most computer-assisted videokeratoscopy is based on Placido-disk principles, although other technologies are rapidly emerging.

Keratoconus has three characteristics seen by videokeratography that are not present in normal eyes: an increased area of corneal power surrounded by concentric areas of decreasing power, inferior-superior power asymmetry, and skewing of the steepest radial axes above and below the horizontal meridian (Figure 8-6). The majority of patients have peripheral cones, with steepening extending into the periphery. The steepening in this group is usually confined to one or two quadrants. A small group of patients has central topographic alterations. Many central cones have a bowtie configuration similar to that found in naturally occurring astigmatism. In the keratoconus patients, the bowtie pattern is asymmetric, with the inferior loop being

Figure 8-7. Typical map for a keratoconus suspect.

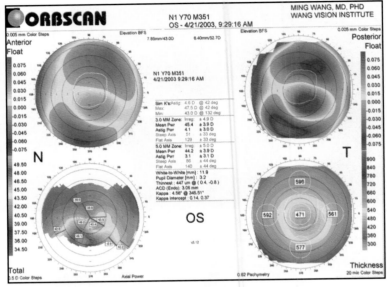

larger in most instances. In contrast to eyes having with-the-rule astigmatism, the steep radial axes above and below the horizontal meridian in keratoconus appear skewed, giving the bowtie a lazy-eight configuration. Another pattern found in central cones is more symmetric steepening without a bowtie appearance. The pattern is usually the same in both eyes, although it may be more advanced in one eye than in the other. Peripheral and central cones probably correspond roughly to the oval sagging and nipple-shaped cones.

A typical map for a keratoconus suspect is shown in Figure 8-7. Currently, there are no specific criteria for categorizing keratoconus suspects. The general rule is that these topography maps closely resemble maps of a mild form of true, clinical keratoconus, yet they do not have any of the traditional, diagnostic criteria for the disease (biomicroscopic appearance of corneal thinning, scissoring of retinoscopic reflex, Munson's sign, etc) nor can they be classified within another category, such as contact lens wearers suffering from warpage. Typically, the keratoconus suspect is similar to the map in Figure 8-7, with the classic appearance of inferior, localized steepening. However, localized steepening in the central or superior cornea is commonly seen, much as one finds clinical keratoconus centrally, or on occasion, superiorly. Suspicious maps are problematic in that they may be signaling the impending development of true, clinical keratoconus, or they may be totally innocuous. While it is advisable to compare maps of fellow eyes to see if ectasias are present in both corneas, the lack of any sign of an ectasia in the fellow cornea does not indicate that the keratoconus suspect will not progress into true keratoconus. At the present time, the ideal course of management would be repeated topographic analysis. Videokeratographic indices are useful to establish quantita-

tive baseline readings of surface irregularity or asymmetry. In addition, videokeratographic-based keratoconus screening programs such as the Klyce/Maeda KCI value or the Rabinowitz I-S measure are helpful in detecting the earliest topographic signs of keratoconus.

An example of mild keratoconus is shown in Figure 8-8. Mild keratoconus is topographically characterized by contour powers that tend to be less than 55 D at any point on the map. Generally there are fewer contours present on the map than cases of moderate or advanced keratoconus, but there are no specific limitations. One reason for this is because if the nasal flattening is pronounced, it may introduce one or two additional contours at the lower end of the power scale. The cone may be located at any position on the surface, but inferior cones tend to be the most common form of ectasia.

An example of advanced keratoconus is shown in Figure 8-9. In cases of advanced keratoconus, maximum contour power is at or above 55 D. However, unlike the continuous color contours in the moderate category, advanced keratoconus does show disruptions of the mire pattern at or near the cone apex, which produces contour discontinuities. Clinicians must be cautious to check that mire disruption is due to the presence of the cone, and not due to some other factor such as tear film drying or mucus strands.

It is important to distinguish keratoconus from other ectatic dystrophies and thinning disorders, such as Terrien's marginal degeneration, keratoglobus, and PMD, since the management and prognosis in these disorders differs markedly from keratoconus. Corneal topography evaluation is helpful to differentiate these disorders in subtle or early cases.

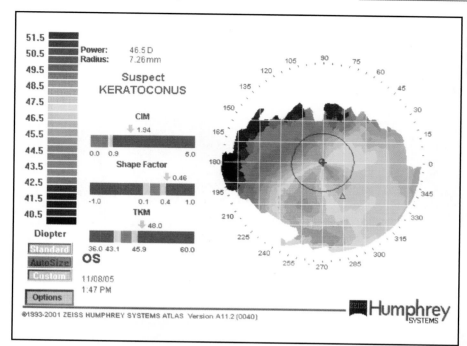

Figure 8-8. Mild pellucid marginal degeneration found to be suspect on the keratoconus detection program.

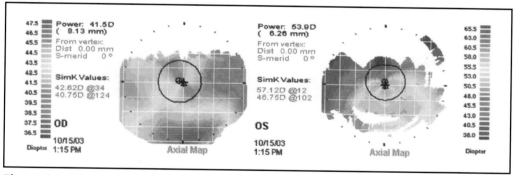

Figure 8-9. More advanced keratoconus. Note the loss of data due to extreme irregularity in curvature.

Terrien's corneal degeneration may affect both the superior and inferior cornea and is accompanied by identifiable signs on biomicroscopy, including lipid deposition and vascular invasion. Peripheral changes in corneal topography may be seen, but central effects are not typically noted on CT. Keratoglobus is seen as an overall enlargement of the cornea.

PMD is sometimes confused with keratoconus because both involve localized steepening of the inferior peripheral cornea. It is quite likely that these two forms of ectasia are closely related and involve some biomechanical factors that govern the location of the ectasia. PMD can usually be distinguished from keratoconus by the extreme peripheral position of the ectasia and its crescent-shaped morphology. The horns of the crescent tend to curve inward toward the central cornea (Figure 8-10). In the vertical axis (or nearly vertical), there is typically a noticeably flat axis

contained within the central region of the cornea. Thus, the inferior aspect of the cornea may have both extremely high and low power contours.

Thinning in PMD occurs in a 1- to 2-mm band, usually in the 4 to 8 o'clock position, located 1 to 2 mm from the inferior limbus. The uninvolved, apparently normal inferior cornea protrudes anteriorly, overhanging the area of thinning. The epithelium is intact, and the cornea above the thinned area is ectatic. The area between the limbus and thinning is clear, without any scarring, lipid deposition, or vascularization. Although PMD classically has been described as an inferior entity, recent reports described the occurrence of isolated superior PMD, the presence of superior corneal thinning in classic PMD, and contiguous extension of the zone of peripheral thinning above the horizontal meridian.[9–11]

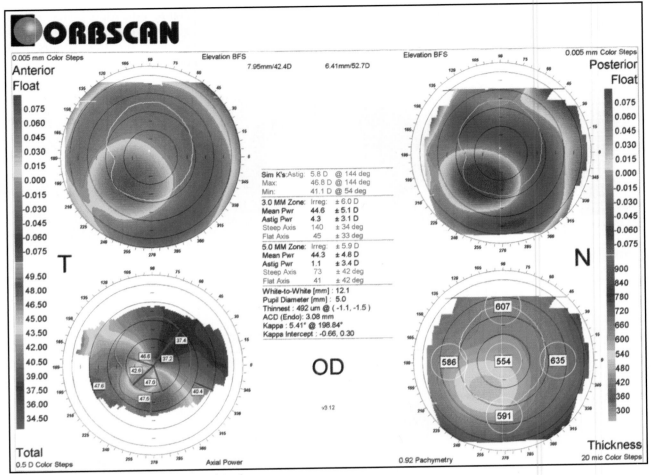

Figure 8-10. Typical PMD topographical map.

Patients usually present in their fourth to fifth decades of life with reduced visual acuity due to high irregular astigmatism, although the patient might have had PMD as early as the age of 8 years.[12] Sridhar et al[12] recently reported 116 eyes of 58 patients with PMD and found that it was seen predominantly in males, with 45 cases (77.6%) and only 13 females (22.4%). All cases were bilateral. In one eye, no clinical features of PMD were seen, but the diagnosis of PMD was made based on the presence of typical topographic features. The degree of astigmatism was < 5.0 D in 19 eyes (19.2%), 5 to 10 D in 36 (36.4%), 10 to 15 D in 23 (23.2%), 15 to 20 D in 15 (15.2%), and > 20 D in 6 (6.1%). Typical inferior PMD was seen in 99 eyes (85.3%), and superior PMD was seen in 17 eyes (14.7%). The thinning was commonly seen from the 5 o'clock to the 7 o'clock positions. Seven eyes (6.0%) had hydrops. The rupture occurred at the site of ectasia superior to the thinning; vascularization was not seen in any of the eyes. In 12 eyes (10.3%), PMD was associated with keratoconus, and in 15 (12.9%), it was associated with keratoglobus. Acute hydrops and spontaneous perforation are the complica-

tions reported.[13–15] Corneal hydrops may be a common phenomenon in patients with keratoconus because of the breaks in the Descemet's membrane. Hydrops reflect a corneal response to progressive thinning, and are seen in various ectatic corneal disorders. Corneal edema with an identifiable break in the Descemet's membrane is the usual presentation. In PMD, the break is usually above the site of crescentic stromal thinning. Lucarelli et al[14] described perforation at the inferior crescent. Resolution of edema occurs by migration of endothelium across the break.

Corneal topography in classic inferior PMD, as depicted by videokeratoscopy, was first reported by Maguire et al.[16] Corneal power is lowest along a narrow corridor of the central cornea, with the axis oriented close to the vertical meridian. Between the lower border of this area and the most peripheral extent of inferior cornea analyzed, corneal power increases rapidly. The area of highest power extends along the inferior cornea, and then turns toward the central cornea along the inferior oblique cornea meridians. The typical topography map of the condition shows marked flattening of the cornea along a vertical axis and a steepening of the inferior cornea peripheral to the site of the lesion. Rao et al[17] reported that corneal topographic changes in atypical PMD are similar to those seen in typical PMD, but corneal changes involve the nasal, temporal, or superior quadrants, or a combination of these.

The correction of irregular astigmatism caused by primary corneal ectasia such as PMD remains a challenge. For correction early in the disease, soft toric lenses are adequate. In moderately severe cases, RGP contact lenses, toric polymethyl methacrylate lenses, and scleral lenses may be useful. A hybrid lens, which has a rigid central portion for obtaining best optics and a soft, hydrophilic peripheral skirt, may also be used. Surgical intervention is delayed as far as possible. It is suggested only when the patient can no longer tolerate contact lens wear. Several surgical procedures have been advocated for visual rehabilitation in PMD. These include large eccentric penetrating keratoplasty, thermocauterization, total lamellar keratoplasty followed by penetrating keratoplasty, epikeratoplasty, crescentic lamellar keratoplasty, corneal wedge excision/resection, and lamellar crescentic resection.[18–24] But we have to understand that most of the reported results are only isolated cases with short follow-up. Any surgical intervention is difficult because of the intraoperative complications faced by the surgeon during the procedure due to the thinning adjacent to the limbus.

Dry Eye Syndromes

Keratoconjunctivitis sicca (KCS), or dry eye, is a disease of the ocular surface attributable to different disturbances of the natural function and protective mechanism of the external eye, leading to an unstable tear film during the open eye state. It is one of the most common complaints seen by ophthalmic specialists, and is commonly seen using topography in the form of focal central irregularities. An example is shown in Figure 8-11. Dry eye is not a trivial complaint, as the symptoms cause considerable discomfort and substantially reduce the sufferer's quality of life. It is now recognized that dry eye is the result of a localized immune-mediated inflammatory response involving both the lacrimal glands and the ocular surface.[25]

Tears are a complex solution composed of water, enzymes, proteins, immunoglobulins, lipids, various metabolites, and exfoliated epithelial and polymorphonuclear cells. The tear film is composed of three main components: mucin layer, aqueous layer, and lipid layer, each of which has been classically described as a separate layer that performs a specific function.

The inner mucin layer is produced by conjunctival goblet cells, conjunctival and corneal epithelial cells. The

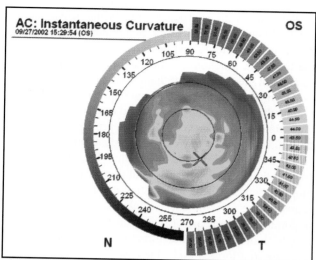

Figure 8-11. Topography in dry eye.

corneal and conjunctival epithelia synthesize a mucin-like glycoprotein (MUC1) at the apical surface of the epithelium to constitute the glycocalyx. This transmembrane mucin has a role in tear film spreading and is essential for proper ocular surface wetting. It prevents adhesion of foreign debris, cells, or pathogens to the ocular surface. The mucinous content of the tear film is mainly produced by the secretions of the goblet cells of the conjunctiva, which open on the ocular surface. The human conjunctiva also expresses the mucins MUC4 and MUC5AC, which may play an important role in forming the tear film layer at the air and ocular surface-epithelium interface. The mucin of the glycocalyx renders the whole of the ocular surface hydrophilic and allows the aqueous layer to spread evenly over the eye. Without the glycocalyx, tears do not properly adhere to the eye and epithelial damage may occur, even with normal aqueous tear production.

The main and accessory lacrimal glands produce the aqueous layer. This layer is quantitatively the most important, and is responsible for creating the proper environment for the epithelial cells of the ocular surface, carrying essential nutrients and oxygen to the cornea, allowing cell movement over the ocular surface, as well as washing away epithelial debris, toxic elements, and foreign bodies. Changes in its composition occur rather quickly in response to environmental or bodily conditions and can influence the health, proliferation, maturation, and movement of the surface epithelial cells. Many of the growth factors that are present in the aqueous phase of the tear film are derived from lacrimal gland tissue. This has been shown for EGF, TGFa, HGF, and others. A significant role of these growth factors in corneal physiology has been suggested. According to current models, decreased aqueous tear production results in a decreased growth factor concentration in the tears, with consequent effects on ocular surface health. Many proinflammatory factors produced locally or by adjacent structures, and located in the aqueous phase of the tear film, function to modulate the eye's response to changes in the condition of the ocular surface.

The meibomian glands, located within the tarsal plates, secrete their oily product onto the lid margins and form the outer lipid layer of the tear film. The principal function of the lipid layer is to prevent the evaporation of tears and enhance the stability of the tear film. The presence of a smooth lipid layer is also essential to provide an excellent dioptric element for light refraction into the eye and sharp retinal image formation. The blink reflex is thought to be important in the release of secretions from the meibomian glands. Indeed, rapid and forceful blinking, such as in response to a foreign body, increases the thickness of the lipid layer.

Deficiencies in any of the tear film layers, defective spreading of the tear film, systemic diseases, and some systemic and topical medications can disturb the ocular surface or tear film and cause dry eye. Dry eye conditions have recently been classified into two main categories: aqueous layer deficiency and evaporative deficiency. Aqueous layer deficiency is the most common cause of dry eye and is usually caused by decreased tear secretion from the lacrimal glands, although increased evaporation of tears may also be involved. Causes of reduced secretion include Sjögren's syndrome; senile hyposecretion; lacrimal gland excision; vitamin A deficiency; immune lacrimal gland damage in sarcoidosis or lymphoma; sensory or motor reflex loss; scarring conditions of the conjunctiva, such as pemphigoid, chemical burns, or trachoma; and contact lens wear. Changes in the composition of the aqueous layer, such as increased electrolyte concentration, loss of growth factors, or presence of pro-inflammatory cytokines, together with a slow tear turnover, are associated with ocular surface damage.

The usual cause of a lipid layer deficiency is obstruction of the meibomian glands. Obstruction may occur spontaneously or be associated with certain forms of skin disease. Deficiency of the lipid layer permits more rapid evaporation of moisture from the eye surface and, in the absence of an adequate increase of tear production by the lacrimal glands, gives rise to an evaporative form of dry eye. Conditions associated with meibomian gland dysfunction include atopic keratoconjunctivitis; blepharitis; generalized dysfunction of sebaceous glands, such as acne rosacea or seborrhoeic dermatitis; and several polluting chemical agents, such as turpentine, often present in the sick building environment. (Sick building syndrome comprises a spectrum of symptoms caused by characteristics of building environments, eg, poor ventilation and chemical and biological contaminants).

Goblet cell deficiency accompanies most forms of dry eye. Certain disorders in particular may precipitate goblet cell loss. These include vitamin A deficiency, as vitamin A is essential for the maintenance of goblet cells and mucin at the ocular surface, and cicatrizing conjunctival disorders, such as Stevens-Johnson syndrome, trachoma, pemphigoid, and chemical burns. Topical medications and preservatives can also damage the ocular surface and goblet cells.

Abnormalities of the eyelids or the ocular surface itself can interfere with the effective spreading of tears across the cornea and cause drying of the ocular surface. This phenomenon is often seen in cases of ectropion or entropion, lid margin irregularity, exophthalmos due to thyroid disease, or corneal scarring.

Collagen vascular disorders (collagenoses) include various autoimmune disorders, such as rheumatoid arthritis. Most patients with rheumatoid arthritis have some degree of dry eye disease. It is thought that lymphocytic infiltration of the lacrimal gland results in reduced tear secretion. Scleroderma sicca syndrome has been described in 70% of patients with scleroderma. Patients with the limited form of the disease (CREST syndrome [calcinosis, Raynaud's phenomenon, esophageal hypomotility, sclerodactyly, and telangiectasia]) tend to have severe sicca symptoms. Lupus erythematosus dry eye disease is the most common ocular finding in this systemic autoimmune disorder, which is characterized by anti-nuclear antibodies. Sjögren's syndrome is a chronic autoimmune disease that affects the major exocrine glands, notably the lacrimal and salivary glands, and thus leads to dryness of the eyes and mouth. The conjunctiva is also infiltrated by inflammatory cells. Dry eye is a common consequence of chronic allergic conjunctivitis due to continuing activation of the local immune system. A vicious cycle of irritation and ocular surface damage may cause dry eye symptoms to persist for months after the allergic episode.

One of the most severe forms of dry eye is seen in the course of Stevens-Johnson syndrome. Chronic mucocutaneous syndromes, such as cicatricial pemphigoid, also often lead to severe loss of goblet cells and dry eye in late stages of the disease. Treatment consists of systemic immunosuppression.

It is often overlooked that systemic drugs can increase the risk of dry eye. These include thiazide diuretics, tricyclic and tetracyclic antidepressants, beta-blockers, anticholinergics, benzodiazepines, anti-Parkinson's drugs, anti-histamines, and antihypertensives.

The causes of increased evaporation of water from the tear film can be found in any of the quantitative or qualitative changes occurring on the ocular surface or in the tear film itself that affect the formation and the spreading of a normal oily layer. This feature does not indicate that a

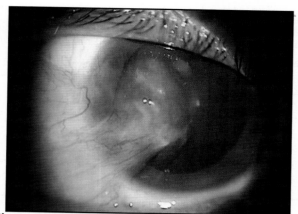

Figure 8-12. Pterygium on clinical exam.

primary abnormality of the oily layer is the only cause of tear film disruption. As indicated, many other factors that are able to destroy the delicate architecture of the tear film will increase evaporation. Results have not been replicated in human eyes. If for any reason the lacrimal glands are not able to maintain an elevated rate of secretion sufficient to compensate for the water lost through evaporation, this results in an increase in osmolarity of the tear film. This, in turn, can be one of the sources of epithelial damage in dry eye disease. It is recognized as evaporative dry eye (EDE).

Goto et al[26] developed a new tear film stability analysis system (TSAS) based on the phenomenon that topographic maps are subject to change because of fluctuation of tear film stability. According to the corneal power change on topographic maps, tear breakup time and tear breakup area were analyzed. The new topographic method feasibly could be used for evaluation of tear film stability as an objective, noninvasive, and reproducible examination with high sensitivity.[27]

Patients with aqueous deficiency have an irregular corneal surface that may contribute to their visual difficulties. The SRI and SAI could be used as objective diagnostic indices for dry eye as well as for evaluating the severity of this disease and the effect of artificial tears.

PTERYGIUM

A pterygium, shown in Figure 8-12, is a fleshy, vascular, triangular, "wing-like" fold of tissue in the interpalpebral fissure (the area defined by the open eyelids). The growth arises from the conjunctiva (the clear tissue layer overlying the white sclera of the eye) and tends to develop on the nasal aspect of the globe (the inner canthus). Occasionally, one sees patients with both inner and outer canthus growths in the same eye. Pterygia are more com-

mon in individuals who spend time outdoors and who live in climates closer to the equator, probably due to UV radiation from the sun. As the pterygium grows, the apex of the fold grows up and over the peripheral cornea and toward the central cornea. The growth is firmly attached to the underlying tissue.

Topographically, the cornea tends to exhibit normal characteristics, such as with-the-rule astigmatism; however, in the direction of the pterygium there is more flattening in the region of the apex of the growth. As more tissue covers the cornea, the topography usually exhibits more flattening and more irregular astigmatism. In Figures 8-13A and 8-13B, the axial maps show irregular with-the-rule astigmatism due to the elevation of the tissue located nasally and temporally. The elevation maps illustrate the growth of the tissue upon the cornea seen nasally and temporally. The loss of data is due to chronic dryness secondary to the irregular surface. Surgical removal of the pterygium after it has grown over the cornea tends to leave behind a flattened irregular region. Ideally, the growth should be removed before it invades the cornea. In the maps, we can see the highly reflective surface of the pterygium covering the sclera on the right (patient's inner canthus). Note the flattening that extends ahead of the pterygium apex.

CONCLUSION

Keratoconus, PMD, dry eyes, and pterygium are the most commonly seen corneal disease entities easily identified using modern corneal topography. Understanding of the clinical interpretation of maps for such diagnoses is especially important for refractive surgeons when patients present without clinical signs seen on biomicroscopy.

REFERENCES

1. Kennedy RH, Bourne WM, Dyer JA. A 48-year clinical and epidemiologic study of keratoconus. *Am J Ophthalmol.* 1986;101:267–273.

2. Nesburn AB, Bahri S, Salz J, et al. Keratoconus detected by videokeratography in candidates of photorefractive keratectomy. *J Refractive Surg.* 1995;11:194-201.

3. Sawagamuchi S, Yue B, Sugar J, et al. Lysomal abnormalities in keratoconus. *Arch Ophthalmol.* 1989;107:1507–1510.

4. Fukuchi T, Yue B, Sugar J, et al. Lysosomal enzyme activities in conjunctival tissue of patients with keratoconus. *Arch Ophthalmol.* 1994;112:1368–1374.

5. Wilson SE, He YG, Weng J, et al. Epithelial injury induces keratocyte apoptosis: hypothesized role for the interleukin

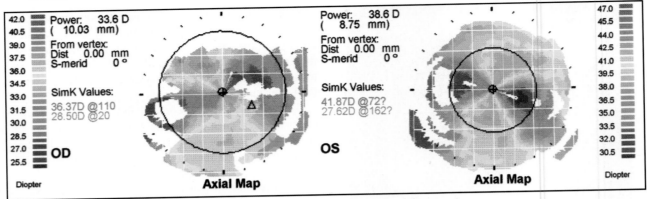

Figure 8-13A. Axial maps for a patient with a large nasal and temporal pterygium.

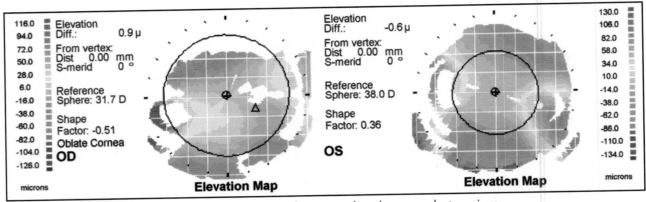

Figure 8-13B. Elevation maps for a patient with a large nasal and temporal pterygium.

1 system in the modulation of corneal tissue organization and wound healing. *Exp Eye Res.* 1996;62:325–337.

6. Amsler M. Le keratocone fruste au javal. *Ophthalmologica.* 1938;96:77–83.

7. Amsler M. Keratocone classique et keratocone fruste, arguments unitaires. *Ophthalmologica.* 1946;111:96–101.

8. Maguire LJ, Bourne WM. Corneal topography of early keratoconus. *Am J Ophthalmol.* 1989;108:107–112.

9. Cameron JA, Mahmood MA. Superior corneal thinning with pellucid marginal degeneration. *Am J Ophthalmol.* 1990;109:486–487.

10. Taglia DP, Sugar J. Superior pellucid marginal degeneration with hydrops. *Arch Ophthalmol.* 1997;115:274–275.

11. Bower KS. Dhaliwal DK, Barnhorst DA, et al. Pellucid marginal degeneration with superior corneal thinning. *Cornea.* 1997;16:483–485.

12. Sridhar MS, Mahesh S, Bansal AK, et al. Pellucid marginal corneal degeneration. *Ophthalmology.* 2004;111:1102-1107.

13. Carter JB, Jones DB, Wilhelmus KR. Acute hydrops in pellucid marginal corneal degeneration. *Am J Ophthalmol.* 1989;107:167–170.

14. Lucarelli MJ, Gendelman DS, Talamo JH. Hydrops and spontaneous perforation in pellucid marginal corneal degeneration. *Cornea.* 1997;16:232–234.

15. Orlin SE, Sulewski ME. Spontaneous corneal perforation in pellucid marginal degeneration. *CLAO J.* 1998;24:186–187.

16. Maguire LJ, Klyce SD, McDonald MB, Kaufman HE. Corneal topography of pellucid marginal degeneration. *Ophthalmology.* 1987;94:519–524.

17. Rao SK, Fogla R, Padmanabhan P, et al. Corneal topography in atypical pellucid marginal degeneration. *Cornea.* 1999;18:265–272.

18. Varley GA, Macsai MS, Krachmer JH. The results of penetrating keratoplasty for pellucid marginal corneal degeneration. *Am J Ophthalmol.* 1990;110:149–152.

19. Biswas S, Brahma A, Tromans C, Ridgway A. Management of pellucid marginal corneal degeneration. *Eye.* 2000;14:629–634.

20. Kremer I, Sperber LT, Laibson PR. Pellucid marginal degeneration treated by lamellar and penetrating keratoplasty [letter]. *Arch Ophthalmol.* 1993;111:169–170.

21. Fronterre A, Portesani GP. Epikeratoplasty for pellucid marginal corneal degeneration. *Cornea.* 1991;10:450–453.

22. MacLean H, Robinson LP, Wechsler AW. Long-term results of corneal wedge excision for pellucid marginal degeneration. *Eye.* 1997;11:613–617.

23. Dubroff S. Pellucid marginal corneal degeneration—report on corrective surgery. *J Cataract Refract Surg.* 1989;15:89–93.

24. Cameron JA. Results of lamellar crescentic resection for pellucid marginal corneal degeneration. *Am J Ophthalmol.* 1992;113:296–302.

25. Stern ME, Beuerman RW, Fox RI, et al: The pathology of dry eye: the interaction between the ocular surface and lacrimal glands. *Cornea.* 1998;17:584–589.

26. Goto T, Zheng X, Klyce SD, et al. A new method for tear film stability analysis using videokeratography. *Am J Ophthalmol.* 2003;135:607–612.

27. Liu Z, Pflugfelder SC. Corneal surface regularity and the effect of artificial tears in aqueous tear deficiency. *Ophthalmology.* 1999;106:939–943.

Chapter 9

Pre-Refractive Surgery Evaluation

Guillermo Avalos-Urzua, MD; Ariadna Silva-Lepe, MD;
Tracy Swartz, OD, MS; and Ming Wang, MD, PhD

As we have seen in previous chapters, corneal topography is a method of corneal curvature examination assisted by computer analysis. Topography is invaluable to preoperative evaluation of patients seeking elective procedures. Corneal maps identify potential obstacles to keratorefractive surgery, such as forme fruste keratoconus (FFKC), contact lens warpage, decentered corneal apex, tear film problems, corneal aberration in dry eye patients, and regular and irregular astigmatism. It is not uncommon for such problems to be present when biomicroscopy fails to identify clinical signs. For this reason, topographic analysis is performed on every keratorefractive surgery candidate.

FORME FRUSTE KERATOCONUS

Despite progress in corneal topography technology and in computer programs with quantitative indices, an exact diagnosis of FFKC is still difficult.[1] Presentation of abnormally steep corneas should raise a few important questions for the surgeon.[2] Patients presenting with steep keratometric readings, unstable or increasing astigmatism, or mild visual distortion may suffer from irregular astigmatism, which is a hallmark of keratoconus and FFKC. Examples of various stages of irregular astigmatism are shown in Figure 9-1.

Varssano et al[3] performed a retrospective evaluation of videokeratographies of previously unoperated refractive surgery candidates. Electronic topography records of 100 candidates were evaluated. The candidates included 41 women and 59 men whose average age was 32 years. Their topographic patterns were described as: spherical (36/200 evaluated eyes), spherocylindrical (60), upper steep (32), lower steep (43), irregular astigmatism (9), decentered (3),

suspected keratoconus (11), and probable keratoconus (6 eyes). More than one-half of corneal topographies of refractive surgery candidates did not comply with the assumed "normal" spherical or spherocylindrical patterns. They concluded that the possible continuum of keratoconus-suspected keratoconus-lower steep pattern raises the question of where to draw the line between "reasonable" and "risky" when considering corneal refractive surgery.

A significant number of keratoconus cases remain undetected with refraction, clinical evaluation, and conventional keratometry, but computed topography reveals a keratoconus-type pattern. This topographic form of keratoconus is known as preclinical, or FFKC. Computer-assisted videokeratoscopes with color-coded maps and topographic indices are the most sensitive and sophisticated devices for confirming the diagnosis of FFKC. Corneas with FFKC may have altered biomechanical properties compared to normal corneas. A review of the peer-reviewed literature revealed preoperative topographic evidence of FFKC in 13 of 27 cases of progressive and visually threatening ectasia following LASIK.[4] FFKC is defined as the lack of clinical signs of keratoconus with two or more of the following corneal topographic data: 1) central keratometry above 47.0 D; 2) superior and inferior keratometric value difference at least of 1.4 D; 3) apex distance from cone to corneal center above 1.0 mm and 4) superior central keratometric difference above 1.0 D between eyes, as shown in Figure 9-2.

Levy et al[4] investigated detection of low-expressivity keratoconus in an effort to improve the diagnosis criteria of FFKC in relatives of familial keratoconus. They found that the uncommon frequency of J or Jinv shapes (detected by the 0.5-D increment scale) suggests that these patterns of steepening, with an S_{rax} over 21 degrees and an Abs(I-S) value over 0.8 D, may correspond to a superior or

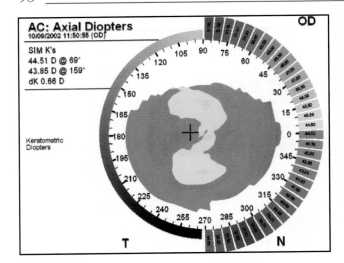

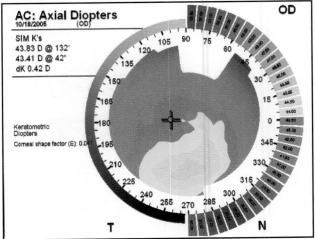

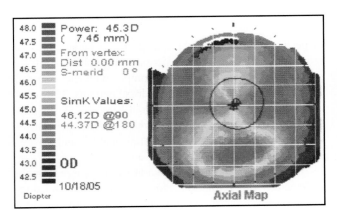

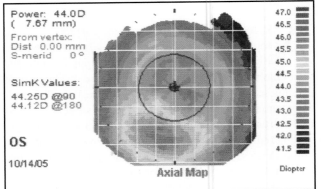

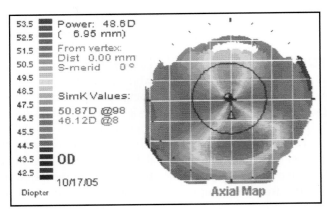

Figure 9-1. Various examples of irregular astigmatism, suspicious for keratoconus.

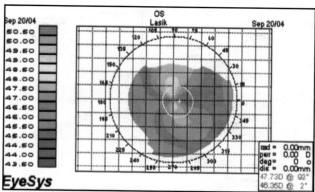

Figure 9-2. Superior central keratometric difference above 1.0 D between eyes may indicate FFKC.

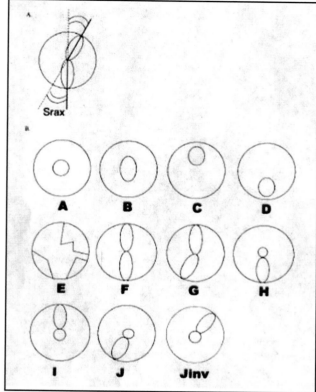

Figure 9-3. Patterns of steepening, with an S_{rax} over 21 degrees and an Abs(I-S) value over 0.8 D, may correspond to FFKC.

inferior FFKC. Example patterns can be seen in Figure 9-3. The observation of such patterns using a 0.5-D increment scale must incite refractive surgeons to be particularly cautious and carefully investigate the familial history of the patient.

Arntz et al[5] evaluated the most effective parameters of a slit scanning corneal topography system for subclinical keratoconus screening. The study included corneas from patients with a clinical diagnosis of keratoconus, patients with subclinical keratoconus, and a control group of myopic subjects. Placement of the apex, anterior and posterior corneal elevation, minimal corneal thickness, anterior chamber depth, and corneal diameter were evaluated. The most frequent location of the apex was the inferotemporal sector (53%). Mean anterior elevation was 56.73 (S.D. 25.95 mm) in group 1 and 20.35 (S.D. 8.04 mm) in group 2. These results are statistically different from the control group. Mean posterior elevation was 126.23 (S.D. 57.7 mm) in group 1 and 54.28 (S.D. 19.55 mm) in group 2, both showing a statistically significant difference from the control group. Minimal corneal thickness and anterior chamber depth also showed statistically significant differences between the three groups.

Rao et al[6] evaluated the relationship between videokeratographic keratoconus screening programs and Orbscan II topography. Sixty consecutive eyes with suspicious videokeratography (TMS-1) were compared to a control group of 50 consecutive eyes without suspicious features by videokeratography. Orbscan II topographies and two keratoconus screening programs, the Rabinowitz method (shown in Figure 9-3) and Klyce/Maeda methods, were performed on these patients. Specific parameters evaluated on the Orbscan II topographies were anterior elevation, posterior elevation, and thinnest pachymetry. Compared with a control group of patients without suspicious videokeratography, there was a statistically significant difference in the mean posterior elevation and mean anterior elevation in the groups with positive keratoconus testing with the Rabinowitz or Klyce/Maeda methods. For patients who met both the Rabinowitz and Klyce/Maeda criteria for keratoconus, the mean posterior elevation was 44 ± 2.5 µm compared with a posterior elevation of 21 ± 0.6 µm for the control group. There was no statistically significant difference in the mean thinnest pachymetry between the control group and all keratoconus suspect groups. They concluded patients with positive keratoconus screening tests have higher anterior and posterior elevation on Orbscan II topography. Thus, when used in combination with Placido-disk videokeratography, the Orbscan II topography system may be helpful in identifying patients who are potentially at high risk for developing ectasia after LASIK, especially those with FFKC. Figure 9-4A shows the graphical analysis of a patient with a difference between the inferior-nasal quadrant (46 D) and the superior-temporal quadrant (41 D). Figure 9-4B shows asymmetric astigmatism with inferior-nasal steepening. LASIK in these patients is controversial, and many would say contraindicated. It is feared that performing LASIK will exacerbate the ectasia, causing the FFKC to progress with subsequent loss of vision.

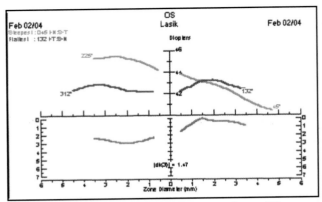

Figure 9-4A. A map of a patient with a difference between the inferior-nasal quadrant (46 D) and the superior-temporal quadrant (41 D).

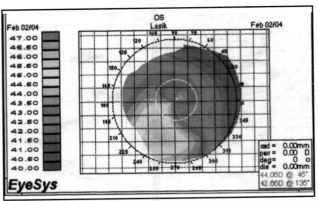

Figure 9-4B. Demonstrates asymmetric astigmatism with inferior-nasal steepening.

Wavefront aberrometers may also aid in the identification of FFKC. Maeda et al[7] compared the ocular wavefront aberrations of normal and keratoconic eyes, describing the characteristics of the higher-order aberrations in eyes with keratoconus. An increase of ocular higher-order aberrations in keratoconic eyes was attributed to an increase of corneal higher-order aberrations. Coma-like aberrations were dominant compared with spherical-like aberrations in keratoconic eyes. The presence of coma and/or significant higher-order aberrations in patients with irregular astigmatism or suspicious topography may be contraindicated for LASIK surgery.

In newly identified FFKC patients, LASIK is avoided and most practitioners recommend contact lens fitting. The majority of patients can be fit with gas permeable contact lenses. Contact lens fitting in these patients is an art form that challenges the skill and patience of the contact lens practitioner. Most patients may be fit with small, steep, gas permeable contact lenses. Double posterior curve lenses, combined soft and hard lenses (piggyback lenses), gas permeable lenses with a peripheral soft lens component, and scleral contact lenses may also be employed.

Patients with FFKC and corneas with preoperative central thickness of less than 500 µm are also at risk for iatrogenic keratectasia, and they should not have LASIK. However, some surgeons feel that photorefractive keratectomy (PRK) can be considered when the patient gives special informed consent about the possible increased risk of irregular astigmatism, progression of the ectasia, decrease in predictability of outcome, increased risk of haze, and increased risk of loss of best-corrected visual acuity (BCVA).

Laser epithelial keratomileusis (LASEK), also known as Epilasik, is a procedure similar to LASIK, but the flap is created differently. In a LASEK procedure, the surgeon temporarily removes only the epithelium (top layer of the cornea) instead of the epithelium and part of the deeper stroma layer

as is done when creating a traditional LASIK flap. The excimer ablation is performed under a hinge flap of corneal epithelium. With this procedure, 35% less tissue is removed. Therefore patients with thin corneas, such as FFKC patients, are now candidates for laser vision correction.

CASE DISCUSSIONS

Case I: A 47-year-old male S/P cataract surgery presented for LASIK evaluation to improve the triple vision noted OD. His refraction OD was –2.00 +6.00 x 180, yielding 20/20– vision with multiple shadows. The refraction of –0.50 +1.50 x 005 allowed him a clear 20/20 OS. His topography is shown in Figure 9-5, illustrating the typical "kissing birds" pattern on the curvature map in the right eye and less irregular astigmatism in the left. INTACS for keratoconus, rather than elective keratorefractive surgery, was recommended for OD, with monitoring of the left for progression.

Case II: A 55-year-old female presented for LASIK wishing to get out of contact lenses. Her refractive error was +2.50 +0.75 x 157 (20/25) OD, +2.00 +2.00 x 31 (20/25–) OS with topography (Figure 9-6A). We followed the patient for a year to determine if the irregular astigmatism was stable or progressive. Her Atlas 1 year later can be seen in Figure 9-6B and shows mild keratoconus complicated by dry eye, as can be seen from the loss of data. Keratorefractive surgery was avoided.

Case III: A 63-year-old female presented for LASIK evaluation wanting to be free of glasses. Her refraction of –4.75 +2.25 x 165 brought her vision to 20/20 OD, and –1.75 +2.50 x 180 allowed her to see 20/20 OS. Ultrasound pachymetry was 625 microns in the center of each eye. Biomicroscopy found moderate punctate epithelial keratitis and mild cataracts OU. Her bilateral curvature

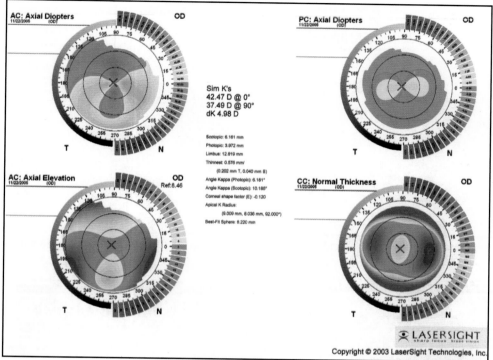

Figure 9-5A. A patient presented for LASIK evaluation having this topography, characteristic of pellucid marginal degeneration. The disease was greater in the right eye (Figure 9-5A) than the left (Figure 9-5B).

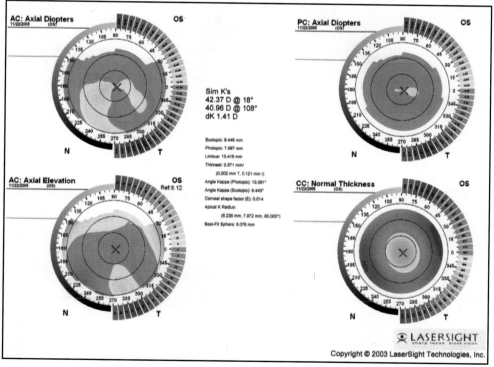

Figure 9-5B. The left eye was less irregular than the right.

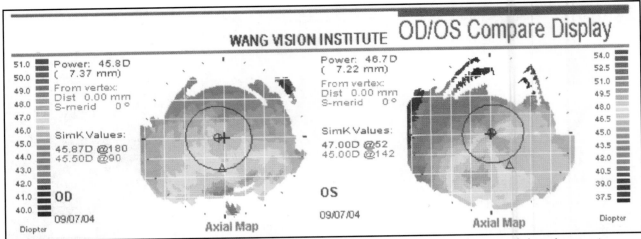

Figure 9-6A. A patient's topographic analysis over time. Mild keratoconus was diagnosed, but dry eye (seen as lost data) complicates interpretation.

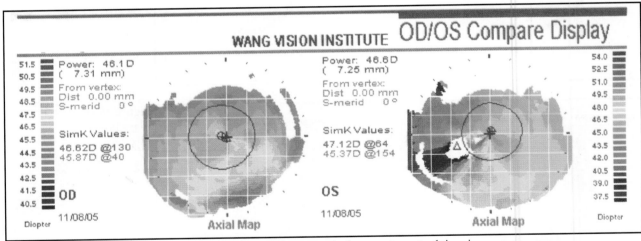

Figure 9-6B. Over time, mild keratoconus was diagnosed after treatment of the dry eye.

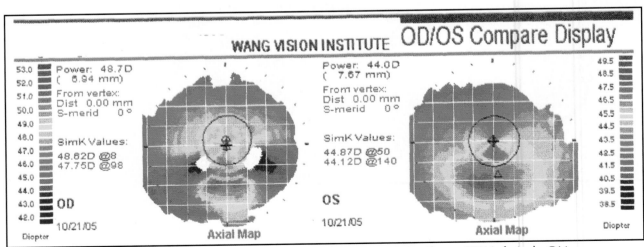

Figure 9-7A. Bilateral curvature maps in a patient with dry eyes and significant SPK inferiorly OU.

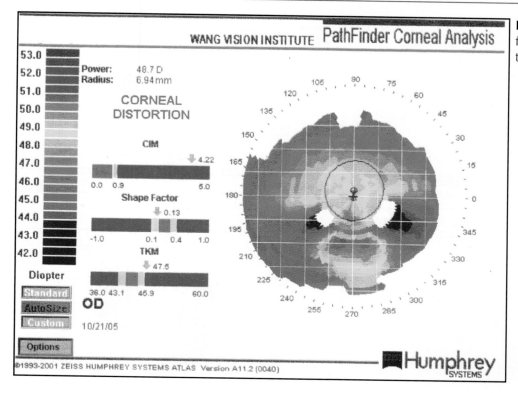

Figure 9-7B. The Pathfinder analysis OD for the same patient.

maps can be seen in Figure 9-7A, and Atlas Pathfinder analysis OD can be seen in Figure 9-7B. Note the lost data caused by the dry eye OD and the pattern of steepening OS, suggesting keratoconus. We instructed the patient to use tears QID OU, and plugged the lower punctum of each eye. When she returned a month later, the irregular astigmatism had markedly improved, and successful PRK was performed.

CONTACT LENS WARPAGE

Hartstein[8] was the first to note contact lens-induced changes in corneal shape and to refer to them as "corneal warpage." More recent publications[9] define the term "corneal warpage" as denoting all contact lens-induced changes in corneal topography, reversible or permanent, that are not associated with corneal edema. Patients with contact lens-induced corneal warpage are commonly asymptomatic. These patients frequently do not use glasses and depend on their contact lenses solely for their refractive error. Some may also notice intolerance to contact lenses or decreased visual acuity with glasses. Approximately 80% of patients presenting for refractive surgery wear contact lenses. It is not uncommon for the refractive surgeon to see such patients with higher frequency then the general practitioner.

Reported signs of contact lens-induced corneal warpage include changes in refraction and keratometric readings (relative steepening of mean corneal curvature in some patients, and flattening in others) and distortion of keratometer or keratoscope mires. But the keratometer evaluates corneal curvature from only four paracentral points, approximately 3 mm apart. The keratoscope provides information from a larger portion of the corneal surface, but the data are qualitative in nature. For these reasons, the best system to study contact lens-induced corneal warpage is computer-assisted topographic analysis of videokeratoscopic images. An example of contact lens warpage is shown in Figure 9-8.

Topographic anomalies induced by contact lenses include[3,10]: central irregular astigmatism as shown in Figure 9-9; loss of radial symmetry, as shown in Figure 9-8; reversal of the normal topographic pattern of progressive flattening of corneal contour from the center to the periphery (absence of the normal prolate pattern), as shown in Figure 9-10; and asymmetric bow-tie patterns or localized corneal steepness as shown in Figure 9-11.

Clinically significant contact lens-induced corneal warpage is seen in a small proportion of soft and gas permeable contact lens wearers. Using computer-assisted topographic analysis, 7 eyes (4 patients) with rigid contact lens-induced corneal warpage were noted to have topographic abnormalities that correlated with the decentered

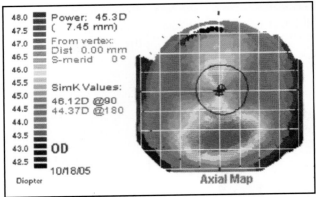

Figure 9-8. Contact lens-induced corneal warpage showing a loss of radial symmetry in a patient who wore gas permeable lenses for 5 years.

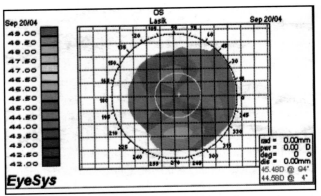

Figure 9-10. Absence of the normal prolate pattern.

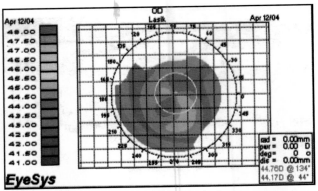

Figure 9-9. Central irregular astigmatism.

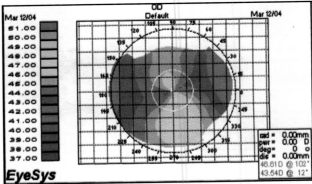

Figure 9-11. Asymmetric bowtie patterns or localized corneal steepness on topographies in patients not strictly meeting the criteria of keratoconus can also present in cases of contact lens warpage, especially in rigid contact lens wearers (keratoconus-like images).

resting position of the contact lens on the cornea by Wilson et al.[11] The warpage pattern on topography for each of these corneas was characterized by a relative flattening of the cornea underlying the resting position of the contact lens. Lenses that rode high, for example, produced flattening superiorly and resulted in a relatively steeper contour inferiorly that simulated the topography of early keratoconus patients who had not worn contact lenses. After discontinuing contact lens use, the corneal topography returned to a normal pattern in five eyes. Two eyes retained asymmetry that is not characteristic of normal corneas. Up to 6 months was required for the corneas to return to a stable topography after contact lens wear was discontinued.

Wilson et al[12] also followed prospectively 21 eyes of 12 patients with contact lens-induced corneal warpage using computer-assisted topographic analysis. Sixteen eyes had worn rigid contact lenses, and five eyes had worn soft contact lenses. Initial corneal topographic patterns were characterized by the presence of central irregular astigmatism, loss of radial symmetry, and frequent reversal of the nor-

mal topographic pattern of progressive flattening of corneal contour from the center to the periphery. A correlation was noted between the initial corneal topography and the resting position of the contact lens on the cornea for 9 of the 16 eyes with gas permeable contact lenses. Initial topography for each of these corneas showed relative flattening of the corneal contour underlying the resting position of a decentered contact lens. Superior-riding lenses produced a topography that simulated early keratoconus. After cessation of contact lens wear, 16 of 21 eyes had a change in corneal shape to a topography that was consistent with a normal pattern. Five corneas stabilized with an abnormal topographic pattern. These studies support the current standard of care regarding the cessation of contact lenses for a significant amount of time prior to surgical vision correction.

Minimum recommendations for discontinuation of contacts vary with lens modality.[13] It is recommended that patients remove soft contact lenses for at least 1 week before assessment, and gas permeable lenses should be removed at least 3 weeks before an evaluation. Typically,

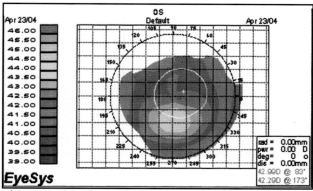

Figure 9-12. The corneal vertex is localized 2 mm below the visual axis.

1 week plus 1 week for every decade of gas permeable or PMMA lens wear is recommended. Soft toric contact lenses seem to behave similarly to gas permeable lenses and their use should be discontinued accordingly.

If topographic abnormalities are detected, contact lens wear should be discontinued and videokeratoscopic examination performed 1 month later. If at 1 month the abnormal topographic pattern remains, the patient should refrain from contact lens wear for a further period and return for examination at monthly intervals. It is not uncommon in patients with rigid lenses to have a 1 D to 2 D increase in myopia during this process, and patients should be educated to expect vision changes. The mean time for contact lens warpage to resolve depends on the type of lens: PMMA (15 weeks), gas permeable (10 weeks), and soft (5 weeks).[3] At least two topographies with the same pattern are recommended in order to decide if the surgery is recommended.

DECENTERED CORNEAL APEX

As discussed by Mandell et al,[14] the diagnosis of asymmetric corneal toricity in videokeratography is based on the occurrence of an asymmetric bowtie pattern in the corneal map, which is usually attributed to corneal radial asymmetry but can be an artifact produced by misalignment of the videokeratograph with the corneal apex. Their study determined whether asymmetric bowtie patterns in 16 subjects (ages 24 to 40 years with corneal toricity of 0.37 to 1.50 D) could be converted to symmetric bowtie patterns by changing the alignment of the videokeratograph so that it was directed at the corneal apex. They found that changing from regular to apex alignment improved the symmetry in 11 eyes, had no change in 3 eyes, and increased asymmetry in 2 eyes. No radius change could be measured centrally, but there were significant changes of greater than 1.00 D in the peripheral

corneal radii of 8 eyes; so this group concluded that an asymmetric or angled bowtie appearance of a corneal map suggests a decentered apex rather than corneal asymmetry and may lead to a misdiagnosis of the type or magnitude of corneal toricity, keratoconus, or other corneal irregularities. Figure 9-12 shows a corneal vertex localized 2 mm below visual axis.

While a decentered apex may be associated with FFKC, it may also be an artifact produced by misalignment of the videokeratograph. In this instance, improvement of the measurement technique resolves the decentration.

TEAR FILM ABNORMALITIES

The tear film is composed of a lipid layer, aqueous layer, and mucous layer. The blinking action is vital for a stable tear film; if absent or improper, dry eye results. During a blink, the overlying aqueous tear film completely wets the mucin-coated epithelium. Between blinks, the tear film thins via evaporation and exits into the fornices, causing the lipid layer to become closer to the mucin layer. When proximity is such that the mucin layer is contaminated by the lipid layer, dry spots form due to the rupturing of the mucin layer. This results in contact between the aqueous layer and the underlying epithelium. Therefore, the mucin layer is essential for maintaining the continuity of the tear film.

Huang et al[15] investigated the effects of artificial tears on corneal surface regularity and visual function in dry eyes. The surface regularity index (SRI), surface asymmetry index (SAI), and potential visual acuity (PVA) were measured by computer-assisted videokeratography (TMS-1). This was done in 40 patients (40 eyes) with dry eyes with (group 1, $n = 15$ eyes) or without (group 2, $n = 25$ eyes) punctate epithelial keratopathy and a normal control group of 20 individuals (20 eyes) with no ocular abnormalities (group 3). Differences in SRI, SAI, PVA, spatial-contrast sensitivity, and glare disability between groups before instillation of tears and within groups after instillation of tears were measured. Compared with group 3, eyes in group 1 had significantly worse SRI, SAI, PVA, and contrast sensitivity (incomplete glare disability data precluded analysis) before instillation of artificial tears. Significant improvement in SRI, SAI, and PVA were observed after instillation of artificial tears in group 1. They reported significant improvement in SRI, SAI, and PVA after instillation of artificial tears in dry eyes with punctate epithelial keratopathy.

Ozkan et al[16] from Turkey compared topographic indices of surface regularity in dry eye patients and in normal subjects (controls) and investigated the short-term effects of lacrimal punctal plugs on these indices in dry eye patients. The SRI and SAI of the TMS-2 corneal topographic modeling system were used to evaluate corneal surface regularity in 20 eyes of 10 dry eye patients before and after the insertion of Herrick silicon lacrimal plugs and in 24 eyes of 12 normal subjects as controls. They concluded that no significant change in the topographic indices of corneal surface irregularity could be detected in severe dry eye patients with lacrimal punctal plugs in the short-term follow-up.

By using high-speed videotopographic measurement of tear film build-up time, Nemeth et al[17] examined 15 eyes of 15 healthy volunteers and 7 eyes of 7 patients with dry eye in their prospective preliminary study. The main outcome measures were changes in SRI, SAI, and corneal power. They found that the corneal surface became more regular in the first few seconds after a blink. In healthy eyes, the SRI improved improved significantly after a blink in 10 of 15 eyes, and the SAI improved in 13 of 15. In the typical cases, the trend line for SRI reached its minimum level, on average, at 7.1 ± 3.9 seconds after a blink and at 5.4 ± 2.7 seconds for the SAI. Similar trends were found in the dry eye group. The changes in keratometric measures were small (mean range, < 1.5% of the absolute value) and showed no definite trends. They concluded that high-speed videotopography provides the possibility of quantitative measurement of tear film dynamics and may have clinical value in the management of ocular surface disorders. After a blink, it takes the tear film approximately 3 to 10 seconds (tear film build-up time) to reach the most regular state. However, despite surface-regularity changes, the measured corneal powers are stable.

It has been shown that patients with ocular irritation have an irregular corneal surface that may contribute to their irritation and visual symptoms. Because of their high sensitivity and specificity, the regularity indices of the Tomey TMS-2N have the potential to be used as objective diagnostic indices for dry eye, as well as a means to evaluate the severity of this disease. This was determined by de Paiva et al[18] when they studied the correlation between the regularity indices of the Tomey TMS-2N computerized videokeratoscopy (CVK) instrument with conventional measures of dry eye symptoms and disease in a retrospective, clinic-based, case-control study. In this study, the SRI, SAI, and IAI were all significantly greater in dry eye patients than normal subjects. These were 0.46 ± 0.36 (normal) versus 1.09 ± 0.76 (dry) for the SRI, 0.30 ± 0.15 (normal) versus 0.90 ± 1.09 (dry) for the SAI, and 0.42 ± 0.28 (normal) versus 0.56 ± 0.24 (dry) for the IAI. The PVA index was significantly lower in the dry eye patients (0.89 ± 0.13) than normal eyes (0.68 ± 0.23). The SRI, SAI, and IAI were positively correlated with total and central corneal fluorescein staining scores. The SRI (≥ 0.80), SAI (≥ 0.50), and IAI (≥ 0.50) had sensitivities in predicting total corneal fluorescein staining (score ≥ 3) of 89%, 69%, and 82%, respec-

tively. The specificity of these indices was 80%, 78%, and 82%, respectively. In all 90 eyes, the mean SRI was greater in subjects older than 50 years compared with younger patients, whereas no age effect was noted in the dry eye patients. The SRI and PVA index showed better correlation with symptoms of blurred vision than the BCVA.

More recently Montes-Mico et al[19] compared ocular wavefront aberrations of normal and dry eyes and described the characteristics of higher-order aberration in dry eyes. They found that total, spherical-like, and coma-like aberrations were significantly greater in dry eyes than in normal controls both for a 4-mm and 6-mm-diameter pupil, and concluded that eyes of dry eye patients showed greater optical aberrations compared with normal control eyes. Increase in higher-order aberrations in dry eyes resulted from increased tear film irregularity.

They also studied the effect of artificial tear instillation on ocular aberrations in dry eye patients,[20] showing that after artificial tear instillation, optical aberrations associated with an increasingly irregular tear film may be improved. Wavefront analysis, as well as computerized videokeratoscopy, facilitate the evaluation of improvement in optical quality after artificial tear instillation in patients with dry eye. The effect of artificial tears is illustrated in Figure 9-13. This patient was S/P myopic LASIK treatment, complaining of blurred vision postoperatively. Figure 9-13A was the initial mapping, and Figure 9-13B was imaged 5 minutes after lubricant instillation.

ASTIGMATISM

Astigmatism occurs when toricity of any of the refractive surfaces of the optical system produces two principal foci, delimiting an area of intermediate focus called the conoid of Sturm. Astigmatism decreases visual acuity by forming a distorted image because light images focus on 2 separate points in the eye.[21,22] Thomas Young in 1801 was the first to describe ocular astigmatism, discovering that his own astigmatism was predominantly lenticular. However, it was some years later before Airy (1827) corrected astigmatism with a cylindrical lens. Corneal astigmatism was characterized by Knapp and also Donders in 1862 after the invention of the ophthalmometer by Helmholtz. In the same year, Donders also described the astigmatism due to cataract surgery. Soon after, Snellen (1869) suggested that placing the incision on the steep axis would reduce corneal astigmatism.[23]

Astigmatism may be naturally occurring, develop after injury, indicate underlying disease such as keratoconus, occur with excessive eye rubbing, and occur after surgery.[24] Astigmatism induces distortion of the image. When the effects of blurring of the image are excluded, the

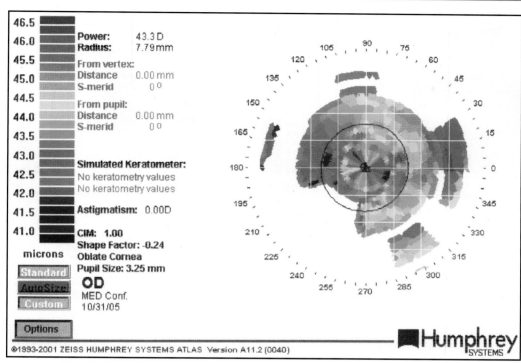

Figure 9-13A. This patient complained of blurred vision S/P LASIK treatment due to dry eyes. This image shows the eye prior to tears.

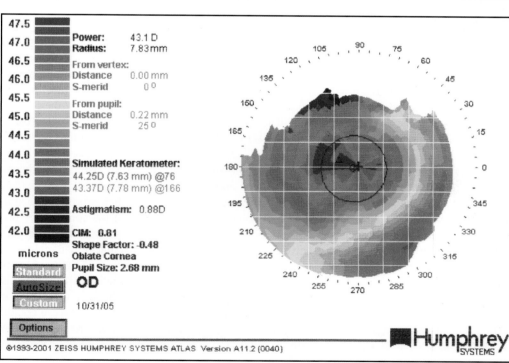

Figure 9-13B. This patient complained of blurred vision S/P LASIK treatment due to dry eyes. This image shows the eye 60 seconds after tear instillation.

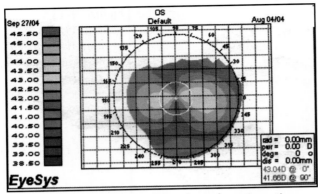

Figure 9-14A. Regular against-the-rule astigmatism.

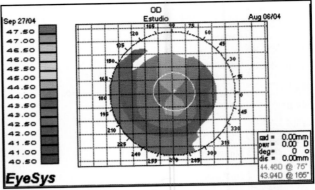

Figure 9-14B. Regular with-the-rule astigmatism.

retinal image in an uncorrected astigmatic eye is distorted because of a differential magnification in the two principal meridians. Expressed as a percentage of the differences in these principal meridians, the image is distorted by about 0.3% per D of astigmatism. In the corrected astigmatic eye, distortion of the sharp retinal image arises from the unequal spectacle magnification in the two principal meridians, which represents about 1.6% distortion per D cylinder in the correction at the spectacle plane. This unequal magnification is manifested by altered shapes and by tilting of vertical lines (the declination error) that occurs maximally when the correcting cylinder is oblique (that is, 45 or 135 degrees). Although oblique astigmatism only produces 0.4 degrees of tilt per D monocularly, it will produce major alterations in binocular perception. Despite the distortion induced by astigmatism, some astigmatism may be of benefit. Various types of astigmatism have different effects on visual perception.

For this reason the concepts of astigmatism "with-the-rule" and "against-the-rule" are clinically relevant. Astigmatism with-the-rule is produced when the corneal curvature is steepest in the vertical meridian. Conversely, astigmatism against-the-rule is produced when the steepest corneal meridian is horizontal.[23] Figure 9-14 shows regular astigmatism, where the surface is smooth, but bent out of shape. Figure 9-15 illustrates irregular astigmatism, where the surface is roughened similar to scratches on glass. This is much more difficult and less predictable to treat.

Tanabe et al[25] assessed corneal regular and irregular astigmatism using Fourier series harmonic analysis of videokeratography data in normal subjects, as well as in subjects with pathologic and postsurgical conditions. They evaluated 200 normal eyes, 58 eyes with keratoconus, 24 eyes with suspect keratoconus, 100 eyes that underwent LASIK, 101 eyes that underwent PRK, and 79 eyes that underwent penetrating keratoplasty (PK). Videokeratography data were decomposed using Fourier analysis into spherical power, regular astigmatism, asymmetry, and higher-order irregularity.

The normal range of the Fourier indices, defined as the mean ±2 standard deviation in the normal eyes, were 40.81 to 47.13 D for spherical power, 0 to 1.04 D for regular astigmatism, 0.02 to 0.68 D for asymmetry, and 0.05 to 0.17 for higher-order irregularity. The keratoconus and suspect keratoconus groups showed significantly greater values in all indices than did the normal group. Eyes that had undergone LASIK and PRK had significantly smaller spherical power and regular astigmatism, and significantly larger asymmetry than the normal eyes.

All indices were significantly greater in the PK group than in the normal group. Among the eyes tested in this study, eyes with keratoconus had the largest asymmetry, whereas eyes that had undergone PK had the most irregular corneas. They defined the normal range for the corneal irregular astigmatism index (asymmetry and higher-order irregularity) which would help to support future studies in this field.

Most people with astigmatism demonstrate differences in magnitude and axis between topographic astigmatism and refractive astigmatism. In other words, refractive power as measured at the surface of the cornea does not coincide with the refractive power that these people perceive as supplying good vision. The phenomenon may be related to the internal optics of the eye and the visual perception of the brain; clinicians sometimes refer to it as "lenticular astigmatism" (related to the lens of the eye). It presents a significant problem to current efforts to couple real-time corneal topography and laser treatment in an effort to "sphericize" the cornea.[26]

Treating refractive astigmatism may do nothing to alleviate topographic astigmatism, and in fact can result in increased corneal topographic astigmatism.

Corneal astigmatism, measured by keratometry or corneal topography, refers to the difference in curvature of the two principal corneal meridians. Lenticular astigmatism, sometimes called internal astigmatism, is generally not measured but calculated as the difference between

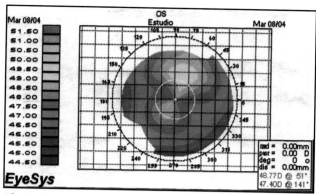

Figure 9-15. Irregular astigmatism.

refractive and corneal astigmatism (RA – CA = LA), an astigmatic error assumed to be within the crystalline lens.[26]

CONCLUSION

In conclusion, it is imperative that all corneal surgery consultations include topography to rule out pertinent corneal disorders prior to elective vision correction procedures such as LASIK. Topographical abnormalities may be the only clinical sign present in some patients, and these subtle changes should be well understood by the surgeon to avoid potential problems postoperatively.

REFERENCES

1. Baruch HR. Reviewed by Emil W. Chynn, MD. *What Every Keratoconus (KC) Patient Should Know About KC and New Laser Treatments for KC.* Available at: http//:www.iwant2020.com. Accessed September 14, 2004.

2. Waheed S, Krueger RR. Steep, flat and irregular corneas in LASIK. *Rev Ophthalmol.* Feb 15, 2003. Available at http://www.revophth.com. Accessed September 15, 2004.

3. Varssano D, Kaiserman I, Hazarbassanov R. Topographic patterns in refractive surgery candidates. *Cornea.* 2004;23(6):602–607.

4. Rao SN, Epstein RJ. Early onset ectasia following laser in situ keratomileusus: case report and literature review. *J Refract Surg.* 2002;18(2):177–184.

5. Arntz A, Durán JA, Pijoán JI. Subclinical keratoconus diagnosis by elevation topography. *Arch Soc Esp Oftalmol.* 2003;78:659–664.

6. Rao SN, Raviv T, Majmudar PA, Epstein RJ. Role of Orbscan II in screening keratoconus suspects before

7. refractive corneal surgery. *Ophthalmology.* 2002;109(9):1642–1646.

8. Maeda N, Fujikado T, Kuroda T, Mihashi T, Hirohara Y, Nishida K, Watanabe H, Tano Y. Wavefront aberrations measured with Hartmann-Shack sensor in patients with keratoconus. *Ophthalmology.* 2002;109(11):1996-2003.

9. Hartstein J. Corneal warping due to wearing of corneal contact lenses. *Am J Ophthalmol.* 1965;60:1103–1104.

10. Wilson SE, Lin DT, Klyce SD, Reidy JJ, Insler MS. Rigid contact lens decentration: a risk factor for corneal warpage. *CLAO J.* 1990;16(3):177–182.

11. Hoyos JE, Cigales M. Topographic and pachymetric changes induced by contact-lenses. *KMSG Journal.* Available at: http://www.kmsg.org/Users/upload/journal/21/index.asp. Accessed September 18, 2004.

12. Wilson SE, Lin DT, Klyce SD, Reidy JJ, Insler MS. Rigid contact lens decentration: a risk factor for corneal warpage. *CLAO J.* 1990;16(3):177-82.

13. Wilson SE, Lin DT, Klyce SD, Reidy JJ, Insler MS. Topographic changes in contact lens-induced corneal warpage. *Ophthalmology.* 1990;97:734–744.

14. Davis EA, Hardten DR, Lindstrom RL. LASIK complications. *Int Ophthalmol Clin Refractive Surgery.* 2002;40:67–75.

15. Mandell RB, Chiang CS, Yee L. Asymmetric corneal toricity and pseudokeratoconus in videokeratography. *J Am Optom Assoc.* 1996;67(9):540–547.

16. Huang FC, Tseng SH, Shih MH, Chen FK. Effect of artificial tears on corneal surface regularity, contrast sensitivity, and glare disability in dry eyes. *Ophthalmology.* 2002;109(10):1934–1940.

17. Ozkan Y, Bozkurt B, Gedik S, Irkec M, Orhan M. Corneal topographical study of the effect of lacrimal punctum occlusion on corneal surface regularity in dry eye patients. *Eur J Ophthalmol.* 2001;11(2):116–119.

18. Nemeth J, Erdelyi B, Csakany B, Gaspar P, Soumelidis A, Kahlesz F, Lang Z. High-speed videotopographic measurement of tear film build-up time. *Invest Ophthalmol Vis Sci.* 2002;43(6):1783–1790.

19. de Paiva CS, Lindsey JL, Pflugfelder SC. Assessing the severity of keratitis sicca with videokeratoscopic indices. *Ophthalmology.* 2003;110(6):1102–1109.

20. Montes-Mico R, Caliz A, Alio JL. Wavefront analysis of higher order aberrations in dry eye patients. *J Refract Surg.* 2004;20(3):243–247.

21. Montes-Mico R, Caliz A, Alio JL. Changes in ocular aberrations after instillation of artificial tears in dry-eye patients. *J Cataract Refract Surg.* 2004;30(8):1649–1652.

22. Hostetter TA. *Soft Contacts: The Hard Facts.* February 2003. Available at: http://www.2020mag.com. Accessed September 18, 2004.

22. Roque MR, Limbonsiong R. *Astigmatism, PRK*. June 2004. Available at: http://www.emedicine.com/oph/topic657.htm. Accessed September 18, 2004.

23. Morlet N, Minassian D, Dart J. Astigmatism and the analysis of its surgical correction. *Br J Ophthalmol.* 2001;85:1127–1138. Available at: http://bjo.bmjjournals.com/cgi/content/full/85/9/1127. Accessed September 18, 2004.

24. Pirnazar JR, McDonnel PJ. Preoperative assessment and patient selection. *Ophthalmic Hyperguides.* Available at: http://www.ophthalmic.hyperguides.com/default.asp?section=refractive&page=preoperative. Accessed September 18, 2004.

25. Tanabe T, Tomidokoro A, Samejima T, Miyata K, Sato M, Kaji Y, Oshika T. Corneal regular and irregular astigmatism assessed by Fourier analysis of videokeratography data in normal and pathologic eyes. *Ophthalmology.* 2004;111(4):752–757.

26. Croes KJ. *Topography Versus Refraction*. Available at: http://www.assort.com/Oldsite/break04.htm. Accessed September 18, 2004.

Chapter 10

Post-Refractive Surgery Topographies

Roberto Pinelli, MD

The analysis of post-refractive surgery corneal topography is fundamental for two reasons: to evaluate the assessment of the eye after surgery and to plan a possible future surgical strategy. All keratorefractive surgery techniques leave a "trace" in the cornea that can be an important indication of surgical effectiveness. The basic premise of refractive surgery is that the cornea's optical properties are intimately related to its shape. Consequently, manipulating corneal shape can change the natural shape of the cornea in an effort to change the refractive status. Ablative procedures, incisional techniques, and intracorneal rings change the natural shape of the cornea in an effort to change the refractive error. We now analyze the characteristics of some corneal maps performed after refractive surgery together with a brief discussion of the clinical histories.

POST-LASIK CORNEAL TOPOGRAPHY

Because excimer laser ablates tissue in the center of the cornea to decrease nearsightedness, the post-op corneal topography appears flatter in the center after treatment. A classical case of LASIK in a myopic patient is illustrated in Figure 10-1. The ablation is well-centered and the keratometry value is lower than average (36.44/35.34 D) denoting a central ablation. The centration of the ablation, compared to the white to white, can be observed in the picture as well.

In this case, the patient showed a preoperative myopia of 10 D and a BCVA of 20/25. After LASIK the patient's UCVA was 20/25, with 0.50 D residual astigmatism remaining. Keratometry in this range has been associated with glare and decreased night vision. Fortunately, this patient's glare disappeared with the correction of –0.50 D of astigmatism (LASIK enhancement).

When treating hyperopia with LASIK, the ablation is peripheral, causing a steepening in the center on topography. In Figure 10-2, the ablation is peripheral and well-centered. The use of an eye-tracking device is fundamental in these cases. The keratometry value (45.98/45.30) indicates steepening of the central cornea, which causes the correction of hyperopia.

When evaluating a postoperative map in a previously hyperopic patient, it is necessary to imagine a surgically-induced corneal prolation. The patient, a 63-year-old male, had 3 D of hyperopia and BCVA 20/20. Following hyperopic LASIK, the UCVA is 20/20.

Discussion of LASIK for astigmatism requires the preoperative analysis to compare to the postoperative result. In the first example shown in the top map of Figure 10-3, the preoperative topography shows a regular astigmatism of +2.40 D at axis 69 degrees. The toric surface of the cornea indicates with-the-rule astigmatism. Note that in the postoperative topography shown in the lower map of Figure 10-3, the astigmatism is corrected. In fact the keratometry values are 43.15 and 42.93, nearly spherical. The smoothing effect of the laser on the corneal surface can be easily observed. This patient was a 36-year-old male with a preoperative BCVA 20/20 with cylinder of +2.25 at axis 70 degrees. Postoperatively, the UCVA was 20/20.

In a second example shown in Figure 10-4, a preoperative 4 D, regular with-the-rule astigmatism is illustrated. The patient, a 28-year-old female, had a BCVA of 20/25 with a refraction of –5.00 –4.00 x 10. The post-LASIK topography for the same eye is shown just below it, where a partial reduction of astigmatism can be seen. Following surgery, 2.50 D of corneal astigmatism

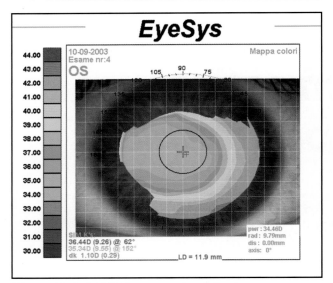

Figure 10-1. LASIK in a myopic patient.

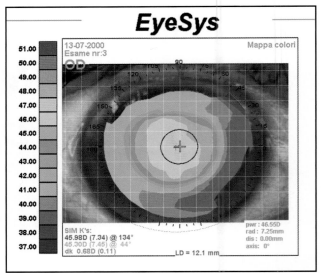

Figure 10-2. LASIK in a hyperopic patient.

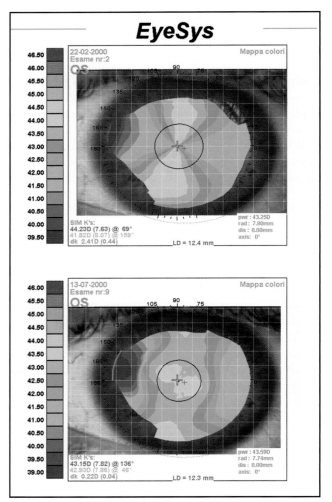

Figure 10-3. LASIK for hyperopic astigmatism. The top map is preoperative, and the bottom map is postoperative.

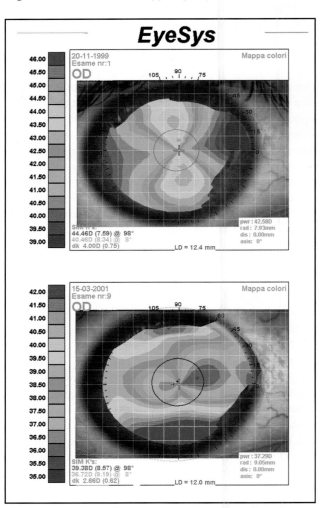

Figure 10-4. LASIK for myopic astigmatism. The top map is preoperative, and the bottom map is postoperative.

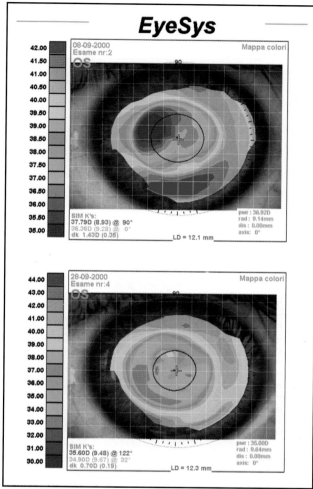

Figure 10-5. A map of a patient complaining of glare and halos after a decentered PRK (top map), whose complaints resolved with a corrective LASIK procedure. The bottom map is S/P the LASIK procedure.

remained. Postoperatively, she had BCVA 20/25 with a refraction of cyl –2.00 x 10. This post-LASIK topography shows a classical case of myopic astigmatism ablation. The difference of K values reflects a flattening (preoperative 44.46/40.46 and 39.38/36.72 postoperative), revealing a myopic-astigmatic ablation. In these cases, if there is enough corneal tissue, the patient's vision can be improved with a LASIK enhancement. Astigmatism over 3 D, especially myopic astigmatism, is difficult to treat completely in a primary procedure because of the scleral effect on corneal astigmatism in these patients. Enhancement is usually an option to correct residual astigmatism. The surgeon should take into consideration the pachymetry before the surgery in order to have enough tissue for the enhancement and to prevent corneal ectasia.

Topography may also lend insight to the etiology of the patient's complaints following keratorefractive surgery. A 32-year-old male patient presented complaining about night vision problems after photorefractive keratectomy (PRK) 2 years prior to his visit. The patient reported halos at night, double images, and poor visual acuity even with spectacle correction. His BCVA was 20/25 with –1.25 D of astigmatism at 180 degrees. The post-PRK corneal topography, shown in Figure 10-5, revealed a nasally decentered ablation shown in the top image. In this case, LASIK was performed to resolve the decentration. The lower map was obtained following the corrective LASIK treatment, which resulted in a reduction of the astigmatism. Postoperative UCVA was 20/25 with resolution of halos and double vision.

Post-presbyopic LASIK (presbyLASIK) topographical maps have only been available recently, after studies on the potentiality of multifocal presbyopic LASIK began. In our daily clinical practice, Presbyopic Multifocal LASIK (PML™) has proven to be a successful technique after 3 years of follow up at the Istituto Laser Microchirurgia Oculare in Brescia, Italy. A gradual multifocality can be seen in these patients when moving from the central cornea to the limbus. The different degrees of green and blue bands indicate gradual, concentric optical zones.

The first case is a 52-year-old woman with a 20/20 preoperative UCVA at distance, and J7 UCVA at near. She preferred an add of +1.75 to read J1. Her postoperative topography is shown in Figure 10-6. Three months after presbyLASIK she had an UCVA of 20/25+ and J1 UCVA at near. The second case shows a 56-year-old male with a 20/20 UCVA at distance, J7 at near unaided. A near vision of J1 was obtained with a +2.00 D lens preoperatively. He obtained 20/20 UCVA and J1 UCVA 3 months after surgery. The topographical map is shown in Figure 10-7.

Post-PRK topographical maps are similar to post-LASIK topographical maps if both techniques are properly performed. Figure 10-8 shows a post-myopic PRK topography. Note the keratometry value is relatively low (34.40/32.83). In this case, the patient was a 32-year-old female with 6 D of myopia. Preoperative central pachymetry was 491 μm (TOMEY), so LASIK was avoided and PRK performed. After 2 months, UCVA was 20/20.

POST-RADIAL KERATOTOMY

Radial keratotomy (RK) incisional surgery was originally designed to weaken the peripheral cornea and cause it to bulge forward, effectively flattening the central cornea to reduce myopia and resulting in a typical presentation as

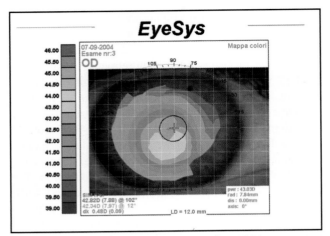

Figure 10-6. Curvature map post-presbyLASIK treatment.

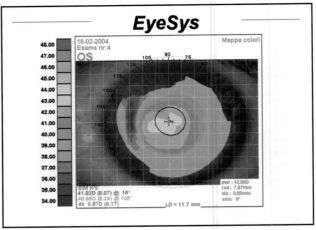

Figure 10-7. Curvature map post-presbyLASIK treatment.

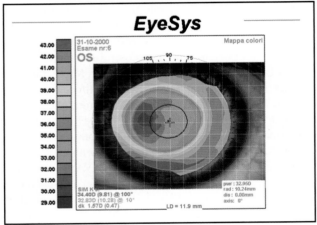

Figure 10-8. Topography post-myopic PRK. These maps are often identical to maps S/P LASIK for the same power.

seen in Figure 10-9. Post-RK patients may ask for excimer laser procedures years after a successful RK procedure due to a hyperopic shift. Peculiar characteristics of post-RK topographies include irregular astigmatism and reduced optical zones compared to modern techniques such as LASIK.

Irregular astigmatism of 2.30 D is shown in the upper image in Figure 10-9, probably resulting from a difference in the tension of the incisions. The lower figure shows a more characteristic map following RK, with residual astigmatism and a slight decentration of the treatment. In these cases, if corneal pachymetry is sufficient and the refraction is stable, LASIK may be performed to resolve the residual refractive error. In rare cases, the incisions become increasingly weak, resulting in ectasia of the cornea. This may manifest as a large shift in the refractive error, irregular astigmatism, and decrease in visual quality with a reduction in BCVA.

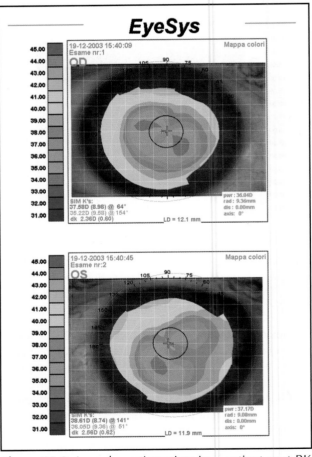

Figure 10-9. Irregular astigmatism in a patient post-RK is illustrated by both the top and bottom figures.

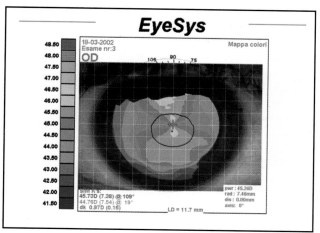

Figure 10-10. A curvature map of a patient post-LTK, resulting in 0.50 D increased myopia.

POST-LASER THERMAL KERATOPLASTY

Laser thermal keratoplasty (LTK) is a technique used to correct smaller amounts of hyperopia. It can be done for distance to correct small hyperopic refractive error, or to induce myopia for monovision correction in presbyopes. In this procedure, the laser creates a series of small superficial leucomas which contract the corneal tissue to create a more prolate shape. The effect corrects small amounts of hyperopia when 8 spots are placed circumferentially at a 7-mm optical zone, and slightly higher amounts of hyperopia when 16 spots are placed at 7 mm and 8 mm circumferentially. In the case shown in Figure 10-10, 0.50 D of myopia was induced to enable the patient to read without a near vision prescription.

Monovision can be created by inducing a small amount of myopia in the nondominant eye. Monovision typically describes presbyopia correction where the dominant eye is corrected for distance and the nondominant eye for reading. Monovision can be created with various types of surgery: PRK, LASIK, LTK, and CK. At the present time, CK is preferred to LTK. This is due to a smaller amount of regression and to the long-term stability of the effect.

POST-CONDUCTIVE KERATOPLASTY

Conductive keratoplasty (CK) represents the last generation of thermokeratoplasty. This technique employs radiofrequency waves delivered to the corneal stroma using a metal, hairlike probe. The burns cause a contracture of the peripheral cornea similar to LTK, inducing an increase in myopia and creating "blended vision" in presbyopes. The aspheric effect of the treatment reportedly produces a more comfortable monovision effect, where the

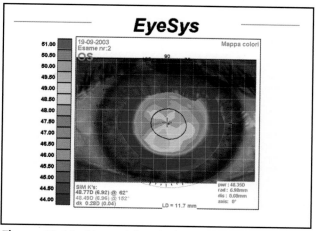

Figure 10-11. Near vision induction using CK radio-wave treatment.

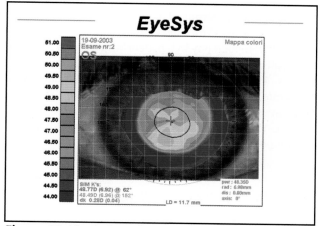

Figure 10-12. Astigmatism resulting from CK, which was later corrected with LASIK.

distance loss is less significant than noted with typical monovision in contacts or post-LASIK.

Corneal topography post-CK is similar to post-hyperopic LASIK in that the cornea becomes more prolate. The more spots delivered, the stronger the effect. The effect of the CK spots (16 in the case of Figure 10-11) is peripheral and prolation is evident. In some cases, low amounts of astigmatism result and, as shown in Figure 10-12, this is retreatable. Both cases are examples of 16 spot treatments in the nondominant eye for blended vision in presbyopic patients.

POST-PENETRATING KERATOPLASTY

Penetrating keratoplasty (PKP) is also a technique easily identified on topography. If the suture is uniform and

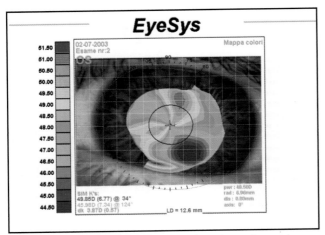

Figure 10-13. Post-PKP topography. Irregular astigmatism is commonly seen.

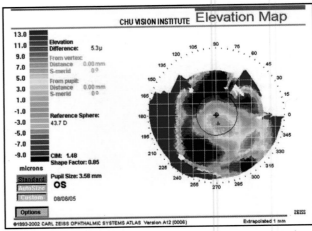

Figure 10-14. Post-ICR topography for myopia reduction. (Courtesy of Ralph Chu, MD.)

well performed (interrupted or continuous) it is difficult to notice astigmatism from topography. Figure 10-13 shows a post-PKP topography in a patient with astigmatism. The astigmatism is irregular, only partially correctable with glasses. This phenomenon was due to the bad quality of the suture, which provoked a difference in tension at axis 60 degrees with respect to the axis 110 degrees. In these cases, LASIK can partially correct the defect with a satisfactory postoperative result.

POST-INTRACORNEAL RINGS

Intracorneal rings (ICR) are indicated in cases of slight myopia, or post-excimer ablations to enlarge small optical zones. In cases of low myopia, intracorneal rings create a "tenting effect," which flattens the center to correct the myopia, as shown in Figure 10-14. In the case of post-excimer laser treatment with a small optical zone, the rings can enlarge the zone to reduce or eliminate visual halos.

Ring segments may also be utilized to stabilize marginal pellucid degeneration, keratoconus, or ectasia in post-RK or post-LASIK patients. In post-ICR topographies, the effect of the ring may appear as a blue arch in the periphery of the cornea or as a loss of data in the map. The number of rings used (1 or 2) is related to the surgical strategy.

POST-SCLERAL EXPANSION BAND IMPLANTATION

The goal of scleral implants is to stimulate the ciliary muscle to work at the presbyopic age. The ciliary muscle becomes less elastic at the age of 40 to 50 years, and expansion bands increase the room available, allowing the muscle to work. Usually the insertion of scleral expansion bands for presbyopia does not induce any significant change in the postoperative topography compared to the preoperative topography. The insertion of these bands in the sclera (especially in the number of 4) seems not to have enough power to create traction on the cornea visible in the topography.

CONCLUSION

In summary, familiarizing yourself with common patterns seen on corneal topography will aid you in the diagnosis and management of clinical cases. A detailed and accurate analysis of maps and topographies after refractive surgery can help the refractive surgeon to plan an effective strategy to correct residual defects, treat decentration, and diagnose and manage irregularity. Topographic analysis is an integral part of the refractive evaluation in order to plan a scientific approach individual to each eye, as well as to manage postoperative complications.

Chapter 11

Posterior Corneal Changes in Refractive Surgery

Amar Agarwal, MS, FRCS, FRCOphth; Sunita Agarwal, MS, DO; Athiya Agarwal, MD, DO;
Soosan Jacob, MS, FRCS, DipNB, FERC; and Nilesh Kanjiani, DipNB, DO, FERC

The development of technology allowing us to visualize the posterior surface of the cornea has been invaluable to our understanding of changes to the normal shape of the posterior cornea. A forward protrusion of the posterior surface, called "ectasia," is an abnormality seen in virgin eyes with keratoconus, pellucid marginal degeneration, and other malformations of the cornea, as well as in eyes following LASIK.

It is known that posterior corneal elevation is an early presenting sign in keratoconus and hence it is imperative to evaluate posterior corneal curvature (PCC) in every LASIK candidate. Unrecognized preoperative forme fruste keratoconus (FFKC) must be identified prior to LASIK. Patients with this disorder are poor candidates for refractive surgery because of the possibility of exacerbating keratectasia.

The development of corneal ectasia is a well-recognized complication of LASIK, when the stromal bed becomes too thin to sustain the normal corneal architecture. Topography is invaluable for preoperative ophthalmic examination of LASIK candidates. Three-dimensional imaging allows surgeons to look at corneal thickness, as well as the corneal anterior and posterior surface, and it can also predict the shape of the cornea after LASIK surgery. Topographic analysis using a three dimensional scanning slit system allows us to identify strong keratorefractive candidates by screening for subtle configurations that may be a contraindication to LASIK.

The Orbscan IIz corneal topography system uses a scanning optical slit scan, making it fundamentally different from corneal topographers that analyze the reflected images from the anterior corneal surface. The high-resolution video camera captures 40 light slits at a 45-degree angle projected through the cornea, similar to a slit lamp examination. The slits are projected on the anterior segment of the eye: the anterior cornea, the posterior cornea, the anterior iris, and anterior lens. The data collected from these four surfaces are used to create a topographic map. Each surface point from the diffusely reflected slit beams that overlap in the central 5-mm zone is independently triangulated to x, y, and z coordinates, providing three-dimensional data.

This technique provides more information about the anterior segment of the eye, such as anterior and posterior corneal curvature, elevation maps of the anterior and posterior corneal surface, and corneal thickness. It has an acquisition time of 4 seconds,[1] which improves diagnostic accuracy. It also has passive eye-tracker from frame to frame, and 43 frames are taken to ensure accuracy. Maps are easy to interpret, with good repeatability.

FFKC

The diagnosis of frank keratoconus is a clinical one. Early diagnosis of FFKC can be difficult on clinical examination alone. Orbscan has become a useful tool for evaluating the disease and, with its advent, abnormalities in posterior corneal surface topography have been identified in keratoconus. Posterior corneal surface data is problematic because it is not a direct measure and there is little published information on normal values for each age group. In the patient with increased posterior corneal elevation in the absence of other changes, it is unknown whether this finding represents a manifestation of early keratoconus. The decision to proceed with refractive surgery is therefore more difficult.

Posterior Corneal Topography

Slit-scanning technology allows evaluation of potential LASIK candidates preoperatively to rule out primary

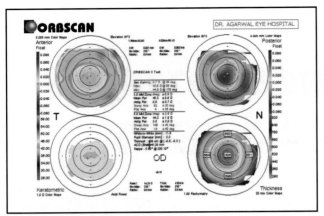

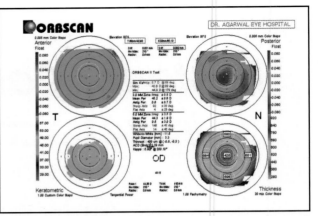

Figure 11-1. A general quad map of an eye with primary posterior corneal elevation. Notice the red areas seen in the top right picture showing the primary posterior corneal elevation.

Figure 11-2. Topographic features shown in a normal band scale map of an eye with primary posterior corneal elevation.

posterior corneal elevation. The quad map shown in Figure 11-1 commonly includes the following maps with the average range listed adjacent to the map:

a. Anterior corneal elevation: normal band = ± 25 μ of best-fit sphere.

b. Posterior corneal elevation: normal band = ± 25 μ of best-fit sphere.

c. Keratometric mean curvature: normal band = 40 to 48 D

d. Corneal thickness (pachymetry): normal band = 500 to 600 μ. Map features within normal band are colored green.

This effectively filters out variations falling within the normal range. When abnormalities are seen on normal band quad map screening, a standard scale quad map should be examined. For those cases with posterior corneal elevation, three-dimensional views of posterior corneal elevation can also be generated. In all eyes with posterior corneal elevation, the following parameters are generated: (a) radii of the anterior and posterior curvature of the cornea, (b) posterior best-fit sphere, (c) and the difference between the corneal pachymetry value in the 7-mm zone and thinnest pachymetry value of the cornea.

PREEXISTING POSTERIOR CORNEAL ABNORMALITIES

Figure 11-2 shows the various topographic features of an eye with primary posterior corneal elevation detected during a pre-LASIK assessment. The general quad map commonly used incorporates the anterior elevation map (upper left), the posterior float (upper right), the kerato-

metric map (lower left), and the pachymetry map (lower right). In Figure 11-2, the pachymetry map shows a difference of 100 μm between the thickest pachymetry value in the 7-mm zone of cornea (613 μm) and thinnest pachymetry value (513 μm). This normal band scale map of anterior surface shows with-the-rule astigmatism in an otherwise normal anterior surface (shown in green). However, the posterior float shows significant elevation inferotemporally. When using the normal band map, only the abnormal areas are shown in red for ease in detection. Figure 11-3 is a three-dimensional representation of the maps in Figure 11-2.

Figure 11-4 shows a three-dimensional representation of with-the-rule astigmatism on the anterior corneal surface with reference sphere. Figure 11-5 shows a three-dimensional representation of the posterior corneal surface showing a significant posterior corneal elevation. Figure 11-6 shows the elevation (color coded) of the posterior corneal surface in microns (50 μm).

In light of the fact that keratoconus may have posterior corneal elevation as its earliest manifestation, preoperative analysis of posterior corneal curvature to detect a posterior corneal bulge is important to avoid post-LASIK keratectasia. The rate of progression of posterior corneal elevation to frank keratoconus is unknown. It is also difficult to specify the exact amount of posterior corneal elevation beyond which it may be unsafe to carry out LASIK. A typical elevation in the posterior corneal map more than 45 μm should alert us against a post-LASIK surprise. Orbscan provides reliable, reproducible data of the posterior corneal surface, and all LASIK candidates must be evaluated by this method preoperatively to rule out "early keratoconus."

Elevation is not measured directly by Placido-based topographers, but certain assumptions allow the construction

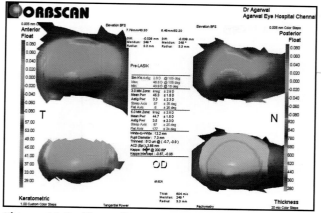

Figure 11-3. Three-dimensional representation of the maps in Figure 11-2 showing posterior corneal elevation of 50 microns (in red). The anterior cornea is normal.

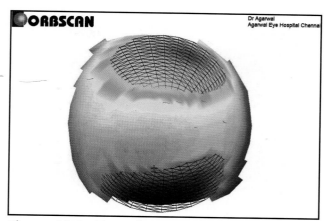

Figure 11-4. Three-dimensional representation of anterior surface of cornea showing with-the-rule astigmatism.

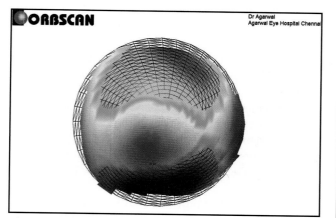

Figure 11-5. Three-dimensional representation showing posterior float. Notice there is marked elevation seen in the red areas.

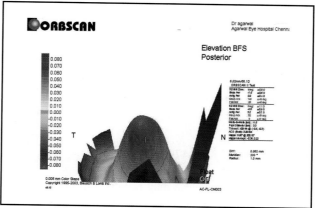

Figure 11-6. Three-dimensional representation showing posterior corneal elevation of 50 microns seen in posterior float.

of elevation maps. Elevation of a point on the corneal surface displays the height of the point on the corneal surface relative to a spherical reference surface. The reference surface is chosen to be a sphere. The best mathematical approximation of the actual corneal surface, called best-fit sphere, is calculated. One of the criteria for defining FFKC is a posterior best-fit sphere of greater than 55 D.

If the ratio of radii of the anterior to posterior curvature of the cornea is 1.21 and 1.27, the patient is considered as a keratoconus suspect. The average pachymetry difference between the thickest and thinnest point on the cornea in the 7-mm zone should normally be less than 100 μm.

Our criteria for diagnosis of the primary posterior corneal elevation include the following:

1. A ratio of the radii of anterior and posterior curvature of the cornea greater than 1.2. Note in Figure 11-2, the anterior curvature radius is 7.86 mm and the radii of the posterior curvature is 6.02 mm. The ratio is 1.3.

2. Posterior best-fit sphere is greater than 52 D. Note in Figure 11-2, the posterior best-fit sphere is 56.1 D

3. Difference between the thickest and thinnest corneal pachymetry value in the 7-mm zone is greater than 100 microns. The thickest pachymetry value, as seen in Figure 11-2, is 651 microns and the thinnest value is 409 microns. The difference is 242 microns.

4. The thinnest point on the cornea should correspond with the highest point of elevation of the posterior corneal surface. The thinnest point as seen in the bottom right picture of Figure 11-2 is a cross. This point or cursor corresponds to the same cross or cursor in top right picture of Figure 11-1, which indicates the highest point of elevation on the posterior cornea.

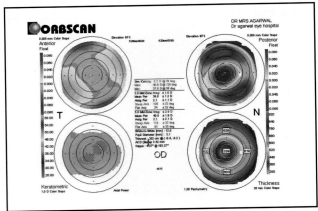

Figure 11-7. This figure shows a patient with iatrogenic keratectasia after LASIK. Note the upper right map showing that the posterior float has thinning. This is also seen in the bottom right map, in which the pachymetry reading is 329.

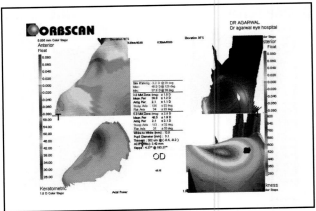

Figure 11-8. This figure shows the same patient as in Figure 11-7, with iatrogenic keratectasia after LASIK in a three-dimensional pattern. Note the ectasia seen clearly in the bottom right map.

5. Elevation of the posterior corneal surface should be more than 45 microns above the posterior best-fit sphere. Note in Figure 11-2, 0.062 mm or 62 microns above the best-fit sphere.

IATROGENIC KERATECTASIA

Iatrogenic keratectasia may be seen following ablative refractive surgery. Examples are shown in Figures 11-7 and 11-8. The anterior cornea is composed of alternating collagen fibrils and has a more complicated interwoven structure than the deeper stroma; it acts as the major stress-bearing layer. Most LASIK flaps are created within this layer, resulting in weakening of the corneal layer that contributes maximally to the biomechanical stability of the cornea.

The residual bed thickness (RBT) of the cornea is the crucial factor contributing to the biomechanical stability of the cornea after LASIK. The flap does not contribute much after its repositioning to the stromal bed. This is easily seen by the fact that the flap can be easily lifted 1 year after treatment. The decreased RBT, as well as the lamellar cut in the cornea, both contribute to the decreased biomechanical stability of the cornea. A reduction in the RBT results in a long-term increase in the surface parallel stress on the cornea. The intraocular pressure (IOP) can cause further forward bowing and thinning of a structurally compromised cornea. Inadvertent excessive eye rubbing, prone position sleeping, and normal wear and tear of the cornea may also play a role. The RBT should not be less than 250 microns to avoid subsequent iatrogenic keratectasias.[2–4] Relift enhancements should be undertaken cautiously in corneas with RBT less than 300 microns. Progressive myopia after successive operations is known as "dandelion keratectasia."

The ablation diameter also plays a very important role in LASIK. Postoperative optical distortions are more common with diameters less than 5.5 mm. Use of larger ablation diameters implies a lesser RBT postoperatively. Considering the formula: ablation depth [μm] = 1/3 (diameter [mm])^2 x (intended correction diopters),[4,5] it becomes clear that to preserve a sufficient bed thickness, the range of myopic correction is limited to approximately 12 D.[6]

Detection of a mild keratectasia requires knowledge about the posterior curvature of the cornea. Posterior topographic changes after LASIK are known. Increased negative keratometric diopters and oblate asphericity of the PCC, which correlate significantly with the intended correction, are common after LASIK leading to mild keratectasia.[6,7] This change in posterior power and the risk of keratectasia was more significant with a RBT of 250 μm or less.[8] The difference in the refractive indices results in a 0.2 D difference at the back surface of the cornea becoming equivalent to a 2.0 D change in the front surface of the cornea.[6] Increase in posterior power and asphericity also correlates with the difference between the intended and achieved correction 3 months after LASIK. This is because factors like drying of the stromal bed may result in an ablation depth more than that intended.[6] Age, attempted correction, the optical zone diameter, and the flap thickness are other parameters that have to be considered to avoid post-LASIK ectasia.[9,10]

The flap thickness may not be uniform throughout its length. In studies by Seitz et al,[6] it has been shown that the

Moria Model One microkeratome (Moria, Inc., Doylestown, Pa.) and the Supratome (Schwind Eye-Tech Solutions, Kleinostheim, Germany) cut deeper toward the hinge, whereas the Automated Corneal Shaper and the Hansatome (Bausch & Lomb, Rochester, NY) create flaps that are thinner toward the hinge. Accordingly, the area of corneal ectasia may not be in the center but paracentral, especially if it is also associated with decentered ablation. Flap thickness has also been found to vary considerably, even up to 40 μm, under similar conditions and this may also result in a lesser RBT than intended.[11–17] It is known that corneal ectasias and keratoconus have posterior corneal elevation as the earliest manifestation.[18] The precise course of progression of posterior corneal elevation to frank keratoconus is not known. Hence it is necessary to study the posterior corneal surface preoperatively in all LASIK candidates.

EFFECT OF POSTERIOR CORNEAL CHANGE ON IOL CALCULATION

IOL power calculation in post-LASIK eyes is different because of the inaccuracy of keratometry, change in anterior and posterior corneal curvatures, altered relationship between the two, and change in the standardized index of refraction of the cornea. Irregular astigmatism induced by the procedure, decentered ablations, and central islands also add to the problem.

Routine keratometry is not accurate in these patients. Corneal refractive surgery changes the asphericity of the cornea and also produces a wide range of powers in the central 5-mm zone of the cornea. LASIK makes the cornea of a myope more oblate so that keratometry values may be taken from the more peripheral steeper area of the cornea. This results in calculation of a lower than required IOL power, resulting in a hyperopic "surprise." Hyperopic LASIK makes the cornea more prolate, thus resulting in a myopic "surprise" after cataract surgery.

Post-PRK or LASIK, the relationship between the anterior and posterior corneal surfaces changes. The relative thickness of the various corneal layers, each having a different refractive index, also changes and there is a change in the curvature of the posterior corneal surface. All these result in the standardized refractive index of 1.3375 no longer being accurate in these eyes.

At present, there is no method of keratometry that can accurately measure the anterior and posterior curvatures of the cornea. The Orbscan also makes mathematical assumptions of the posterior surface rather than direct measurements. This is important in the LASIK patient because the procedure alters the relationship between the anterior and posterior surfaces of the cornea, as well as changes the curvature of the posterior cornea.

Thus, direct measurements such as manual and automated keratometry and topography are inherently inaccurate in these patients. The corneal power is therefore calculated by the calculation method, the contact lens over-refraction method, and by the computerized video keratography (CVK) method. The flattest K reading obtained by any method is taken for IOL power calculation; the steepest K is taken for hyperopes who had undergone LASIK. One can still aim for 1.00 D of myopia rather than emmetropia to allow for any error, which is normally in the hyperopic direction post-myopic LASIK patients. For best results, a third- or fourth-generation IOL calculating formula should be used for such patients.

REFERENCES

1. Fedor P, Kaufman S. Corneal topography and imaging. *eMedicine Journal.* 2001;2(6).

2. Seiler T, Koufala K, Richter G. Iatrogenic keratectasia after laser in situ keratomileusis. *J Refract Surg.* 1998 May-June;14(3):312–317.

3. Seiler T, Quurke AW. Iatrogenic keratectasia after laser in situ keratomileusis in a case of forme fruste keratoconus. *J Refract Surg.* 1998;24(7):1007–1009.

4. Probst LE, Machat JJ. Mathematics of laser in situ keratomileusis for high myopia. *J Cataract Refract Surg.* 1998;24(2):190–195.

5. Mc Donnell PJ. Excimer laser corneal surgery: new strategies and old enemies {review}. *Invest Ophthalmol Vis Sci.* 1995;36:4–8.

6. Seitz B, Torres F, Langenbucher A, et al. Posterior corneal curvature changes after myopic laser in situ keratomileusis. *Ophthalmology.* 2001;108(4):666–672.

7. Geggel HS, Talley AR. Delayed onset keratectasia following laser in situ keratomileusis. *J Cataract Refract Surg.* 1999;25(4):582–586.

8. Wang Z, Chen J, Yang B. Posterior corneal surface topographic changes after laser in situ keratomileusis are related to residual corneal bed thickness. *Ophthalmology.* 1999;106(2):406–409.

9. Pallikaris IG, Kymionis GD, Astyrakakis NI. Corneal ectasia induced by laser in situ keratomileusis. *J Cataract Refract Surg.* 2001;27(11):1796–1802.

10. Argento C, Cosentino MJ, Tytium A, et al. Corneal ectasia after laser in situ keratomileusis. *J Cataract Refract Surg.* 2001 Sep;27(9):1440–1448.

11. Binder PS, Moore M, Lambert RW, et al. Comparison of two microkeratome systems. *J Refract Surg.* 1997;13:142–153.

12. Hofmann RF, Bechara SJ. An independent evaluation of second generation suction microkeratomes. *Refract Corneal Surg.* 1992;8:348–354.

13. Schuler A, Jessen K, Hoffmann F. Accuracy of the microkeratome keratectomies in pig eyes. *Invest Ophthalmol Vis Sci.* 1990;31:2022–2030.

14. Behrens A, Seitz B, Langenbucher A, et al. Evaluation of corneal flap dimensions and cut quality using a manually guided microkeratome [published erratum appears in *J Refract Surg.* 1999;15(4):400]. *J Refract Surg.* 1999;15(2):118–123.

15. Behrens A, Seitz B, Langenbucher A, et al. Evaluation of corneal flap dimensions and cut quality using the Automated Corneal Shaper microkeratome. *J Refract Surg.* 2000;16:83–89.

16. Behrens A, Langenbucher A, Kus MM, et al. Experimental evaluation of two current generation automated microkeratomes: the Hansatome and the Supratome. *Am J Ophthalmol.* 2000;129:59–67.

17. Jacobs BJ, Deutsch TA, Rubenstein JB. Reproducibility of corneal flap thickness in LASIK. *Ophthalmic Surg Lasers.* 1999;30:350–353.

18. McDermott GK. Topography's benefits for LASIK. *Rev Ophthalmol.* 2003;9(3). Available at: http://www.revophth.com/index.asp?page=1_55.htm. Accessed January 25, 2006.

SECTION III

TOPOGRAPHY-BASED CUSTOM TREATMENT

Chapter 12

Corneal Topography and Wavefront Sensing: Complementary Tools

Gustavo E. Tamayo, MD and Mario G. Serrano, MD

With the latest advances in diagnostic ophthalmology tools, particularly in refractive surgery, we have come to a point of excellence in the knowledge of the cornea, the optics of the eye, and the change we can produce both in the morphology and refractive ability of the eye. Thorough comprehension of physiological optics and ocular anatomy is indispensable when proceeding with refractive surgery.

The cornea is the major refractive surface of the eye, due to its high curvature as well as the refractive index change that occurs at the level of the air/anterior tear film interface. The change to this curvature and in the shape of the anterior corneal surface is therefore one of the most important changes resulting from corneal refractive surgery.[1]

The eye is a complex optical structure where all its external and internal structures may play a role in visual quality. With this in mind, we know today that the role of the most important refractive structures of this system—the cornea and the lens—must be measured separately in order to clearly differentiate their roles before surgery.[2] Therefore, evaluation of the optical properties of the eye as well as the shape of the cornea must be carried out before refractive surgical correction on the cornea takes place. Optics are measured by wavefront technology, and shape by corneal topographic systems. Both evaluations are not only necessary but also complimentary in the refractive surgery armamentarium and, even more, their combination is essential to customized laser ablation as it is performed today.

WAVEFRONT SENSING AND ITS LIMITATIONS

There are two very distinct ways to measure the aberrations of the eye: outgoing wavefront aberrometry employed by the Hartmann-Shack device,[3] and incoming devices such as the Tscherning wavefront sensor spatially resolved refractometer[4] and ray tracing technology.[5] Each of these techniques has its own limitations on sampling, density, and reconstruction. An example of the Hartmann-Shack method is the VISX WaveScan (VISX, Inc., Santa Clara, Calif.), shown in Figure 12-1. An example of ray tracing methodology is shown in Figure 12-2.

The purpose of aberrometry is to measure the slope of the wavefront deviated from the normal pattern, using a number of points (sampling points) from which the shape of the wavefront is calculated. Those sampling points are distributed across a grid that covers the pupil in shapes that differ with each system in use. If undulations in the wavefront vary slowly as compared to the space among the sampling points, the wavefront error can be accurately and repeatedly measured—as is the case with normal optical systems.[6] However, when the wavefront error varies greatly among grid points (highly irregular optical systems), the information about the shape of the wavefront may be incorrect, inprecise, and unrepeatable.

Aliasing is an optical phenomenon that can occur with aberrometers, because they measure the aberrations at discrete locations within the pupil. The sampling theory states that any fluctuation in the wavefront error faster than the spacing between the samples results in an image that is not of optimal quality or accuracy because the aberrometer mistakenly produces an alias image that is different than the original.

Once the slope information error has been detected by the aberrometer, reconstruction of the wavefront has to be done utilizing straightforward matrix calculations. The most common method of reconstruction involves fitting the data to a set of polynomials, typically Zernike or Taylor polynomials. Those sets have been selected because they are used very often in ophthalmic optics, but

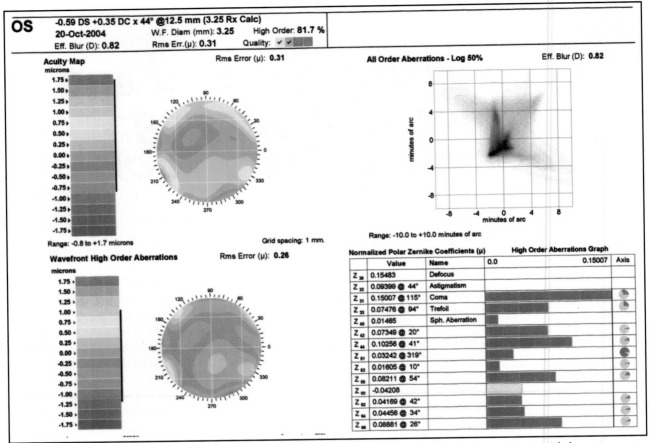

Figure 12-1. An example of the Hartmann-Shack method is the VISX WaveScan in a patient with keratoconus.

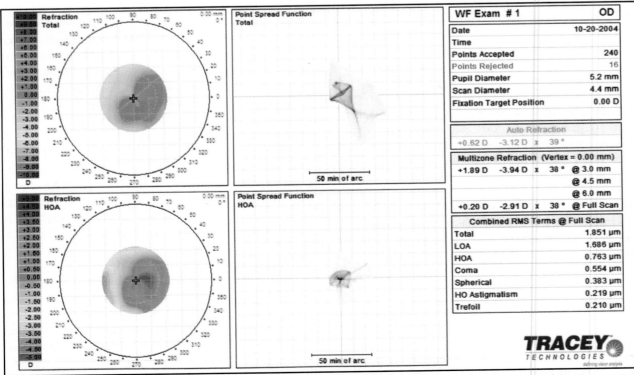

Figure 12-2. An example of ray tracing methodology is the iTrace. This is the same eye examined in Figure 12-1.

they are not the only ones. The result of the fitting data is a least square technique that minimizes the absolute error between the sample points and the reconstructed wavefront. However, since there are usually many more sample points than there are polynomials to fit the wavefront, an exact solution to the equation cannot be produced. Instead, in the process of determining the weighting coefficient required to describe a given aberration map, a least square curve-fitting solution is calculated (Zernike decomposition).[7]

WAVEFRONT DEFICIENCIES

The reconstruction process has two very important problems. First, it does not take into account the quality of each individual spot but rather displacement from each spot's "ideal" location. However, as clinicians, we have learned that a blurred spot has the significance of a rather large aberration overlapped by the neighboring spots. Similarly, a very small irregularity can scatter light and blur the spot.[8] The second problem is that the reconstructed wavefront is not a perfect mirror image of the real aberrated map, but instead, a "best-fitted calculation" due to the fact that Zernike polynomials do not use all data points measured from the wavefront slopes. These problems have become significant enough that manufacturers like VISX have changed from Zernike to Fourier-based algorithms, other polynomials that use all available data points for a superior characterization of the actual wavefront that exits at the patient's pupil.

The technical deficiencies described above translate into clinical deficiencies we see in practice:

1. Wavefront devices can overlook small irregularities, particularly at the corneal level, because the sample density is sometimes small. On the other hand, topographers have a much higher sample density that allows detection of even the smallest irregularities.

2. Wavefront devices measure the complete refractive state of the eye and do not differentiate the effect of internal structures of the eye, such as the lens and the posterior surface of the cornea. However, corneal topographers give direct information regarding the status of the cornea and, with appropriate mathematical calculations, can also produce a calculated corneal wavefront.

3. Wavefront sensing devices only sample the pupillary zone. Therefore, areas peripheral to the pupil and the center of the cornea are not measured. A wavefront map misses areas of the pupil that only participate in vision under low light conditions. It does not measure changes that occur at the periphery of the cornea after a central ablation, for example, or the changes induced by peripheral treatments such as certain hyperopic and presbyopic ablations. Topography, on the other hand, is not dependent on pupil size and therefore measures more peripheral areas of the cornea, in some instances out to 9.0 mm of corneal surface.

4. In some sense, wavefront devices are highly sampled autorefractors and are therefore sensitive to accommodation. If accommodation occurs, the resultant aberrated wavefront map is altered from the map without accommodation. In younger people, accommodation introduces a source of error to wavefront measurements, whereas topographies are independent of both pupil size and accommodation and are therefore highly repeatable.

5. Wavefront sensing devices have to send and receive light from the retinal surface without significant interference from tissue. When the cornea is highly deformed, such as in keratoconus or S/P refractive surgery, the incoming light no longer forms a well-formed spot. In situations like this, good wavefront maps are no longer possible. Topography does not have this limitation, as reflection occurs at the anterior ocular surface. Topographic maps can be obtained even in highly irregular corneas, and topography-guided ablation can be still performed successfully.

THE INDISPENSABLE NATURE OF CORNEAL TOPOGRAPHY

Since the development of refractive surgical techniques that alter corneal shape, topographic maps have become an indispensable tool for refractive surgeons. The refractive power of the cornea comes from two optical contributions: the change of index of refraction at the anterior surface (change from air to tear film) as well as corneal curvature. Since the index of refraction cannot be changed, we concentrate refractive surgical efforts on altering the shape of the cornea in order to correct the optical defects of the eye. Therefore, measurement of corneal shape has become indispensable when considering refractive surgery. Today, we have two predominant means of measuring shape: keratometry and corneal topography. Keratometry is limited to measuring only the central 3.0 mm zone with the analysis of only two major meridians, whereas corneal topography is indispensable when it comes to making a complete topographic analysis of an eye.[9]

However, corneal curvature analysis is not the best evaluation when we are going to change the refractive status of the eye via corneal surgery. Precise measurement of the elevation of the corneal surface is the most important data we can obtain for this type of treatment, particularly when customized corneal ablation is going to be attempted. The reason for reliable elevation analysis much more than curvature analysis is clearly understood when we see the way wavefront-guided ablations are performed, particularly when we make a careful evaluation of the way the laser beam ablation is going to be delivered to the corneal surface.

The treatment of aberrations in excimer laser corneal surgery is done based on the difference in OPL (optical path length) between the actual wavefront and some ideal wavefront. Therefore we use distance measurement, in the form of elevation changes of a surface. The aberrated wavefront exiting from the eye through a pupil deviates from the ideal in that all its component rays do not exit at the same time. In a very simple way, if we have information on time, location, distance, and position of every wave (OPL), we can mathematically change this information into microns. Therefore, when calculating a treatment, we can consider the change in elevation (resection of microns of predetermined areas) to produce a wavefront in which all the components exit at the same time (an ideal or flat wavefront).

DIFFERENCES AND CORRELATIONS IN WAVEFRONT AND CORNEAL TOPOGRAPHIC FINDINGS

In order to evaluate the possible role of corneal topography and its correlation with wavefront analysis of an optical system, we have to compare both methods relevant to refractive surgery:

1. Corneal topography allows for evaluation of the cornea with respect to curvature and elevation. Wavefront data refers exclusively to the optical properties of the eye.

2. Topography measures a large area of the cornea, and not only the pupillary area. It can extend its analysis to the far periphery of the cornea, depending on the type of system. Wavefront only analyzes the pupil area.

3. Corneal topography is independent of accommodation and other refractive states. Wavefront is still influenced by accommodation.

4. Most commonly, corneal topographers sample the cornea with concentric rings; they measure at the limits between light and dark areas or average the areas illuminated by the ring. This produces a higher sample density than the one produced by wave-

front aberrometers. This fact makes topography more sensitive to small irregularities than wavefront.

5. Topography maps images of the corneal surface. Wavefront devices cannot differentiate the location of aberrations.

6. As corneal topography gives direct information on the shape of the cornea, it can be used to predict the effect of corneal ablative procedures on the anterior surface. Using elevation presurgical data, software programs enable the ablation pattern to be subtracted to produce a new corneal shape. Wavefront predictions are presently not possible.

7. Following the ability to predict postsurgical corneal shape, topography elevation maps can be used to simulate different ablation patterns, illustrating different potential outcomes. This provides the ability to customize already custom procedures. The surgeon has the ability to discern which of the proposed ablation patterns will have the desired effect.

8. In cases in which the cornea is compromised to the extent of interference with incoming light for wavefront analysis, corneal shape can still be measured with topography. Even in the presence of significant irregularities, a surgical plan can be produced when a wavefront-guided ablation is not possible.

9. Corneal topography can produce difference maps to graphically show the difference between two corneal surfaces. These are used to monitor the changes induced by the treatment and the changes produced by time during the healing process.

10. The final important advantage of topography is the evolution of the "corneal aberrometry map."

CORNEAL WAVEFRONT ABERRATIONS

Today it is possible to calculate corneal aberrations with the use of the corneal shape as measured with submicron precision by the topography units, regardless of the system used by those videokeratoscopes. However, most topographers today employ Placido-disk principles. A camera captures images coming from the anterior surface of the cornea, following the reflective properties of the cornea. The surface geometry is obtained in each meridian from the ring spacing. There are several calculations and procedures to determine the corneal aberrations, derived from the topography map obtained from a given cornea.

One simple approach to calculate wavefront aberrations from corneal topography is to obtain a lens by subtracting

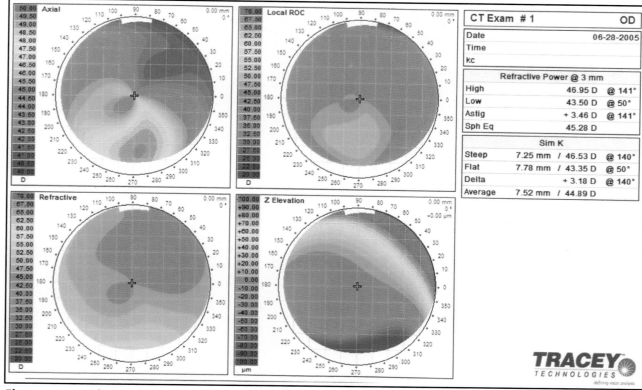

Figure 12-3A. The iTrace is able to perform topographical analysis to determine aberrations attributed to the cornea.

the best-fitted conic surface to the measured cornea and calculating the aberrations by multiplying it by the refractive index difference. Another more complicated but widely used method is to have the corneal elevation map provided by videokeratography fitted to a Zernike polynomial expansion. Then, through ray tracing, the wavefront aberration associated with the corneal surface is obtained as the difference in OPL between the principal ray that passes through the center of the pupil and a marginal ray. Several studies have confirmed the precision for this method to calculate the aberration in small to medium pupil sizes (from 4.0 to 6.0 mm diameter).[10] An example of using ray tracing and Placido-disk principles to determine the corneal aberrations is shown in Figure 12-3. Figure 12-3A shows the topographical analysis of a patient with pellucid marginal degeneration. Figure 12-3B shows the total aberrations (top) and higher-order aberrations (lower) in the same eye. Figure 12-3C shows the combined analysis. The four maps in this figure include the internal aberrations (top left), the corneal aberrations (bottom left), and the total aberrations (top right).

CORNEAL ABERRATIONS VS OPTICAL ABERRATIONS

Once we have wavefront aberrations of the whole eye and the aberrations produced by the cornea, contribution of the corneal aberrations can be evaluated. Theoretically, we subtract aberrations from the cornea to total aberration and obtain aberrations corresponding to the posterior surface of the cornea and crystalline lens. However, ocular aberrations and corneal aberrations originate from two different systems.[11] This produces a problem in registration, because corneal and ocular aberrations are obtained centered in different locations of the pupil, many times at different pupil sizes. Subtraction of those different maps will produce an incorrect estimate of internal aberrations. They are different and because of the difference in centration during acquisition, they are not comparable. As clinicians, we know that decentration induces significant changes in aberrations—a completely different map in fact.[12]

Although decentration is a source of error when combining ocular and corneal aberrations, we have another problem for registration. Wavefront devices use the visual axis as an alignment axis. Topographers do not; they use the vertex instead. This difference produces a corneal aberration map with a different angle than the wavefront map of the whole eye. These two problems could be solved by mathematical calculations—by assuming the geometric center of the pupil in both maps, particularly if the two maps are acquired by the same system. However, despite technical difficulty, the combination of these two different maps has been done successfully and results have proven to be consistent.

In the great majority of refractive problems we treat today, the differentiation of those aberrations may not be vital. But the ability to know the relevance of aberrations in the quality of vision may help find those so-called "good aberrations" and may help explain the dynamics of better vision. In patients over 50, it may play an important role in identifying which aberrations proceed from the lens and which ones are from the cornea. Without any doubt, in the future of refractive surgery a combination map will always be a part of the examination and, therefore, the role of corneal topography will be crucial again.

CONCLUSIONS

Wavefront sensing and corneal topography are complementary tools in the diagnosis and management of refractive problems. They have very strong differences: different equipment, different technology, and different functions. Corneal topography measures shape, and wavefront measures optics. Topography measures a large area of the cornea, while wavefront is limited to the pupillary area. Due to the strong differences between the two systems, they do not exclude each other. On the contrary, they have to be used together in order to fully understand the complex problems of visual quality in order to truly evaluate a refractive problem.

With technological sophistication, not only are topography and aberrometry complementary tools but they are used together in a "corneal aberrometer." Aberrations from the cornea are calculated from a topographic elevation map, and are subtracted from the total wavefront aberrations to provide corneal contribution to total wavefront error. In the near future, we will see a single unit taking both measurements at the same time. Such units will identify where each aberration originates within the eye. Understanding this will help improve outcomes of refractive surgery, correct resultant refractive defects, and clarify which aberrations are beneficial and should remain and which are debilitating and should be eliminated.

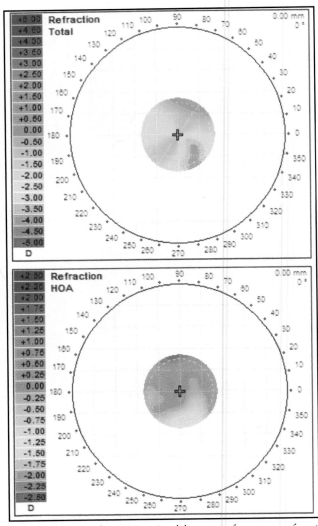

Figure 12-3B. The iTrace is able to perform wavefront analysis to determine aberrations attributed to the cornea.

REFERENCES

1. Munnerlyn CR, Koons SJ, Marshal J. Photorefractive keratectomy: a technique for laser refractive surgery. *J Cataract Refract Surg.* 1988;14(1):46–52.

2. Campbell FW, Gubish RW. Optical quality of the human eye. *J Physiol.* 1996;186:558–578.

3. Liang J, Williams DR. Aberrations and retinal image quality of the normal human eye. *J Opt Soc Am A.* 1997; 14(11):2873–2883.

4. Mrochen M, Kaemmerer M, Seiler T. Wavefront-guided laser in situ keratomileusis: early results in three eyes. *J Refract Surg.* 2000;16:116–121.

5. Molebny VV, Panagopoulou SI, Molebny SV, Wakil YS, Pallikaris IG. Principles of ray tracing aberrometry. *J Refract Surg.* 2000;16:S570–S571.

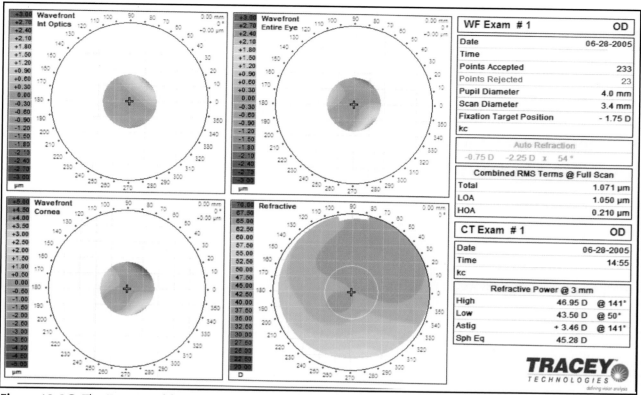

Figure 12-3C. The iTrace is able to perform combined analysis to determine aberrations attributed to the cornea.

6. Liang J, Grimm B, Goelz S, Bille JF. Objective measurement of wave aberrations of the human eye with the use of a Hartmann-Shack wavefront sensor. *J Opt Soc Am A.* 1997;14(11):2873–2883.

7. Wang JY, Silva DE. Wavefront interpretation with Zernike polynomials. *Applied Optics.* 1980;19(9):1510–1518.

8. Thibos LN, Hong X. Clinical applications of the Shack-Hartmann aberrometer. *Optom Vis Sci.* 1999;76:817–825.

9. Seiler T, Reckmann W, Maloney RK. Effective spherical aberration of the cornea as a quantitative descriptor in corneal topography. *J Cataract Refract Surg.* 1993;19:155–165.

10. Schwiegerling J, Greivenkamp JE. Using corneal height maps and polynomial decomposition to determine corneal aberrations. *Optom Vis Sci.* 1997;74:906–916.

11. He JC, Gwiazda J, Held R, Thorn F, Ong E, Marran L. Wavefront aberrations in the cornea and the whole eye. *Invest Ophthalmol Vis Sci.* 2000;41:S104.

12. Endl MJ, Martinez CE, Klyce SD, et al. Irregular astigmatism after photorefractive keratectomy. *J Refract Surg.* 1999:S249–S251.

Combined Wavefront and Topography Approach to Refractive Surgery Treatments

Noel Alpins, FRACO, FRCOphth, FACS and George Stamatelatos, BscOptom

Recent advances in refractive surgery and diagnostic technology, together with the introduction of wavefront treatments, have given doctors a more thorough understanding of the eye's refractive characteristics than ever before. The excellent results attained with this new technology have shown the capabilities of wavefront-guided treatments in effectively reducing spherical aberration.[1-3] However, wavefront-assisted laser surgery does not address the intraocular (noncorneal) astigmatism that remains on the cornea postoperatively. With this approach, topographic values are not taken into account.

At the other end of the treatment scale, state-of-the-art topographers have allowed for an increase in the amount of data captured. However, they do not consider the fact that the amount of astigmatism at the corneal plane often differs from the refractive (second-order) astigmatism. As a result, treatments based solely on the map generated from a topographer, or aberrometer, do not usually have optimum outcomes.

Surgeons now have at their disposal a large amount of preoperative data, which would be helpful to them if they could fully integrate this into their treatment plan. Currently, they cannot take full advantage of this using refraction alone. However, by incorporating both the refractive and corneal measurements in the treatment paradigm, this may allow for improved visual outcomes.[4,5]

UNDERSTANDING REFRACTIVE VS CORNEAL ASTIGMATISM

Astigmatism treatment is prevalent in more than 60% of refractive surgery cases. By targeting zero corneal astigmatism, as well as zero refractive astigmatism, overall visual outcomes can be improved. While zero overall astigmatism is ideal, usually this result is unattainable due to the inherent differences in magnitude and/or orientation of corneal (topographic) and refractive (wavefront) astigmatism. The intraocular (noncorneal) astigmatism is gauged by the ocular residual astigmatism (ORA).[5,6] This is the vectorial difference calculated between the measured corneal and refractive astigmatism.

The ORA value is the amount of astigmatism that will remain in the eye if only refractive astigmatism is corrected. The ORA is calculated, using trigonometric principles, by doubling the angles of the refractive and corneal astigmatic axes to determine the difference between the two (Figure 13-1). The astigmatic magnitudes remain unchanged. The resultant ORA axis on the double-angle vector diagram is then halved to convert it back to a polar diagram, which represents the parameters on the eye.[4,5,7,8]

Using this approach, the maximum amount of astigmatism is treated. The distribution of any remaining ORA needs to be considered carefully. Do we leave this totally on the cornea by treating with manifest wavefront refraction, as is customary practice, or is it better to distribute the astigmatism between the two in a "favorable" optimized manner?

Certainly, it would be advantageous to be able to reduce a greater amount of corneal astigmatism by directing the treatment closer to the principal meridia, creating less "off-axis" effect and reduced torque[9] without compromising the refractive outcome. Using the vector planning technique, this is achievable and can result in a better refractive outcome associated with reduced second-order aberrations.

LIMITATIONS OF WAVEFRONT-GUIDED OR TOPOGRAPHIC-GUIDED TREATMENTS ALONE

While wavefront- and topographic-guided treatments both have much to offer, when it comes to astigmatism, neither can offer the complete picture alone. Wavefront aberrometry devices measure lower- and higher-order aberrations of the eye's optical system. The refractive guidance provided by wavefront technology to reduce spherical aberrations by achieving the most effective prolate aspheric profile may be significant and the benefits clear.[10]

However, for astigmatism, the treatment issues are more complex. There is a perceptual component to consider, which is not taken into account by the wavefront-guided approach. There is no consideration of the patient's subjective appreciation of astigmatism, which is related to the visual cortex of the brain. The visual cortex may "accept" some, or all, of the astigmatism resulting from the wavefront refraction and, as a result, the patient does not perceive any visual problem. This "acceptance" of the wavefront refraction by the visual cortex is best reflected in the manifest refraction. The inclusion in the treatment of a patient's conscious perception of his or her astigmatism is likely to lend to satisfaction.[11,12]

Another drawback of the wavefront-guided approach is that if practitioners attempt to correct all ocular aberrations at the corneal surface, it would result in corneal surface irregularities.[11] In order to obtain the best possible astigmatic outcome, it would be advantageous to have a regular cornea with orthogonal and symmetrical orientation.[4] It is important to note that even eyes with normal (emmetropic) vision can suffer from aberrations that affect functional vision.[13]

Manifest refraction also needs to be brought into the picture. By measuring manifest refraction, we incorporate input from the visual cortex as well as the contribution from corneal astigmatism and internal optics (lens) of the eye. In most cases, the refractive cylinder is different in orientation and/or magnitude from the corneal astigmatism, as measured by topography. If treatment were performed by refraction parameters alone, an excessive and unnecessary amount of corneal astigmatism would be left behind. Consequently, lower second-order astigmatic aberrations and third-order coma would not be minimized by treatment. This would potentially compromise visual acuity and contrast sensitivity outcomes.

Meanwhile, topography-guided ablations are derived from an objective measurement of the corneal astigmatism. One problem, however, is that treatment directed principally on this basis does not take into consideration

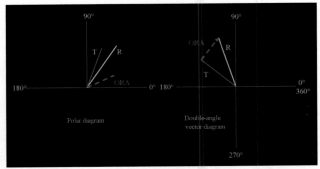

Figure 13-1. Polar and double-angle vector diagrams showing ORA vector.

the likely difference in astigmatism magnitude and/or axis from that present on the manifest or wavefront refraction. However, corneal topographic analysis is essential not only as a diagnostic tool for detection of irregular or keratoconic corneas, but also for determining where the total treatment is applied. Incorporation of the corneal status into the treatment plan provides potential for improvement in BCVA.

It is important to note that directly combining the wavefront-guided approach and disregarding the topographic surface is not a favorable option. If we try "sculpting" one cylinder (refractive astigmatism) onto a second cylinder (corneal astigmatism) of different magnitude and/or axis, this can result in a third cylinder with greater magnitude than the original preoperative astigmatism.[5,9]

COMBINING WAVEFRONT AND TOPOGRAPHIC DATA USING VECTOR PLANNING

With the vector planning method, both wavefront and topographic information can be taken into account. The advantages of addressing both corneal and refractive astigmatism preoperatively are clear—this approach can improve visual outcomes of spherocylindrical treatments by combining the topographic and refractive astigmatic components. A reduced level of astigmatism is left on the cornea compared to using refractive parameters alone and, as a result, fewer second- and third-order aberrations may remain.[4,5,7,14]

The calculations performed in this chapter utilize the ASSORT program (Alpins Statistical System for Ophthalmic Refractive Surgery Techniques) developed by Dr. Alpins. The program uses vector planning and analysis in a paradigm that favors with-the-rule astigmatism. With this method, corneal astigmatism is taken into account and reduction in postoperative refractive astigmatism is optimized.[4,5,7,8,14]

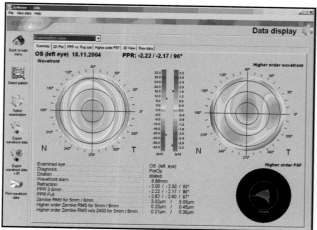

Figure 13-2. Wavefront analysis display.

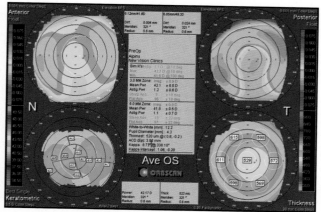

Figure 13-3. Topographical analysis display.

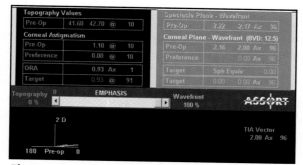

Figure 13-4. The ASSORT surgical planning module with emphasis to 100% reduction of refractive astigmatism.

Consider the following example:

Figure 13-2 shows a wavefront data display. The spherocylindrical refraction as measured by the wavefront device at the spectacle plane is –2.22 –2.17 x 96 (corneal plane is –2.16 –2.00 x 96 with BVD 12.5 mm). The aberrations are quantified as root-mean-square values at the bottom of the display. Higher-order aberrations comprise 0.45 microns of the total aberrations (5.05 microns), indicating that the majority of the treatment lies in correcting (second-order) spherical and cylindrical components.

Figure 13-3 displays the topographic data of the same astigmatic eye. The "keratometric" map in the lower left corner shows the typical bowtie appearance of the regular corneal against-the-rule astigmatism. The simulated keratometry values show 1.10 D of astigmatism at the steepest meridian of 10 degrees.

Combining this topographic information into the treatment module of the ASSORT program allows us to view the optimal treatment and resultant spectacle and corneal astigmatic targets for which we are aiming (Figure 13-4).

The topography-simulated K values are displayed on the left, and the wavefront refraction is on the right. The amount of uncorrectable astigmatism in this patient's eye is 0.93 x 001 (ORA). The distribution of this is reflected in the "Emphasis" bar, where 100% indicates treatment of refractive astigmatism alone and 0% shows the contribution of topographic astigmatism to the treatment.

If we treat conventionally, that is with 100% second-order wavefront refraction, all of this residual astigmatism will remain on the cornea. This is shown as the "Target" 0.93 D at a near vertical meridian of 91 degrees, which is 90 degrees away from the ORA axis to neutralize the internal (noncorneal) error and results in zero astigmatism in the postoperative refraction (shown as the light blue "Target"). The target-induced astigmatism vector (TIA) being employed is 2.00 D x 96.

At the other extreme, if we treat this eye by topography values alone, –0.93 DC x 91 will remain in the postoperative refraction. Incorporating a proportion of each into the overall treatment, by shifting the emphasis for astigmatism reduction "to the left" and increasing the proportion of corneal astigmatism correction, results in the treatment being more closely aligned to the principal corneal meridian, more flattening effect, and reduced corneal astigmatism and torque.[9] Figure 13-5 shows the emphasis placed at 40% topography and 60% refraction.

The patient's ORA is still 0.93 D, but it is apportioned between the refraction and the cornea. Here, less corneal astigmatism is targeted, with 60% of 0.93 D (0.56 D) targeted at the same meridian of 91, and the remaining 40% (0.37 D) of the emphasis placed refractively in a spherical equivalent of zero (+0.19 –0.37 x 91). This remaining refractive astigmatism is not perceptually evident.

When measurements were in fact taken at 2 months postoperatively, simulated keratometry showed 0.50 D @ 85 degrees, while wavefront refraction measured –0.24 DC x 49. This minimal amount of astigmatism was not detected by the perceptive system as the manifest refractive astigmatism was plano, gaining less overall astigmatism.

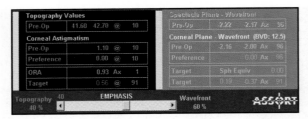

Figure 13-5. The ASSORT planning module with emphasis placed at 40% topography and 60% refraction.

TABLE 13-1		
FORME FRUSTE AND MILD KERATOCONUS OUTCOMES		
Mean Astigmatism	**Preoperative**	**Postoperative (3 months)**
Corneal	1.92D ± 1.44	1.11D ± 0.72
Refractive	1.65DC ± 1.25 (corneal plane)	0.51DC ± 0.56

Mean ORA = 1.22 D ± 0.85
Mean postoperative spherical equivalent was 0.00 D ± 0.62.
N = 33

The fact is that even though all the astigmatism could not be removed from the system, with some apportioned to the refractive astigmatism and the rest to the remaining corneal astigmatism, results with this technique were still significantly better than they would have been by employing wavefront parameters alone. The overall astigmatism was reduced from 3.10 D (1.10 D corneal +2.00 DC wavefront) to 0.74 D (0.50 D corneal –0.24 DC wavefront refraction). This is lower than the uncorrectable amount of 0.93 D calculated by the ORA. The data also showed that by taking care of corneal astigmatism as well, there was a large reduction in remaining lower-order aberrations, with a RMS of 0.94 microns.

STUDY USING COMBINED TOPOGRAPHIC AND REFRACTIVE DATA TO TREAT ASTIGMATISM

To determine if this vector planning approach could benefit patients, a study was recently launched. A group of 33 eyes with subclinical (forme fruste) or mild keratoconus (nonprogressive) were treated using the Alpins method of vector planning. Due to the irregular shape of these corneas, as reflected in asymmetry of greater than 1.50 D on topography and higher than average ORA values (0.73 D[4] and 0.81 D[5]), photoastigmatic refractive keratectomy (PARK) was performed in each case (Table 13-1).

All treatments were optimized to leave minimum remaining corneal astigmatism toward with-the-rule orientation, with 40% of the emphasis placed on topography and 60% on refraction. Postoperative results at 3 months showed that, on average, the corneal cylinder was reduced by 0.75 D, compared to results that would have been attained by treating refractive values alone. This was done without compromising the refractive outcome.

In the future, we envision developing software to use this method of vector planning and to optimize treatment for each separate hemi-division of the cornea in cases of irregular astigmatism. This should result in a more orthogonal, regular cornea[4,15,16] with its ensuing benefits to vision.

SUMMARY

The Alpins method of vector planning utilizes information from both corneal topography and manifest refraction/wavefront data to target less postoperative corneal astigmatism and reduced torque. Using this combined approach, second- and third-order (coma and trefoil) astigmatic aberrations are minimized. As a result, there is the potential for improvement in BCVA and contrast sensitivity.

Neither of these two approaches, either topographic or refractive alone, can attain the same results in most astigmatic patients. Topographic-guided lasers play an important role in customizing treatments for irregular postoperative or traumatized corneas—enabling comprehensive mapping in situations where subjective wavefront refractions may be inadequate to provide a smoother corneal surface.

Wavefront-guided laser refractive surgery has certainly been of benefit in correcting aberrations of the eye, in particular helping to maximize low-light and night vision. However correction of the second-order astigmatic aberrations needs to be more fully explored to increase overall patient satisfaction.

Together, using the vector planning technique, information from these two approaches can help to minimize astigmatism from the system and ultimately to optimize results in many cases.

REFERENCES

1. Carones F, Vigo L, Scandola E, et al. Expanded range custom cornea algorithms for myopia and astigmatism: one-month results. *J Refractive Surg.* 2004;20(5):S619–S623.

2. Winkler von Mohrenfels C, Huber A, Gabler B, et al. Wavefront-guided laser epithelial keratomileusis with the wavelight concept system 500. *J Refractive Surg.* 2004; 20(5):S565–S569.

3. Mastropasqua L, Nubile M, Ciancaglini M, et al. Prospective randomized comparison of wavefront-guided and conventional photorefractive keratectomy for myopia with the Meditec MEL 70 laser. *J Refractive Surg.* 2004;20(5): 422–431.

4. Alpins NA. Astigmatism analysis by the Alpins method. *J Cataract Refract Surg.* 2001;27:31–49.

5. Alpins NA. New method of targeting vectors to treat astigmatism. *J Cataract Refract Surg.* 1997;23:65–75.

6. Duke-Elder S (ed). *System of Ophthalmology. Vol 5: Ophthalmic Optics and Refraction.* St Louis, MO: Mosby; 1970:275–278.

7. Alpins NA. A new method of analyzing vectors for changes in astigmatism. *J Cataract Refract Surg.* 1993; 19:524–533.

8. Alpins NA, Goggin M. Practical astigmatism analysis for refractive outcomes in cataract and refractive surgery. *Surv of Ophthal.* 2004;49:109–122.

9. Alpins NA. Vector analysis of astigmatism changes by flattening, steepening, and torque. *J Cataract Refract Surg.* 1997;23:1503–1514.

10. Munger R. New paradigm for the treatment of myopes by refractive surgery. *J Refractive Surg.* 2000;16:S651–S655.

11. Alpins NA. Wavefront technology: a new advance that fails to answer old questions on corneal vs. refractive astigmatism correction (editorial). *J Cataract Refract Surg.* 2002;18:737–739.

12. Kohnen T. Combining wavefront and topography data for excimer laser surgery: the future of customized ablation? (editorial). *J Cataract Refract Surg.* 2004;30:285–286.

13. Williams D, Yoon GY, Porter J, Guirao A, Hofer H, Cox I. Visual benefit of correcting higher-order aberrations of the eye. *J Refract Surg.* 2000;16:S554–S559.

14. Alpins NA, Walsh G. Aberrometry and topography in the vector analysis of refractive laser surgery. In: Boyd BF, Agarwal A, eds. *Wavefront Analysis, Aberrometers and Corneal Topography.* Panama: Highlights of Ophthalmology;2003:313–322.

15. Goggin M, Alpins N, Schmid L. Management of irregular astigmatism. *Curr Opin Ophthal.* 2000;11:260–266.

16. Alpins NA. Treatment of irregular astigmatism. *J Cataract Refract Surg.* 1998;24:634–646.

Chapter 14

LaserSight Alternatives in Topography-Based Custom Ablation

Aleksandar Stojanovic, MD

The concept of customized ablation (CA) developed in the mid-nineties was corneal topography-based. Treatment of irregular astigmatism (IA) was its primary aim,[1–4] but due to the complexity of the task, as well as underdeveloped diagnostics and treatment equipment, the initial results were below expectations.[5,6] Introduction of wavefront technology around the year 2000, backed by an enormous marketing effort, led to a paradigm shift in CA, turning its focus to virgin eyes.[7-10] The historical background and obvious commercial advantage of an immensely larger virgin eye market seems to have influenced research and development policy. It led to the development of their own LaserSight's "Custom Eyes" solution, based on the AstraMax diagnostic workstation and AstraPro ablation planning software (primarily designed for vision correction in virgin eyes) and turning away from an already mature third party CA system based on Orbscan diagnostics and CIPTA (Ligi, Taranto, Italy) software, despite the latter systems' unique and unsurpassed results in treatment of IA.[11,12]

AstraMax Workstation

The two widely available corneal topography technologies ("Placido disk" and "slit scanning") were not originally designed for use in CA. It requires higher precision and accuracy of corneal elevation mapping than the current instruments can provide. Monocular Placido disk-based topographers that register cornea curvature information were developed primarily for contact lens fitting. The Orbscan slit-scanning topographer, although registering the corneal height information, was not designed with CA in mind either and lacks the necessary precision for the task. Monocular Placido-based systems rely on information from one camera, one angle, and "one shot." Under such circumstances, direct measurement of height information for a single independent point on the corneal surface is not possible. The mathematically calculated height of each point using the arc step method depends on neighboring points, and an artifact can easily lead to a cumulative error, significantly affecting the accuracy of the system.

Height measurements of the Orbscan's slit-scanning system are more accurate due to the use of the triangulation method. However, they lack the necessary precision due to a relatively long data acquisition time that requires eye movement compensation and causes errors due to abnormal light scattering on a dry corneal surface, as well as any other type of blocking of light transmission including corneal scarring, irregular epithelium, edema, irregular corneal collagen, or interface fluid.

AstraMax is a "checkerboard disk," three-camera–based topographer. It is the only topography system designed from inception to provide triangulation-based corneal elevation information for use in CA. It generates anterior and posterior corneal height maps and spatial pachymetry, as well as scotopic and photopic pupillometry including the registration of pupillary center with respect to the anterior surface intercept of the visual axis (which is the center of its topography map by default). The projection of the pupil on the anterior surface of the cornea is measured under different lighting conditions with an infrared instrument, providing both the surgical registration data used for automatic centration of the ablation (achieved by the laser's eye-tracker) as well as the scotopic pupil diameter used for ablation size planning. The reflected corneal surface image of the checkerboard "polar grid" target (Figure 14-1) is acquired by use of a three-camera system (Figure 14-2). This system employs an advanced surface reconstruction algorithm designed to

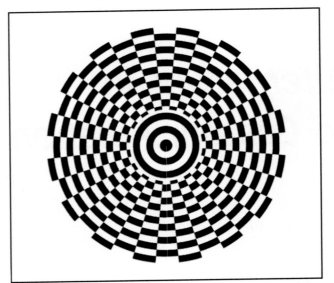

Figure 14-1. Checkerboard, polar grid target of the AstraMax.

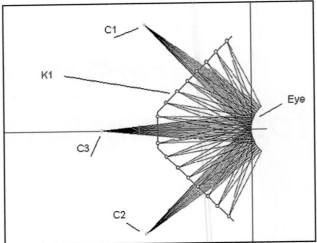

Figure 14-2. Use of three-camera system for data acquisition.

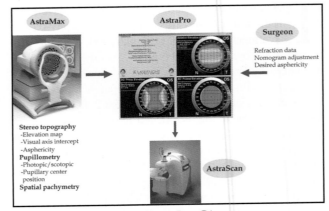

Figure 14-3. AstraMax/AstraPro CA system.

provide accurate and precise height maps, as well as accurate sensing of corneal asphericity. This is possible even in cases of irregular corneas with significant discontinuities of shape. A laser cross can be projected for measurement of the posterior corneal surface and optical pachymetry. All measurements are taken simultaneously with respect to a single axis in only a fraction of a second, providing robust data without having to attempt to compensate for eye movements. This instrument is still under development, and its hardware capabilities are only partially exploited at this time.

In its original incarnation, the AstraMax/AstraPro system has been primarily designed for CA treatment of virgin eyes, and it seems to provide its users with outcomes comparable to any current wavefront-based system. AstraMax data, including the first surface higher-order aberrations (HOAs), pupillometry, and the ablation registration information, is fed to the AstraPro ablation planning software, combined with the surgical information concerning the desired spherocylindrical correction and targeted asphericity. Registration of the ablation center is achieved by registration of the pupillary center with respect to the center of the topography map which, in the AstraMax, represents the first corneal surface intercept with the visual axis. The amount of light used for the acquisition of registration can be set to the level approximating the amount of light during the surgery, in order to prevent error caused by drift of the pupillary center if different lighting conditions are used during the surgery. Finally, the surgeon provides the patient's refractive data and nomogram adjustment, as well as the desired postoperative asphericity value. This is illustrated in Figure 14-3. Cyclotorsional registration is achieved by manual marking.

AstraMax/AstraPro System in Treatment of Myopia and Astigmatism in Virgin Eyes

The author performed a prospective, randomized, double-masked study comparing the outcomes from the AstraMax/AstraPro CA with standard LaserSight treatments. One hundred and twenty eyes of 60 patients were treated for myopia with or without astigmatism with bilateral LASIK. One eye was treated with CA and the fellow eye with standard treatment. Virgin eyes with best spectacle-corrected visual acuity (BSCVA) of 20/25 or better, with myopic astigmatism, with sphere up to –10 D and cylinder up to –3 D were included in the study. Baseline refraction is shown in Table 14-1. One year after the surgery, 50 out of 60 patients were available for evaluation. Two standard eyes and one Astra eye lost one line of BSCVA, 46% of the standard eyes gained lines of BSCVA,

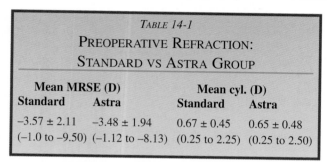

TABLE 14-1			
PREOPERATIVE REFRACTION:			
STANDARD VS ASTRA GROUP			
Mean MRSE (D)		**Mean cyl. (D)**	
Standard	**Astra**	**Standard**	**Astra**
–3.57 ± 2.11	–3.48 ± 1.94	0.67 ± 0.45	0.65 ± 0.48
(–1.0 to –9.50)	(–1.12 to –8.13)	(0.25 to 2.25)	(0.25 to 2.50)

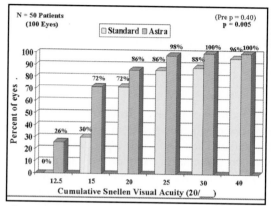

Figure 14-5. Efficacy of Astra versus standard treatments 6 months after surgery.

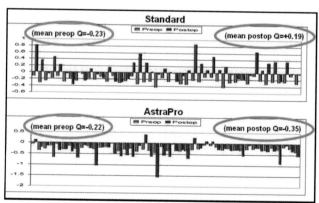

Figure 14-7. Asphericity change in Astra and standard treatments from preoperative to 6 months after surgery.

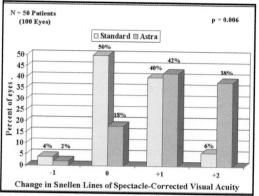

Figure 14-4. Safety of Astra versus standard treatments 6 months after surgery.

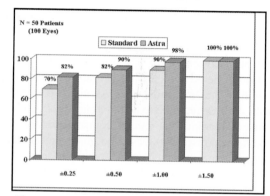

Figure 14-6. Predictability of Astra versus standard treatments 6 months after surgery.

while 80% of Astra eyes gained lines and almost half of those gained 2 lines or more. The difference between the standard and AstraPro eyes was statistically significant (Figure 14-4). The difference between the two groups was also statistically significant concerning the achieved UCVA (Figure 14-5). Ninety percent of the Astra eyes versus 82% of the standard eyes were within 0.5 D of emmetropia (Figure 14-6). Asphericity indexes for the two groups went in opposite directions. Standard eyes changed from prolate to oblate asphericity while Astra eyes main-

tained their prolate shape, shown in Figure 14-7. The patients graded the quality of their postoperative vision on a scale from 1 to 10. The difference in favor of Astra eyes was statistically significant, and is shown in Figure 14-8.

This double-masked comparative study showed statistically significantly better outcomes with Astra treatments compared to the standard. When we looked for the possible reasons for the inferior outcomes of standard treatments, the most apparent was the induction of spherical aberration and coma, both of which could be traced to changes in corneal topography. Induction of spherical aberration was attributed to the new oblate shape. This may result from the noncompensated laser energy reduction toward the periphery (cosine effect), as well as by the corneal biomechanical response to creation of the LASIK flap.[13] The induction of coma-like HOAs could be attributed to asymmetric corneal optics due to displacement of the ablation with respect to the optical center of the cornea, as well as cyclotorsional registration errors. Thus, the reason for superior results with Astra treatments is most likely the correction of these shortcomings of standard treatments. Most of all, the preserved preoperative prolate asphericity, resulting in less induced spherical aberration and better quality of vision in low light. The correct centration and registration with respect to cyclotorsion resulted in less-induced asymmetric coma-type HOAs. Especially since generally no significant reduction of the amount of preoperative HOAs has been registered with CA on virgin eyes, the question remains how much, if at all, the correction of the HOAs in virgin eyes contributes to the superior outcomes with AstraPro, or any type of current CA, including the wavefront aberrometry based CA. The author is concerned that an attempt to correct HOAs in virgin eyes might actually introduce an unnecessary risk of induction of iatrogenic HOAs due to the artifacts produced by limited precision and accuracy of current diagnostic devices.

If we define the aim for treatment of virgin eyes as elimination of a need for spectacles and/or contact lenses, as well as preservation of the preoperative quality of vision, then correction of low-order aberrations without induction of new HOAs should be our goal. That implies that neither the first surface HOAs nor wavefront aberrometry data are required to achieve our goals. Asphericity optimized ablation (that ideally compensates for corneal biomechanical response), based on precise measurements of preoperative sphere and cylinder and perfectly centered on the corneal optical center with a perfectly registered astigmatism axis, should not lead to induction of iatrogenic HOAs.

ORBSCAN AND *CIPTA* IN CUSTOM ABLATION FOR IRREGULAR ASTIGMATISM

The LaserSight platform currently provides its mainstream users with its own AstraMax/AstraPro CA technology, while the systems sold in Italy and the selected few systems in the rest of the world, were modified to enable the use of CIPTA CA software. CIPTA uses Orbscan-generated information for compiling its CA.

An issue in CA treatment of IA that has not been discussed much is evaluation of different ablation-planning strategies, something that the CIPTA system provides. It seems that the CA plans based on data confined to the eye's visual optics (commonly used in CA treatments of virgin eyes) and the plans based on the eye's geometrical optics can be very different for eyes with IA. The principal elements of the optical system of the eye (cornea, pupil, and the crystalline lens) are not centered with respect to each other. Additionally, the eye's neural axes (visual axis and the line of sight) and optical axis do not coincide because of the eccentric placement of the fovea. Consequently, the target object can be placed on the fovea

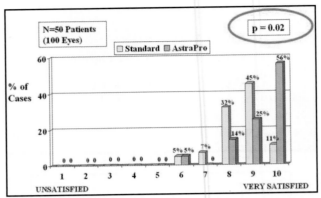

Figure 14-8. Subjective quality of vision score, Astra vs. standard treatments 6 months after surgery.

only by rotation of the eye. Hence the corneal optics can be considered and analyzed from both geometrical (morphological) and neural (visual) aspects.

Ablation planning in excimer laser corneal refractive surgery has traditionally been based on measurements that in one way or another reflect the eye's visual function. Wavefront aberrometry, autorefractometry, Placido-based corneal topography, and even manifest refraction are all dependent on patient fixation during the examination. Consequently, the data or maps acquired under such circumstances are referenced to the rotational position of the fixating eye. The concept of using the measurements that reflect the eye's visual function seems logical in refractive surgical ablation planning, since the goal of the refractive surgery is improvement of the existing visual function. Such a concept has also proved to be very successful in standard and customized excimer laser treatments of virgin eyes. Unfortunately, the same reasoning cannot be applied to treatment of cases with visual disturbances secondary to induced asymmetric corneal irregularities after refractive surgery, other eye surgery, corneal injuries, etc. Decentered corneal optics radically change the eye's visual optics, forcing the visual axis "to move" from its original (physiologic) position to a new one. The eye then adapts to the changed optical circumstances by assuming a new rotational position in an attempt to place the targeted image on the fovea. Hence an ablation plan that uses topography or aberrometry information referenced to the visual axis (or line of sight) would attempt to optimize the corneal optics on the basis of a pathological rotational position.

The author investigated the influence of centration and orientation of the ablation profile using simulated outcomes of customized treatments. Cases of irregular astigmatism due to decentered ablations were treated with respect to the amount of tissue removal and the smoothness of transition zone. The ablations based on the corneal

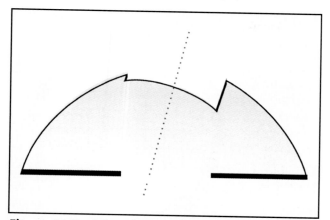

Figure 14-9. Schematic presentation of visual axis strategy.

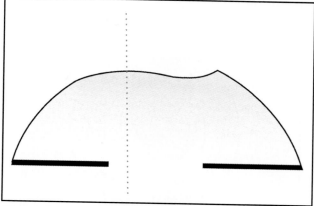

Figure 14-10. Schematic presentation of morphological axis strategy.

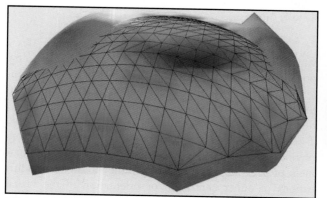

Figure 14-11. Three-dimensional map of a decentered LASIK case.

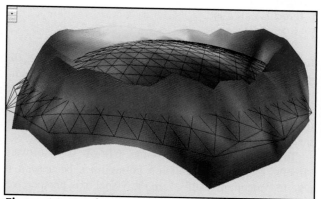

Figure 14-12. Three-dimensional map of a simulated outcome with visual axis strategy.

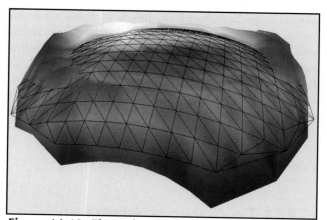

Figure 14-13. Three-dimensional map of a simulated outcome with morphological axis strategy.

morphological axis resulted in significantly shallower ablations, and smoother transitions compared to the ablations based on visual axis.[14] Figures 14-9 and 14-10 show schematics of the two customized ablation strategies. The same targeted surface was fitted perpendicularly to the visual axis, which is defined as a line drawn between the topography camera and the patient's macula (Figure 14-9), and to the CIPTA proprietary corneal "morphological" axis that approximates the best match between the axis of symmetry of the ideal shape and that of the current shape of the cornea (Figure 14-10). The visual axis strategy uses local corneal morphology around the visual axis as a foundation for computation of its ablation, without considering the cornea beyond the ablation area, while the corneal morphological axis strategy is based on a global three-dimensional assessment. It uses the morphology of the entire corneal surface as a foundation for its ablation in attempt to restore the damaged symmetry of the cornea. Figure 14-11 shows preoperative topography for the simulation, while Figures 14-12 and 14-13 show postoperative simulations based on visual and corneal morphological axes for a case of irregular astigmatism after a decentered LASIK. These figures show that the treatment simulations based on the visual axis attempt to optimize the primary decentered treatment area: increasing the corneal asymmetry even

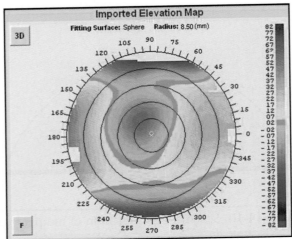

Figure 14-14. Floating elevation map of a decentered LASIK case.

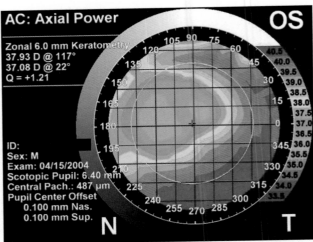

Figure 14-15. Axial curvature map of a decentered LASIK case.

further and creating an abrupt transition toward the untreated area (Figure 14-12), while the treatment simulations based on the corneal morphological axis attempt to "recenter" the primary treatment by placing the ablation on the previously untreated area which should have been treated during the primary surgery (Figure 14-13).

To our knowledge, only the CIPTA CA software "freely" explores the ablation possibilities because it is able to "uncouple itself" from the visual axis perspective. It can globally evaluate the raw elevation data and consider the corneal shape from a purely morphological aspect. This opens a possibility for a free, three-dimensional fitting of the desired targeted surface, providing infinitely more ablation alternatives than the systems referenced to the visual axis. The AstraPro customized ablation system bases its ablation planning on the corneal elevation data referenced to the visual axis and places its targeted surface perpendicular to that axis. Such an approach results in deep ablations in cases with irregular astigmatism.

AstraPro provides a solution to that problem by employing so called "advanced" ablation planning alternatives. The software automatically adjusts the ablation center (but keeps the ablation axis orientation unchanged) until the targeted surface is fitted to a position that requires the least amount of tissue removal. The T-cat customized ablation system (WaveLight Laser Technologies, Erlangen, Germany) uses Placido disk-based topography information. Curvature data referenced to the visual axis is converted to elevation data and decomposed into orthogonal Zernike polynomials. Since this approach, like AstraPro and the visual axis strategy of CIPTA, results in deep ablations in treatments of irregular astigmatism, T-cat provides an ablation planning alternative where the tilt component can be removed from the ablation plan. This

way the orientation of the fitting axis is changed to a new position that results in reduced tissue removal, but the centering of the ablation axis is kept intact (ie, still attached to the intercept of the "pathological" visual axis).

In their default constellation, both the AstraPro and T-cat systems base their ablation on the visual axis. They obviously recognize the problem of that approach in treatment of irregular astigmatism, and they allow for modifications of either centration or orientation of the visual axis. Unlike CIPTA, neither of the two systems leaves the visual axis completely.

Ablation simulations on the three aforementioned systems were performed for an eye with a decentered ablation causing irregular astigmatism. Targets included a 6.5-mm optical zone, 7.5-mm total ablation diameter, a curvature corresponding to the curvature of the flattest preoperative meridian, and asphericity with a Q-index value of –0.30. The preoperative floating elevation is shown in Figure 14-14. The axial curvature map is shown in Figure 14-15. Two ablation maps (one using the visual axis, the other using the system specific solution for treatment of IA) were generated for each of the three systems and are shown on Figures 14-16 through 14-21.

CIPTA TREATMENT OF IRREGULAR ASTIGMATISM

An ongoing prospective study for the evaluation of customized treatments for irregular astigmatism causing visual disturbances after previous LASIK or PRK is being performed by the author using the CIPTA morphological axis strategy. The study has been conducted at the eye department

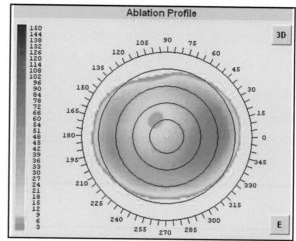

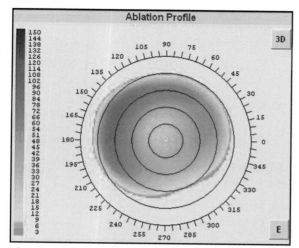

Figure 14-16. CIPTA ablation map using visual axis strategy.

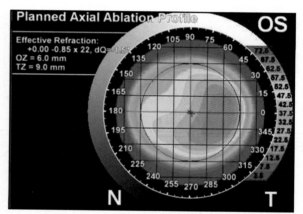

Figure 14-17. CIPTA ablation map using morphological axis strategy.

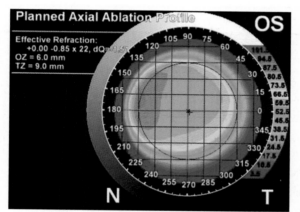

Figure 14-18. AstraPro ablation map using standard (visual axis) mode.

Figure 14-19. AstraPro ablation map using "advanced mode."

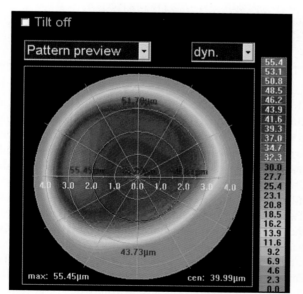

Figure 14-20. T-cat ablation map using "tilt on" mode.

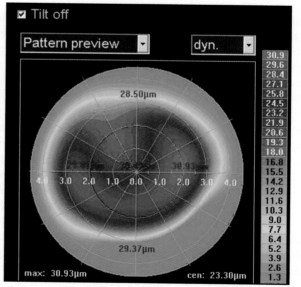

Figure 14-21. T-cat ablation map using "tilt off" mode.

TABLE 14-2			
PREOPERATIVE REFRACTION AND VISUAL ACUITY OF CIPTA TREATMENTS			
Mean MRSE (D)	**Mean cyl. (D)**	**Mean BSCVA**	**Mean UCVA**
−0.95 ± 1.65	1.37 ± 1.46	20/25	20/60
(−2.88 to +2.25)	(0.25 to 6.50)	(20/60 to 20/20)	(20/400 to 20/25)

TABLE 14-3			
PREOPERATIVE VISUAL DISTURBANCES RELATED TO TOPOGRAPHIC FEATURES			
Visual disturbancy	Topographic feature		
	Decentered ($n = 12$)	Insuff. abl. diameter ($n = 4$)	Irregular surface ($n = 4$)
Multiple images/ contours ($n = 13$)	12	0	1
Night driving problems ($n = 17$)	10	4	3
Decreased BSCVA ($n = 11$)	8	1	2

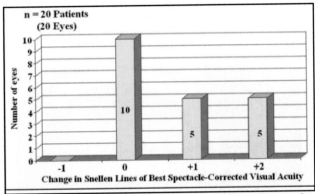

Figure 14-22. Safety of CIPTA treatments of irregular astigmatism 6 months after surgery.

TABLE 14-4					
POSTOPERATIVE VISUAL DISTURBANCES					
Preoperative visual disturbancy		Postoperative 6 months			
	n	Worse	Unchanged	Improved	Cured
Multiple images	13	0	0	6	7
Night driving problems	17	0	0	8	9
Decreased BSCVA	11	0	1**	5	5*

*If postoperative BSCVA ≥ primary preoperative BSCVA, than the "decreased BSCVA" was considered cured.

** BSCVA < 20/25 before surgery

of the University of Tromsoe in Norway since March 2002. The primary aim of the treatment was to alleviate the patient's visual disturbances, such as multiple images, halos, glare, and night vision problems, and improvement of visual acuity using spectacles or soft contact lenses. The secondary aim was correction of any existing spherocylindrical refractive error. These goals were addressed by regularizing the corneal surface, optimizing the corneal asphericity, and changing the corneal base curve in order to eliminate the spherocylindrical error. Regularizing the corneal surface would address the first surface HOAs responsible for multiplopia, halos, and similar visual disturbances. Optimizing the corneal asphericity would address the spherical aberration of the whole eye responsible for low-light visual disturbances and low contrast sensitivity. Aiming for a certain corneal curvature would address the correction of the manifest sphere and cylinder.

Forty eyes of 40 patients with visual disturbances and corneal irregularities after previous LASIK or PRK were enrolled. Twenty patients to date were available for evaluation 6 months after surgery. Preoperative spherical equivalent was relatively low, while the cylinder ranged up to 6.5 D and the mean BSCVA was reduced to 20/25 (Table 14-2).

If one correlates the topographic changes to the visual complaints, patients with decentered ablations mainly complained of multiplopia and most of them had night driving problems with reduced BSCVA. The patients with insufficient ablation diameter mainly complained of night driving problems (Table 14-3). At 6 months after surgery, no eyes lost lines of BSCVA while 50% gained lines. Twenty-five percent gained 2 lines or more. Safety index, the ratio between postoperative and preoperative BSCVA, was 1.21. This is shown in Figure 14-22. The measure of efficacy of the treatment for this group of patients is the amount of visual disturbances after the surgery. Table 14-4 shows that the preoperative visual disturbances were either reduced or eliminated at 6 months after surgery.

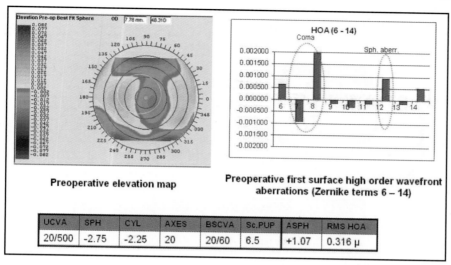

Figure 14-23. Floating elevation topography, HOAs, and clinical data in a decentered LASIK case.

Preoperative elevation map

Preoperative first surface high order wavefront aberrations (Zernike terms 6 – 14)

UCVA	SPH	CYL	AXES	BSCVA	Sc.PUP	ASPH	RMS HOA
20/500	-2.75	-2.25	20	20/60	6.5	+1.07	0.316 μ

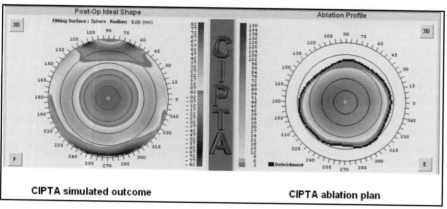

Figure 14-24. Ablation map and simulated topographic outcome.

CIPTA simulated outcome

CIPTA ablation plan

CASE STUDIES

A 40-year-old female with a preoperative refractive error of –11.00 D, BSCVA 20/30, and 6.5-mm scotopic pupils, was treated using LASIK OD in 1996. After surgery, BSCVA fell to 20/60 and the patient was disturbed by multiplopia, halos, glare, and night driving problems. Corneal topography showed a nasally and inferiorly decentered and very narrow ablation. The asphericity was oblate with a Q-value of +1.07. First surface Zernike analysis showed a significantly increased coma (8th and 7th terms) and, as expected, an increased positive spherical aberration. This is shown in Figure 14-23. The patient's elevation data as well as the patient's refractive data were input into the CIPTA ablation planning software. Transepithelial PRK was performed on top of the flap due to the limited amount of stromal tissue available for the ablation. Mitomycin C was used prophylactically. Figure 14-24 shows the ablation map and the simulated outcome.

Six months after surgery, most of the visual disturbances improved, with a significant improvement in visual acuity and minimal residual refractive error. Postoperative topography showed a well-centered and widened ablation. Asphericity went from oblate to prolate. First surface Zernike analysis showed a significant decrease of terms from 6 to 14, and especially the coma. A significant decrease in spherical aberration occurred as well. This can be seen in Figure 14-25.

The CIPTA approach showed a high level of safety and efficacy. Most importantly, the preoperative visual disturbances were decreased or eliminated. Topographies were vastly improved and the first surface HOAs were significantly reduced. The author has used CIPTA software for treatment of other types of corneal irregularities as well. It seems that with use of its "morphological axis" strategy, the challenging cases (like those with high-grade irregular astigmatism after cornea transplantation and significant irregularities due to corneal scarring after injuries or keratitis) are no longer beyond the reach of laser refractive surgery.

Figure 14-25. Floating elevation topography, HOAs, and clinical data after CIPTA retreatment of a decentered LASIK case.

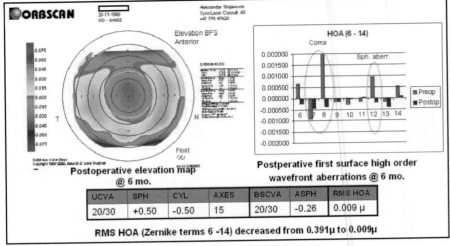

Postoperative elevation map @ 6 mo.

Postperative first surface high order wavefront aberrations @ 6 mo.

UCVA	SPH	CYL	AXES	BSCVA	ASPH	RMS HOA
20/30	+0.50	-0.50	15	20/30	-0.26	0.009 μ

RMS HOA (Zernike terms 6 -14) decreased from 0.391μ to 0.009μ

GENERAL CONCLUSIONS

A topography-based CA that uses corneal surface information independent of the visual axis seems to be the best treatment modality for IA, while an ideal treatment of virgin eyes might be achieved by correction of low-order aberrations (sphere and cylinder) and by the optimization of corneal asphericity and perfect ablation registration. A CA plan that includes correction of higher-order aberrations in virgin eyes (with no preoperative visual disturbances) might be counterproductive because of the possibility of introduction of new, iatrogenic aberrations using currently available preoperative diagnostics. Between the CIPTA system (admittedly used only within a limited number of clinics) for treatment of IA and the AstraPro for treatment of virgin eyes (especially with a newly added option of removal of correction of the first surface HOAs from the ablation plan—while keeping the asphericity and registration customization information from the AstraMax), the LaserSight platform can at this moment provide a more complete CA solution than most of the competing systems.

REFERENCES

1. Seitz B, Langenbucher A, Kus MM, Harrer M. Experimental correction of irregular corneal astigmatism using topography-based flying-spot-mode excimer laser photoablation. *Am J Ophthalmol.* 1998;125(2):252–256.

2. Weisinger-Jendritza B, Knorz MC, Hugger P, Liermann A. Laser in situ keratomileusis assisted by corneal topography. *J Cataract Refract Surg.* 1998;24:166–174.

3. Dausch D, Schroder E, Dausch S. Topography-controlled excimer laser photorefractive keratectomy. *J Refract Surg.* 2000;16:13–22.

4. Alessio G, Boscia F, La Tegola MG, Sborgia C. Topography-driven photorefractive keratectomy. *Ophthalmology.* 2000;107:1578–1587.

5. Alio JL, Belda JI, Osman AA, Shalaby AMM. Topography-guided laser in situ keratomileusis (TOPOLINK) to correct irregular astigmatism after previous refractive surgery. *J Refract Surg.* 2003;19:516–527.

6. Hjortdal JO, Ehlers N. Treatment of post-keratoplasty astigmatism by topography supported customized laser ablation. *Acta Ophtalmologica Scandinavica.* 2001;79:376–380.

7. Lawless MA, Hodge C, Rogers CM, Sutton GL. Laser in situ keratomileusis with Alcon CustomCornea. *J Refract Surg.* 2003;19:691–696.

8. Cosar CB, Saltuk G, Sener AB. Wavefront-guided laser in situ keratomileusis with the Bausch & Lomb Zyoptix system. *J Refract Surg.* 2004;20:35–39.

9. Vongthongsri A, Phusitphoykai N, Naripthapan P. Comparison of wavefront-guided customized ablation vs. conventional ablation in laser in situ keratomileusis. *J Refract Surg.* 2002;18(3 Suppl):332–335.

10. Dausch D, Dausch S, Schroder E. Wavefront-supported photorefractive keratectomy: 12-month follow-up. *J Refract Surg.* 2003;19:405–411.

11. Alessio G, Boscia F, La Tegola MG, Sborgia C. Topography-driven excimer laser for the retreatment of decentralized myopic photorefractive keratectomy. *Ophthalmology.* 2001;108:1695–1703.

12. Alessio G, Boscia F, La Tegola MG, Sborgia C. Corneal interactive programmed topographic ablation customized keratectomy for correction of postkeratoplasty astigmatism. *Ophthalmology.* 2001;108:2029–2037.

13. Roberts C. The cornea is not a piece of plastic. *J Refract Surg.* 2000;16:407–413.

14. Stojanovic A, Suput D. Strategic planning in topography-guided ablation of irregular astigmatism after laser refractive surgery. *J Refract Surg.* 2005;21(4):369–376.

Chapter 15

Topography-Guided Corneal Refractive Treatment: The VISX Model

Rejean Munger, PhD and Bruce Jackson, MD

The advent of wavefront-guided refractive surgery has raised the bar for outcome expectations from vision researchers, clinicians, and most importantly, patients. Now patients with significant clinical symptoms resulting from optical problems, even when best spectacle corrected, come to the clinic seeking relief through refractive surgery. For many reasons, some patients cannot be treated reliably through wavefront-guided refractive surgery. For these patients, we believe that corneal-topography-driven treatments or treatments based on the integration of both ocular wavefront and corneal topography measurements can be a treatment solution.

Furthermore, evidence shows that even in normal eyes, there could be some optical benefits to integrating corneal shape to optimize the treatment of optical aberrations using refractive surgery.[1] Figure 15-1 shows that reshaping the cornea is not equivalent to treating with an optical correction. Shaded symbols represent results following a wavefront-guided surgery; nonshaded symbols represent a theoretically perfect optical correction. Different eye models use different techniques to change the ocular aberrations, CR (corneal radius of curvature), CQ (corneal asphericity), EL (eye length), LT (lens tilt), and LD (lens displacement). Correction efficacy depends on the anatomy of the eye model, but consistently, the optical correction of the eye model is much closer (better than 98%) to a perfect correction than corneal reshaping using wavefront guided excimer refractive surgery. Results for four clinically significant aberrations critical to quality of vision are shown here: spherical and astigmatic defocus as well as coma and spherical aberrations.

This chapter details an approach that uses a new software tool, the Advanced Custom Ablation Planner (ACAP) (VISX, Inc., Santa Clara, Calif.), to provide refractive surgery treatment solutions that can take advantage of corneal surface shape information to produce improved outcomes.

USING CORNEAL TOPOGRAPHY AS REFRACTIVE SURGERY INPUT DATA

Although the optical properties of the cornea are critical to the optical performance of the eye, they are not the only important factor. The crystalline lens is also a critical component. The other media in the eye (aqueous and vitreous) can have an impact on optical performance as well. Because of these factors, it is not a simple matter to look at the optical properties of the cornea and infer the impact on the patient. Furthermore, the optical properties of the eye as a visual system do not depend only on the optical properties of the cornea and crystalline lens individually, but on their optical interaction as well.

For example, changing the spherical aberration (SA) of the cornea does not result in an equivalent change in SA for the whole eye. The amount of change is dependent on the optical properties of the crystalline lens, as shown in Figure 15-2. The preoperative cornea (Figure 15-2A) and postoperative cornea (Figure 15-2B) have different refractive properties. This means that rays entering the two corneas at the same height (h) will take different pathways through the crystalline lens (different point of entry, p and p'). The lens aberrations encountered by the postoperative cornea are not the same as those of the preoperative cornea, and thus, the postoperative eye is not aberration free.

Corneal topographers and equivalent technologies measure the shape of the anterior surface of the cornea, not its optical properties. At this time, no technology is

Figure 15-1. Reshaping the cornea is not equivalent to treating it with an optical correction. The shaded symbols represent results following a wavefront-guided surgery; non-shaded symbols represent a theoretically perfect optical correction.

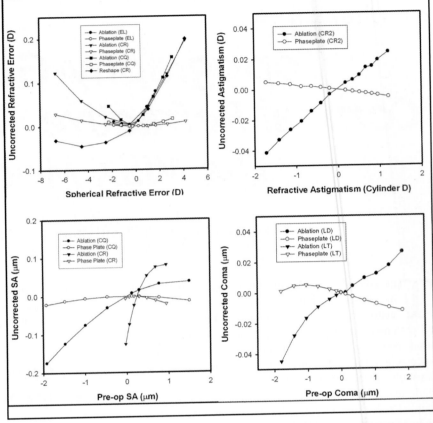

available that can reliably provide shape or optical information for the posterior corneal surface. These additional issues make the task of clinical inference and refractive treatment planning from corneal topography that much more difficult.

The goal of any corneal-shape-driven refractive treatment is to convert shape information into more clinically relevant data that result in better treatments and outcomes.

In the absence of ocular wavefront measurements, the refractive treatment planning software must provide tools that allow clinicians to understand the impact of corneal shape on corneal optical properties. In the presence of ocular wavefront measurements, the software should integrate both corneal and ocular data in order to better anticipate outcomes of any selected treatment.

The ACAP is designed to integrate seamlessly with VISX technology for wavefront-guided treatments. This includes the WaveScan (VISX, Inc.) ocular wavefront sensor, the variable spot scan (VSS), and WaveStar (VISX, Inc.) technology. The ACAP uses the information obtained through this technology to convert requested treatments into a treatment table for the laser.

The ACAP runs as a stand-alone software and can be installed on any computer to allow for treatment planning away from the clinic. Ocular wavefront data can be read directly from the WaveScan database or as a file exported

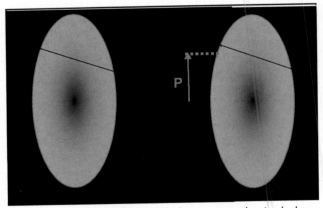

Figure 15-2. The amount of change in spherical aberration with custom ablation is dependent on the optical properties of the crystalline lens.

by WaveScan software. Corneal surface data must currently be obtained from the Zeiss-Meditec corneal topography system (Humphrey Zeiss, Dublin, Calif.), but no technical limitations exist in the ACAP that exclude the use of other devices in the future.

After importing the required input data from the WaveScan and/or the corneal topographer, the ACAP provides the operator with the opportunity to define multiple

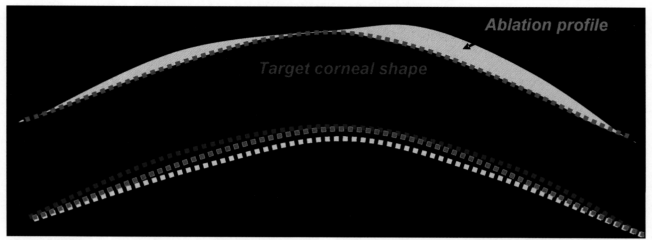

Figure 15-3. Treatment is calculated as the difference between the preoperative corneal shape and the desired corneal shape, which defines the amount of material to be removed at each location across the cornea. Different shapes can be used to obtain the desired refractive effect.

treatment plan possibilities, called exam sets. Exam sets are independent of each other so that treatment planning can be based on different combinations of ocular and/or corneal data. A set of visualization tools is then available to the operator to allow for better assessment of the potential outcomes of each treatment plan. Some visualization tools will be discussed in the following sections, showing how these tools provide a better understanding of the ACAP's approach to topography-driven treatments. The ACAP can then quickly generate a treatment table that is compatible with the VISX laser for any of the exam sets.

If no ocular wavefront data is available, the ACAP treatment options and visualization tools are limited to the properties of the cornea. This approach is discussed in detail in section 2. If both ocular and corneal topography are available, the ACAP integrates the two data sets into a predictive model that simulates potential ocular outcomes. This approach is discussed in detail in section 3.

For many reasons, there are patients for whom no ocular wavefront is available. For these patients, the only information available to plan a refractive surgery is the corneal topography. The ACAP is designed to provide the clinician with a range of visualization tools that quantify the optical properties of the cornea. These can then guide the clinician toward the best treatment plan.

One approach when using corneal topography to plan treatment is first to define the desired shape of the cornea following surgery. This is called the target surface. The planned treatment is then calculated as the difference between the preoperative corneal shape and the desired corneal shape, which defines the amount of material to be removed at each location across the cornea. This plan is illustrated in Figure 15-3. The treatment (ablation profile) is defined as the height difference between the actual ante-

rior cornea surface and the target corneal surface (shape of the postoperative cornea) selected by the surgeon. The issue is how to select a corneal shape for the cornea following surgery. The same change in power can be obtained using different corneal shapes that have different levels of asphericity. In order to correct most ocular aberrations, the preferred shape would have opposite spherical aberration to the rest of the eye. The difficulty with this approach is selecting an appropriate corneal target surface. Each human eye is a unique optical system, and a good corneal surface for one patient can lead to an unacceptable increase in ocular aberrations in another.

Another approach is to define the desired optical properties of the cornea following the surgery. This is called the optical target. Because the cornea is an optical element, it is easier to relate an optical target to visual performance than to a surface target. Furthermore, ACAP software is designed to fully integrate the wavefront-guided refractive surgery technology from VISX. The algorithms that are used to control the VISX excimer laser require wavefront error maps (as generated by the WaveScan) as input to calculate the ablation profile and generate a treatment table for the laser. ACAP depends on the optical target approach to treatment planning.

In ACAP, the optical properties of the preoperative cornea are obtained by tracing light rays through the corneal surface and calculating the wavefront error map using the optical path difference in the entrance pupil of the eye. Figure 15-4 shows how rays are refracted through the cornea to the plane of best focus, producing the smallest optical blur. The optical path length of each is calculated to the plane of best focus, and the deviation from the perfect imaging system (equal path length for each ray) is calculated with respect to the pupil plane. The result is the

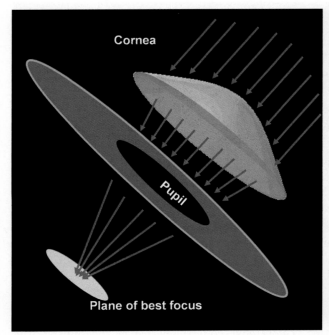

Figure 15-4. Rays are refracted through the cornea to the plane of best focus, producing the smallest optical blur.

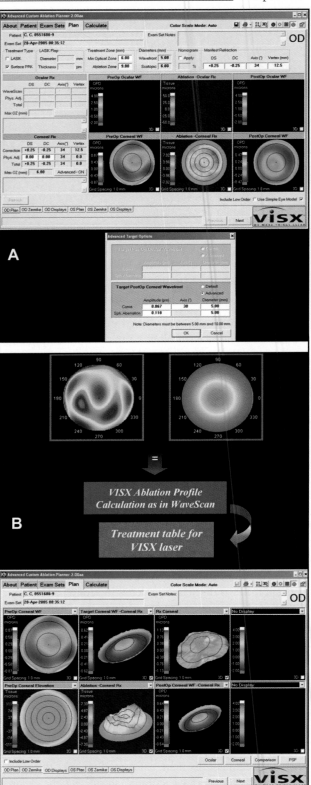

Figure 15-5. (A) The operator defines an optical target for the postoperative cornea. (B) The treatment is calculated as the difference between the target wavefront and the preoperative corneal wavefront.

wavefront error map in the pupil plane of the eye, which can then be used by the VISX algorithm to produce a cornea surface correction based on the corneal topography.

The operator then defines an optical target for the postoperative cornea, as shown in Figure 15-5A. In ACAP, the optical target is defined using a treatment window. This window shows the ocular wavefront data in the top row if it is available (unavailable in this case) and the corneal data in the lower row, if available. For cornea-based treatments, the operator can program the low-order terms (refractive correction) of the optical target through the manifest refraction. The high-order terms (coma and spherical aberration) of the optical target can be specified through the advanced button in the same row as the corneal data. The software provides the operator with three views of each data set. In the lower row (corneal data), the left graphic window is the data set as imported from an elevation map for the cornea. The middle graphic window is the wavefront error map for that cornea, and the right graphic window shows the corneal map after alignment of the ocular and corneal data (if both are displayed) to validate the treatment plan. More visualization tools for the validation of the treatment are available through the OS/OD Zernike and OS/OD Displays tabs. The low-order aberrations are selected through the choice of the manifest refraction for the treatment, which can be set to any value that is within the limits set by VISX in WaveScan.

By default, the high-order aberrations of the optical target are set so that the spherical-like aberrations of the preoperative cornea (Zernike coefficients 4,0 and 6,0) are retained after the surgery while all other high order aberrations are eliminated or set to zero. This is done in order to maintain the natural balance of spherical aberration between the cornea and the crystalline lens. If there is evidence that the spherical aberration of the postoperative cornea needs to be changed, the operator can do this by altering the default value. The only other high-order aberration of the optical target that can be modified from its default target value is coma (default value is zero). If the default values for coma and spherical aberrations are changed, the operator must provide a value (based on a Zernike expansion) and a pupil size for both aberrations. This is critical because the Zernike coefficients depend on the pupil size; both parameters are required to uniquely define the optical aberrations of the target.

Finally, the treatment is calculated as the difference between the target wavefront and the preoperative corneal wavefront, as depicted in Figure 15-5B. The treatment ACAP is calculated as the difference between the corneal wavefront map and the target wavefront map, which is used to generate a wavefront correction map. This map information is then implemented into the VISX software for wavefront guided corrections, and a treatment table is produced that can be used by the excimer laser to ablate the cornea. Figure 15-5B depicts some of the displays available through the ACAP OD/OS Display window to assess the treatment plan. In the top row from left to right are the preoperative corneal wavefront, the optical target, and the wavefront correction to be achieved. In the bottom row are the corneal preoperative elevation map, the treatment to be performed (actual tissue to be removed), and the predicted wavefront map of the cornea following treatment.

CLINICAL EXAMPLES

Before the development of ACAP, VISX had made available the Custom Ablation Planner (CAP). This software tool allowed an operator to construct complex ablation patterns by grouping together a number of standard treatments such as ellipses and cylindrical corrections. A comparison of treatment plans created using the VISX CAP tool and ACAP for two symptomatic patients is shown in Figure 15-6. Patients were treated based on the CAP plan and significant improvements (better than two lines of BSCVA) were obtained although both patients were less than 20/40 BSCVA after the treatment. The achieved treatment (change in corneal topography) resulting from the CAP treatment plan is also shown for comparison. Clearly, the ACAP treatment is more comprehen-

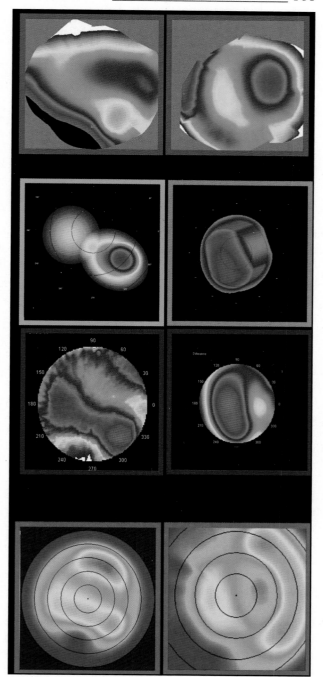

Figure 15-6. Comparison of treatments designed using custom software based on CAP and ACAP for the same eye.

sive because it treats the whole cornea as opposed to only the highly abnormal areas targeted by the CAP treatment. Furthermore, the ACAP treatment is generated automatically, whereas the CAP treatment requires that the operator deduce the shape, location, and amplitude of each of the small ablations—information needed to obtain the required treatment profile.

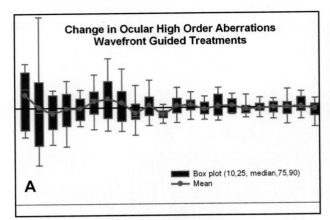

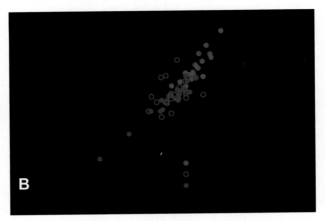

Figure 15-7. Results from the first 23 subjects treated at the University of Ottawa Eye Institute. All patients were at least 6 months postoperative, and none had optical symptoms, other than refractive error, before surgery. (A) Clinical results using wavefront-guided surgery have shown a clear improvement over standard refractive surgery, but clearly, we are not effective at correcting high-order aberrations. (B) Comparison of the main high-order aberrations, spherical aberration and coma, before surgery (shown on the horizontal axis) and after surgery (shown on the vertical axis).

The treatment has to be designed by the operator one ablation at a time until the target surface or a close approximation is obtained. This limits the treatments to localized areas on the cornea and the use of spherical or elliptical ablation profiles, leaving many high-order aberrations uncorrected. Figure 15-6 shows treatments designed by us using custom software based on the CAP (and treated using this solution) as well as the treatment designed by ACAP (optical target) for the same patients. In each case, the correction suggested by ACAP (optical target, VSS technology) matches the corneal irregularity much better than what was achievable with CAP. Furthermore, the ACAP solution considers the optics of the whole cornea; CAP could not.

Clinical results on wavefront-guided surgery have shown a clear improvement over standard refractive surgery, but clearly, we are not very effective at correcting high-order aberrations[2] (Figure 15-7A). Furthermore, there is a strong correlation between the aberrations before and after the refractive surgery. Comparison of the main high-order aberrations, spherical aberration and coma, before (shown on the horizontal axis) and after (shown on the vertical axis) surgery, is illustrated in Figure 15-7B. Clearly, none of the patients obtained a significant reduction in his or her high-order aberrations. The line is a guide to the eye showing no change in aberration following surgery.

It is very likely that physiological mechanisms, such as healing, as well as mechanical forces, such as stress release in the collagen matrix following ablation of tissues, account for some of the reduced efficacy in correcting HOAs. However, the similarity between the preoperative and postoperative aberrations suggests that some optical issues: the treatment pattern is incorrect, the pattern is not the targeted value, etc. Treatment models have shown[3] that there are optical errors built into the basic assumption that laying the ocular wavefront error directly on the cornea, as is done in wavefront guided refractive surgery, will correct the optical aberrations perfectly. Furthermore, there could be some other optical errors built into the current wavefront-guided treatments that have yet to be fully explored.[4] To correctly address optical issues requires that both the corneal topography and the ocular wavefront measurements be considered simultaneously.

When dealing with optical errors, the ACAP builds a custom model that can predict refractive surgery outcomes for each patient. The designed treatment is then applied to the patient's custom model, and the predicted optical outcome is calculated. The main challenge in this approach is in building a custom model that will accurately represent the outcomes following the surgery.

BUILDING A PREDICTIVE MODEL

The best possible predictive model would be an exact replica of the patient's optics, including all the correct surface shapes, distances, and positions. This custom eye model would also include any misalignments and the gradient of refractive index (GRIN) of the crystalline lens. To date, such models cannot be constructed because the GRIN of the lens has not yet been measured, and tools providing the biometric information necessary to fully quantify the alignment and distances among the optical components are not available.

In the ACAP, the predictive model is constructed to maximize the value of the available data: the corneal topography and the ocular wavefront. Starting with the preoperative eye, the ocular aberrations can be defined as the sum of the aberrations from the anterior surface of the cornea, as measured in the entrance pupil, and the "internal aberrations," including the contribution of all other optical surfaces measured in the entrance pupil plane.[1] The ACAP integrates the corneal topography and ocular wavefront data, when both are available, by constructing a phase plate model of optical properties of the patient's eyes (Figure 15-8).

In most eyes, internal aberrations are dominated by the optical properties of the crystalline lens, though they also include the optical contributions of the posterior surface of the cornea. It is possible to define an optical element positioned in the entrance pupil plane with no physical thickness but containing all of the internal aberrations as a phase plate. This provides a simple method to build a model of any preoperative eye. The preoperative ocular aberrations are the sum of the corneal wavefront (in the entrance pupil) and the preoperative phase plate (PrePP).

The phase plate model is at the core of two different predictive models used by the ACAP to calculate optical outcomes following refractive surgery. The underlying methodologies used to develop these models and their use in the ACAP are discussed in the following two sections.

By definition, the PrePP includes all aberrations of an eye with the exception of the anterior corneal surface. A first order predictive model for the postoperative eye assumes that the internal aberrations are not affected by the refractive treatment, which is expected to reshape the anterior surface of the cornea and nothing else. Under this assumption, the postoperative phase plate (PosPP) is equal to the PrePP, and the postoperative aberrations are simply the sum of the wavefront of the postoperative cornea in the pupil plane of the eye and the aberrations of the PrePP.

This simple model correctly suggests that when following wavefront-guided refractive surgery, the postoperative ocular aberrations are not fully corrected. Comparing the postoperative aberrations predicted by modeling wavefront-guided surgeries in an optical design software (methodological details are available[1]) shows that optical outcomes based on the current wavefront-guided approach are not optimal because this approach cannot take into account the effect of the optical interaction between the corneal shape and the crystalline lens post-operatively. A more complex predictive model is required to improve the accuracy of the optical outcome predictions.

A better predictive approach can be constructed with a small modification of the simple model. Since the wavefront of the postoperative cornea is obtained from ray tracing through its surface, the wavefront is not likely to be the

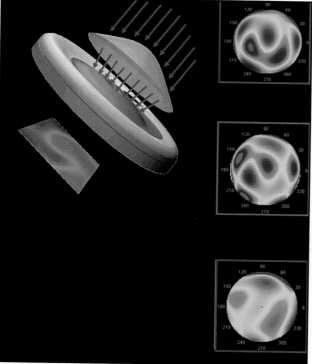

Figure 15-8. The ACAP integrates the corneal topography and ocular wavefront data, when both are available, by constructing a phase plate model of optical properties of the patient's eyes. The phase plate is defined as an optical component placed in the eye's entrance pupil such that the sum of its aberrations and those of the cornea in the pupil plane give the ocular wavefront of the eye.

source of error of the simple phase plate model. This suggests that the source of the error is the assumption that the internal aberrations of the preoperative eye are the same as those of the postoperative eye. The complex interaction between the corneal surface and the crystalline lens changes when the anterior surface of the cornea is reshaped, resulting in a different set of internal aberrations for the postoperative eye.[2] The phase-plate approach discussed previously can be maintained if it is possible to define a new PosPP not equal to the PrePP. The issue is to find a method of constructing the PosPP from the available clinical information.

To develop a method for constructing customized PosPP for human eyes, a large set of different eye models with aberrations similar to those seen in human eyes was constructed in a commercial optical design software package. Each eye model was treated according to the current wavefront-guided refractive surgery paradigm, and the postoperative ocular aberrations were measured. From

Figure 15-9. Software models enabled construction of PostPP (postoperative ocular—postoperative cornea wavefront) that correctly predicted the optical aberrations of the eye models following wavefront-guided refractive surgery. The four plots show the relationship between the aberrations of the predicted and modeled phase plates.

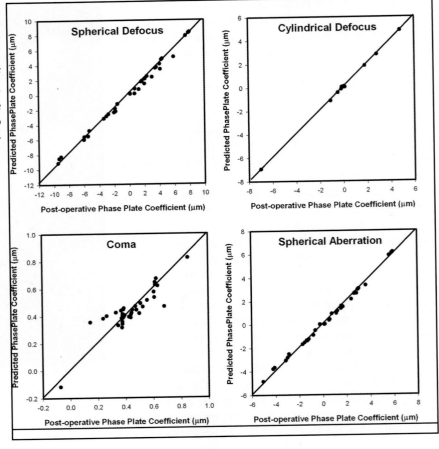

each eye model, a PrePP (preoperative ocular—postoperative cornea wavefront) and a PosPP (postoperative ocular—postoperative cornea wavefront) was obtained.

We then constructed a regression model that allowed us to construct the PosPP from the available clinical data. In this way, we were able to construct PosPP that correctly predicted the optical aberrations of the eye models following wavefront-guided refractive surgery (Figure 15-9). To predict postoperative optical outcomes, it is essential to create a PosPP using the clinically available data. To develop a method for creating this phase plate, eye models were created with a wide range of optical properties. Each model was treated in software using the wavefront-guided paradigm and the PosPP obtained. Once the method to generate the PosPP was developed, the predicted phase plate values were compared with the phase plate from the modeling. The four plots in Figure 15-9 show the relationship between the aberrations of the predicted and modeled phase plates.

The postoperative optical outcomes can now be calculated for any eye by adding the postoperative cornea wavefront and the new PosPP. From the outcome information obtained

for this model, the clinician can now compare the predicted outcomes for ocular wavefront- or cornea-driven treatments in order to make more informed clinical decisions.

CLINICAL EXAMPLES

Three patients with visual complaints (with best correction) following a primary refractive treatment were examined using the ACAP. A treatment based on the ocular wavefront and a treatment based on the corneal wavefront were calculated, and PreVue (VISX, Inc., Santa Clara, Calif.) lenses were generated for each treatment (Figure 15-10). Visual acuity was then measured (ETDRS) for each correction, and the patient was asked which correction provided the best subjective quality of vision.

For two of the patients, the treatments based on the ocular and corneal data were very similar (Figure 15-10A and 15-10B). For the third patient, the two treatments differed significantly (Figure 15-10C). For all patients, PreVue lenses generated from wavefront treatments and topography treatments both improved BCVA and visual symptoms. For

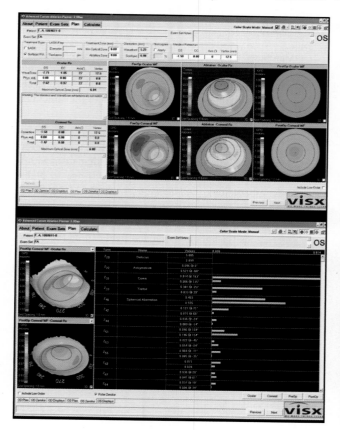

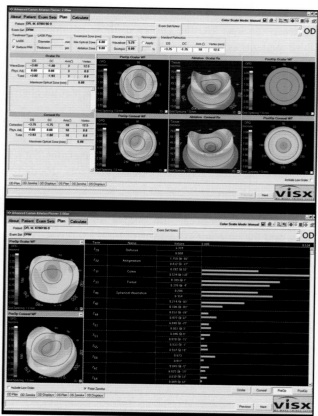

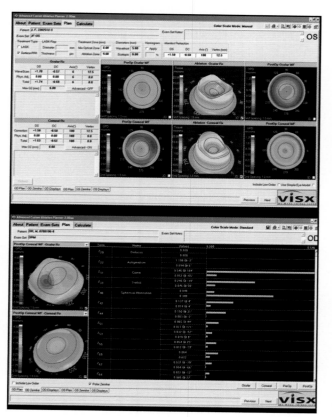

Figure 15-10. The top window is the ACAP treatment plan window used to produce both ocular-wavefront- and corneal-topography-based preview lenses for three patients with visual symptoms, (A) patient 1, (B) patient 2, and (C) patient 3. The bottom windows show the predicted corneal aberrations following both treatment types: ocular wavefront treatment in green and topography treatment in blue. Also included is the visual data of each patient obtained with and without each of the preview lenses. Notice that for patient 1, two testing conditions were used with the topography preview lens. This was due to a large discrepancy between the wavefront-based refraction and the manifest refraction in this patient. The addition of a +1.50 D spherical correction produced equivalent conditions for the two previews lens tests.

patients 1 and 2, wavefront-guided treatment was the preferred correction. For patient 3, the treatment based on the corneal data was preferred.

Also included in Figure 15-10 are the predicted aberrations of the postoperative cornea following surgery. In patients 1 and 2 who preferred the ocular treatment, the corneal treatment resulted in greater reduction in aberrations of the cornea than the ocular treatment. This indicates that there was significant compensation of aberrations between the lens and the cornea in these patients. In the third patient, who preferred the corneal correction, the opposite situation is true. The ocular wavefront treatment left the cornea with significant uncorrected aberrations that are not compensated for by the eye's internal aberrations.

The ACAP is a new refractive-surgery-planning tool that provides clinicians with the capability to fully integrate corneal topography and ocular wavefront data to optimize the treatment of optical problems. Predictive models, optical prediction technology to modify wavefront-guided treatments and account for the impact of optical interactions between the cornea and the crystalline lens, and the outcomes of wavefront-guided refractive surgery will improve in the near future.

REFERENCES

1. Marchese LE, Munger R, Priest D. Wavefront-guided correction of ocular aberrations: are phase plate and refractive surgery solutions equal? *J Opt Soc Am.* 2005;22(8):1471–1481. Available at: http://josaa.osa.org/abstract.cfm?id=84676.

2. Kohnen T, Bühren J, Kühne C, Mirshahi A. Wavefront-guided LASIK with the Zyoptix 3.1 system for the correction of myopia and compound myopic astigmatism with 1-year follow-up: clinical outcome and change in higher order aberrations. *Ophthalmology.* 2004;111(12):2175–2185.

3. Munger R, Marchese L, Priest D. Equivalency of optical aberrations for light entering and light exiting the human eye. *Invest Ophthalmol Vis Sci.* 2005;46(E-Abstract).

4. Artal P, Guirao A. Contributions of the cornea and the lens to the aberrations of the human eye. *Optics Letters.* 1998;23(21):1713–1715.

SECTION IV

SPECIFIC TOPOGRAPHIC SYSTEMS

Chapter 16

The Magellan Mapper

Michael Endl, MD; Claus Fichte, MD; and Jason Zornek

Over the past decade, the number of corneal refractive procedures has reached an all-time high. Increasingly, eye care providers have become aware of potential postoperative complications. One of the most feared outcomes following excimer laser procedures is the development of progressive corneal ectasia. If the physician is to fulfill his primary goal of "do no harm," prevention is key.

Unfortunately, preoperative screening for corneal ectasia presently has no standardized detection method. Clinicians currently rely on keratometric, slit lamp, and standard topographic "red flags" when evaluating the candidacy of a keratorefractive patient. Although these remain the gold standard, corneal topographers—like the new Magellan Mapper from Nidek (Fremont, Calif)—may provide refractive surgeons with a helpful tool to avoid unwanted complications.

The Magellan features new software that includes a neural network application capable of predicting various corneal diseases and postsurgical outcomes. Based on corneal statistics derived from topographic data, the software classifies and predicts the probability of several categories in an easy-to-read bar graph below the traditional axial map. This is the first application of an artificial intelligence system that utilizes a previously trained set of logic rules "learned" from sets of ectatic and normal patient topographies.[1]

Unlike previous keratoconus screening programs, the Magellan is able to differentiate between astigmatism, keratoconus suspects, true keratoconus, and pellucid marginal degeneration. In addition, the mapper's neural network is able to assign a percentage of probability, or grade, to these disease states. This will potentially allow users to better document and follow their patients for progression over time. Lastly, the software can also detect the proba-bility of previous myopic and hyperopic refractive surgeries, as well as penetrating keratoplasty.

Another feature of the Magellan software is the high resolution of the map displays, made possible through improvements in the dual-edge ring finding algorithms. As a cone-based Placido system, the mapper enjoys a smaller working distance, improving corneal coverage. The cone features a streamlined 30-ring projector. However, the system can locate both edges of each ring, which allows the Magellan's new algorithm to detect 60 rings of data. This provides an astounding 21,600 data points. As these are evenly distributed across the cornea, that translates to twice the resolution of traditional topographers.

Figure 16-1 illustrates a typical Magellan printout with the traditional axial map, a grouping of indices, and their values. In addition, an easy-to-interpret bar graph with classification categories is displayed that includes a percentage of that category's probability. Furthermore, the user can place the computer mouse over any of the abbreviated indices or classifications for a full explanation of the title and its significance.

CLINICAL APPLICATIONS

Any information that can help the refractive surgeon avoid the dreaded postoperative complication of progressive corneal thinning is beneficial. Keratoconus prevalence has been reported in the range of 50 per 100,000.[2] However, as these patients are often dissatisfied with their glasses or contact lenses, the incidence is significantly higher for the refractive surgeon.

There remains no substitute for a complete medical history and full slit lamp examination to best evaluate a preoperative patient's potential risk for ectasia following excimer

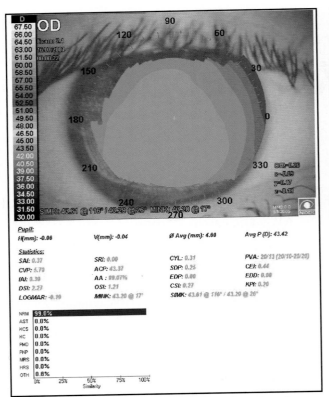

Figure 16-1. This topographical map has the characteristics of a normal cornea (99.0%).

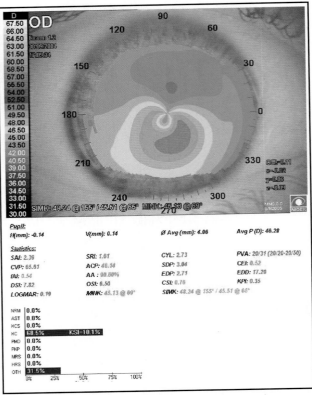

Figure 16-2. This topographical map has the characteristics associated with clinical keratoconus (68.5%) with a severity index of 10.7%. This map also contains features characterized as unclassified variations (31.5%).

laser surgery. Although pachymetry and preoperative keratometry readings are an essential part of every refractive surgery evaluation, corneal topography has become the "standard of care" when it comes to identifying irregular corneal astigmatism and disease states.

Despite advances in instrumentation and graphics, most modern kerato-mapping systems lack the ability or programming to help identify early progressive disorders such as keratoconus or pellucid marginal degeneration. Most practitioners are comfortable recognizing advanced thinning and irregular or asymmetric maps. However, detecting early changes or possible forme fruste keratoconus remains a clinical dilemma.

The advanced resolution and user friendly bar graphs of the Magellan mapper provide a much needed screening tool for the identification of abnormal corneal shape preoperatively. Utilizing this statistical information may help prevent undesirable postoperative outcomes by recommending against surgery for patients with evidence of progressive ectatic disease. Figure 16-2 shows a Magellan printout of a patient having properties consistent with keratoconus. Note also the indices listed in red are abnormal.

Alternatively, patients classified with mild characteristics that are consistent with keratoconus suspect or KCS on the bar graph may be treated best by surface ablation or photorefractive keratectomy. It should be noted that any removal of corneal tissue could theoretically accelerate the progression of early ectatic disease. Most experts agree that surface ablation poses a far lower risk than the creation of a 130- or 160-micron corneal flap plus ablation depth. Moreover, recent studies of up to 12 years[3] have demonstrated the long-term safety and refractive stability of PRK.

Figure 16-3 shows a preoperative map that registers properties associated with suspect keratoconus in a patient that later underwent uncomplicated surface ablation rather than LASIK. The same patient's preoperative Orbscan, shown in Figure 16-4, did not display any of the classic "red flags" associated with early ectasia. Such red flags include pachymetry readings with a thinnest point less than 470 microns or more than 100 micron difference from thinnest point to the 7 mm zone; posterior elevation greater than 40 microns (compared to best fit sphere); high irregularity indices at 3 mm and 5 mm zones; and (perhaps most important) the overall correlation of the highest/thinnest point

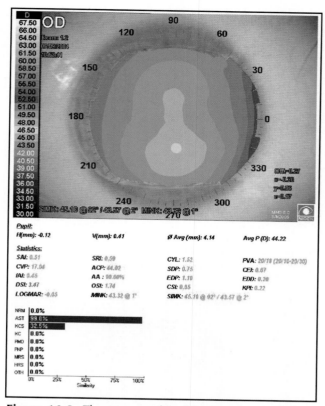

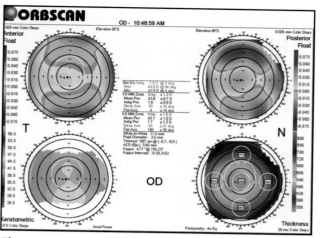

Figure 16-4. The preoperative Orbscan map of the same eye shown in Figure 16-3. Note there is no indication of ectasia.

Figure 16-3. The topographical image shows characteristics associated with a cornea with 1.52 D of cylinder (99.0%), and suspect keratoconus (32.5%).

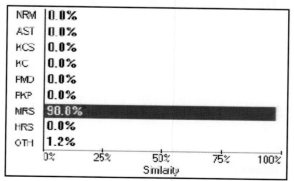

Figure 16-5. The indicated map has the characteristics associated with myopic refractive surgery (98.8%).

coinciding on the anterior, posterior, and pachymetry maps.[4]

Figure 16-5 shows the postoperative Magellan classification graph consistent with characteristics of myopic refractive surgery (MRS). This case may represent a patient that was spared the increased risk of postoperative

progressive irregular thinning brought on by the creation of a microkeratome cut.

It should be noted that the previously mentioned characteristics for Orbscan screening compliment the outlined Magellan statistical classification. This is illustrated in Figure 16-6 and 16-7. Both show cases where the Magellan topographical maps are consistent with mild KCS, while the Orbscan maps appear unassuming at first glance. Upon further review, the "hottest" region on the Orbscan posterior float (upper right of quad map) is greater than 40 microns from the best fitting sphere and the difference between the thinnest region and the 7-mm zone on corneal pachymetry is >100 microns. Again, these are two characteristics that are consistent with early keratoconus-like changes,[4] and this is a patient that perhaps should be followed prior to pursuing LASIK until further information is gathered.

As refractive technology continues to evolve, wavefront-based excimer ablations are emerging as the procedure of choice for optimum visual quality. In order for these types of customized treatments to work, a match must be made between the wavefront data and the pattern to be traced on the patient's cornea.

Since the preoperative wavefront information is the entire basis for the ablation profile, the capture of a patient's true corneal shape has become more important than ever. One cannot expect a perfect outcome if the data used to create the treatment plans is less than optimal. The Magellan mapper's statistical corneal analysis is designed to differentiate between classic ectasia signs and other abnormal shapes that may be more likely to appear with extended contact lens wear and corneal warpage.[1]

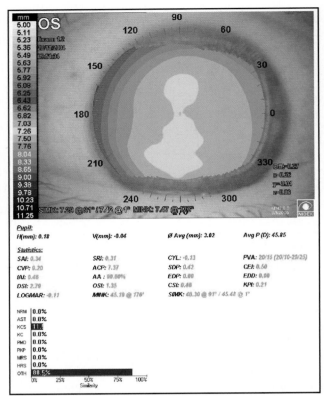

Figure 16-6. This map shows characteristics associated with unclassified variations (88.5% likelihood), and keratoconus suspect (11.5%).

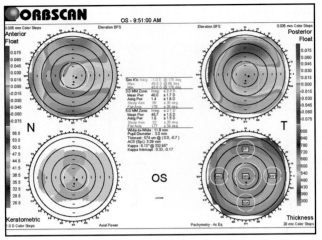

Figure 16-7. Orbscan map of the eye shown in Figure 16-6. Note the elevation on the posterior float.

Most refractive surgeons recommend discontinuation of soft lenses at least 2 weeks prior to wavefront measurement, and hard lenses or rigid gas permeable (RGP) lenses a minimum of 1 month before refractive evaluation. As contact lens warpage from RGP lens use has been noted to produce an irregular corneal shape for up to 6 months,[5] any axial maps that appear asymmetrical on preoperative evaluation should be followed and correlated with clinical history before considering surgery.

Figure 16-8 shows an axial map of a refractive surgery candidate that on initial exam displayed some mild irregular astigmatism. The Magellan classifier registers in the "other" category. Note that no ectatic characteristics were triggered. Upon further history, this patient had been out of her extended wear soft contact lenses for just 1 week. Figure 16-9 shows her follow-up exam after being out of lenses for over a month. We now see a more regular axial map with the reclassification of only "normal" and "astigmatism."

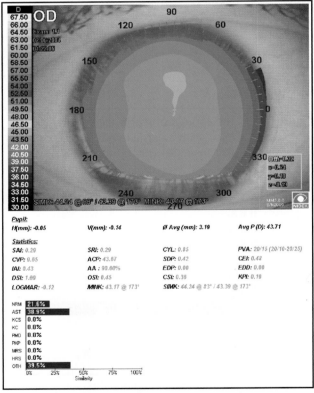

Figure 16-8. This axial map has the characteristics associated with unclassified variations (OTH = 39.5% likelihood), 0.85 diopters of cylinder (AST = 38.9%), and normal topography (21.6%).

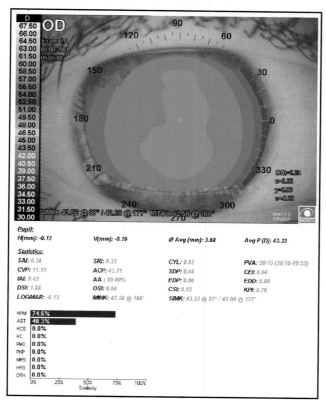

Figure 16-9. This map shows characteristics associated with a normal cornea (74.6%), as well as features of a cornea with 0.82 diopters of cylinder (AST 10.3%).

The previous case is a perfect example of subtle contact lens warpage detected by the Magellan that might otherwise be overlooked. These findings allow the refractive surgeon to collect more accurate wavefront information and thus produce better postoperative results.

In conclusion, the Magellan Mapper and its novel classification system can provide clinicians with accurate, easy-to-read topographies that compliment any refractive evaluation. The high resolution maps and expanded range of indices make this topographer an invaluable tool for pathology detection and management.

REFERENCES

1. Personal communication with Dr. S. Klyce and Dr. M. Smolek. November 5, 2004.

2. External Disease and Cornea: Basic and Clinical Science Course, Section 8. American Academy of Ophthalmology. 2001–2002:305.

3. Rajan MS, Jaycock P, O'Brart D, et al. A long term study of photorefractive keratectomy: 12 year followup. *Ophthalmology*. 2004;111:1813–1824.

4. Orbscan Keratoconus Screening Indices: Operators Manual and Procedural Recommendations. Rochester, NY: Bausch & Lomb; July 2004.

5. Wilson SE, Lin DTC, Klyce SD, et al. Topographic changes in contact lens-induced corneal warpage. *Ophthalmology*. 1990;97:734.

Chapter 17

The iTrace Combination Corneal Topography and Wavefront System by Tracey Technologies

Joe S. Wakil, MD; Tom D. Padrick, PhD; and Sergey Molebny, MS

The iTrace system, manufactured by Tracey Technologies (Houston, TX), is uniquely designed to combine full surface Placido corneal topography with the advantages of ray tracing aberrometry—a new and robust wavefront technology to measure quality of vision in a rapid and comprehensive manner. The iTrace incorporates the Vista corneal topography hardware manufactured by EyeSys Vision, Inc. (Houston, TX) with an integrated software application produced by Tracey Technologies to deliver complete corneal topography and total eye aberrometry data acquisition and analysis.

At the core of this instrument is unique technology providing optical ray tracing of the eye, as is evidenced by the product name—iTrace. A sequential series of thin, infrared beams or rays of light on the order of 100 microns each is projected into the entire entrance pupil of the eye using a programmable scanning pattern that measures hundreds of points within milliseconds. Each of these points represents the entrance of parallel, sampling light rays into the eye, which become refracted by the eye's optical power and eventually focus on the retina. By locating the spot on the retina where each thin beam of light is focused, a direct aberration measurement is made. This leads to calculations for a complete aberration profile and optical performance examination of the eye.

This technology stems from former Soviet military applications, and was developed by the scientist Vasyl Molebny, PhD and his team of engineers in Kiev, Ukraine in collaboration with ophthalmic surgeon Ioannis Pallikaris, MD and his colleagues in Crete, Greece. The combination of this aberrometry information with corneal topography provides valuable clinical information regarding the ocular sources of aberrations: corneal or lenticular.

iTRACE DESIGN PHILOSOPHY

Important in any system design is the philosophy behind it and the utility goals for its practice and use. The iTrace features a dual-purpose system with full corneal topography and wavefront capabilities, along with integrated software analysis, on a single computer platform. This device demonstrates the great power of bringing these two technologies together in diagnosing refractive disorders and ocular disease states. The dual sliding mount hardware places the Placido-based EyeSys Vista corneal topographer side-by-side with the Tracey ray-tracing aberrometer on top of a standard manual slit lamp base (Figure 17-1), enabling the aberrometer to maintain a slim profile. This allows the eye under measurement to fixate directly through the instrument's transparent optics at a target well beyond 20 feet (for example, through an office window at a tree across the street) while the fellow eye has an unobstructed view of the same target. This helps provide a binocular open field fixation of a real object at distance, much greater then 20 feet, during wavefront measurement. This feature realizes true, natural binocular vision to overcome the menace of instrument myopia, where monocular fixation on an optically simulated "far" target plagues all conventional autorefraction systems in measuring younger patients. Effectively obtaining objective distance refraction with this feature and avoiding accommodation may also greatly reduce the need for performing cycloplegic refractions.

Additionally, this dual-mount system easily allows for the Vista corneal topographer to be detached and utilized with a computer laptop as a stand-alone, portable, handheld corneal topography unit with the full software benefits of the EyeSys system. The EyeSys system was developed in 1986 and has been an industry leader in the corneal topography field, including the well-known Holladay Diagnostic Summary. The EyeSys Vista corneal topographer is designed for convenient handheld use and has special electronic features, such as auto-capture and tilt sensors, to ensure accurate and precise corneal topography and keratometric data on par with any tabletop unit. This includes using the system in a vertical mode on supine patients during surgery; for example, to document flap orientation and condition at the end of standard LASIK procedures. With integrated or detachable corneal topography, the iTrace is truly two instruments in one—multiplying its clinical utility.

REVIEW OF THE FUNDAMENTALS OF CORNEAL TOPOGRAPHY

Computerized corneal topography has become a logical advance from the basic principles of keratometry over the past two decades. However, the actual term *corneal topography* is misleading as it denotes measurement of the cornea in terms of its sagittal height and other three-dimensional qualities of shape, similar to geographical topography with the elevation of mountainous terrain. This poor descriptive term for the field has been, and continues to be, a source of confusion in interpreting clinical data about the cornea and in understanding the importance of the cornea's dual roles: corneal shape (in terms of its curvature) and corneal optics (in terms of its optical performance in vision).

For over a century, the keratometer has been promoting this confusion by analyzing the cornea as a fixed combination of both curvature in terms of millimeters radius of curvature, and refractive power in terms of diopters with its over-simplified keratometric or sphere-fitting formula. Although manual and automatic versions of the keratometer have been valuable instruments in providing reasonably accurate and repeatable results on central corneal curvature measurements, there are indisputable shortcomings in truly describing corneal optics and shape for today's world of refractive correction. Primary shortcomings of the keratometer are listed here:

The keratometer derives its two readings by averaging the values across two perpendicular chords, approximately 3 mm apart, on a single ring mire that is reflected off the anterior tear film of the cornea. One pair of points is aligned along the steepest axis of the corneal surface, with the second pair forcibly along the axis 90 degrees away for the flattest axis. These two readings yield radius of curvature values that are used to approximate the cornea's central refractive power (K values).

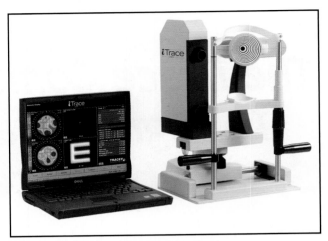

Figure 17-1. The iTrace system.

The resultant K values are reported, assuming the surface of the cornea is an orthogonal symmetric spherocylindrical surface. This is not consistent with known asymmetries of the cornea and its actual aspheric shape.

The keratometer cannot measure corneal curvature inside or outside of the annular mire upon which the two pairs of points lie.

To overcome these issues, photokeratoscopy based on full surface Placido imaging of the cornea became popular beginning in the 1960s. This provided a qualitative method for detecting the variations and asymmetries of the cornea across most of its surface area. With the advent of the personal computer in the 1980s, computerized videokeratoscopy became an available diagnostic instrument to quantify corneal topography measurements and present them in the form of color maps. Since that time, a number of digital imaging improvements and mathematical algorithms have been applied to fully describe and measure many aspects of the cornea's shape and optics, leading to the new generation of diagnostic instruments available today.

The iTrace utilizes a large Placido format based on the hardware made popular by EyeSys Technologies as one of the largest installed bases of corneal topographers in the world since the late 1980s. The EyeSys Placido is noted for using edge detection of the Placido mires to provide precise determination of ring location for highly accurate corneal topography measurements. The Placido design of the Vista is the same as that of the larger EyeSys 2000 system, covering the central cornea at around 0.6 mm to over 10 mm in the normal peripheral cornea. This larger Placido design provides for a longer working distance than smaller cylindrical Placido cones. The longer working distance has the advantage of being less sensitive to positional errors in focusing and alignment, which significantly improves the reproducibility and accuracy of the system.

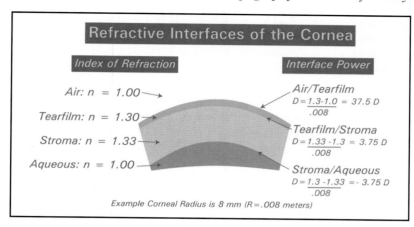

Figure 17-2. The refractive power is determined by each of the interfaces in the normal cornea.

The EyeSys Vista hardware has this advantage working in its favor under both conditions, mounted on the slit lamp base and when used as a handheld. The reproducibility results are impressive at under ±0.125 D in the hands of an experienced user.

It is important to always remember that with corneal topography measurements one is measuring the anterior tear film surface of the cornea. This is the refractive surface that provides the vast majority (>75%) of the eye's refractive power. Please note that although some topography systems emphasize that the cornea has anterior and posterior surfaces that this can be misleading, since optically with tear film on the living cornea there are actually three refractive interfaces: air/tear film, tear film/corneal stroma, and corneal stroma/aqueous humor. Figure 17-2 shows the refractive power ($D = (n2 - n1) / R$) determined by each of these interfaces in the normal cornea. The index of refraction change is approximately 10 times greater on the anterior tear film at 0.3 than in the other interfaces.

Effectively, nature has provided for these last two refractive interfaces of the cornea to practically cancel each other out, leaving the anterior tear film as the effective refractive power interface of the cornea. Considering the optics just described, the cornea serves two roles to fulfill its optical purpose in the visual process:

1. The cornea must be transparent to let light pass unhindered toward the retina, maximizing contrast sensitivity.

2. The cornea must give the proper curvature to the tear film where light is primarily refracted to focus upon the retina.

Keeping the above in mind when analyzing corneal topography and aberrometry lends insight into the sources of aberrations in the eye between the cornea and lens. This will assist greatly in the process of selecting the best refractive correction therapy for each patient. To ensure ideal visual correction, matching the available surgical procedures or corrective lens choices to address each patient's visual deficits depends heavily on correct diagnosis of the aberration sources in each patient's eyes. The iTrace is designed to meet this goal for every patient in an easy-to-use and comprehensive format, creating a new standard of visual function analysis well beyond the antiquated Snellen refraction.

CORNEAL TOPOGRAPHY FEATURES OF THE iTRACE SYSTEM

The corneal topography calculations and displays are generated from the EyeSys Vista Placido image of the cornea and are fully customizable in the iTrace software. Using advanced edge detection software, the Placido image of the cornea is analyzed across all the ring edges from center to periphery. Along with patient name and identification number, OD/OS label, and time of exam, standard keratometric readings are generated at the 3-mm zone of the cornea to accurately measure its central curvature and simulate keratometer measurements for routine use. These K readings are provided with every corneal topography display.

Additionally, a refractive power reading of the cornea is calculated for the 3-mm zone in similar fashion to the K readings, but is based on Snell's law of refraction to more accurately describe the refractive power of the central cornea. A single effective refractive power reading is given for the entire central 3-mm zone of the cornea, to be used primarily for IOL calculations. This number has been popularized by Jack Holladay, MD, as an improvement in understanding central corneal refractive power contribution to more accurately calculate IOL power for eyes post-refractive surgery. The Holladay Diagnostic Summary available with the compatible EyeSys software package to the Vista hardware has become an industry standard, single-page display that provides additional corneal indices to comprehensively analyze the cornea and simplify corneal diagnosis, particularly for early keratoconus. These indices include: the inferior-superior (I-S) index; a corneal uniformity index (CUI); an aspheric Q factor of the cornea; and the unique potential corneal acuity (PCA) measurement that provides a direct objective measure of mire quality related to the tear film of the eye, in effect helping measure potential dry eye problems.

Beyond the numeric data of K readings, refractive power readings, and other corneal indices, color maps are provided to depict the unique features of each cornea. For both two- and three-dimensional color maps, there are a number of algorithms available that provide complete corneal analysis. These include the axial map, local radius of curvature map, refractive map, Z elevation map, and wavefront map.

The standard axial color map is based on the keratometric formula, wherein the curvature of the cornea is presented with respect to the optical axis of the instrument. This color map has been commonly used over the years as an extension of the keratometer to the entire corneal surface. However, in applying the simple keratometric formula, this map only provides accurate curvature data and corneal refractive power data in the central corneal region. The data outside of the 3-mm zone is simply not accurate in terms of either the true curvature of the cornea or the refractive power generated in the peripheral cornea. Due to these misrepresentations, the axial color map is becoming less popular and will most likely be phased out, as the local radius of curvature map and the refractive map provide more accurate and complete information in terms of corneal shape and corneal optics, respectively.

The local radius of curvature map, known as the tangential map or instantaneous radius of curvature map in other systems, is used to accurately depict the true corneal shape in terms of millimeter radius of curvature from center to periphery. This map is a mathematical derivative of the axial color map and can be most useful in appreciating the detail of corneal surface features both centrally and peripherally. Contact lens fitters will derive more accurate curvature measurements in the periphery to better fit contact lenses, while refractive surgeons will better appreciate the sharpness of transition zone edges from excimer laser ablations that commonly generate halos and glare to postsurgical eyes with small effective optical zones using this map. Also, for the critical diagnosis of keratoconus, the local radius of curvature map will emphasize the true size and nature of an ectasia as observed in the slit lamp microscope. This is very important to note, as it is necessary to know the actual apex location and severity of curvature generated by the keratoconus to treat it appropriately. The local radius of curvature map is typically the best source of information for such corneal shape information.

The refractive map accurately calculates the refractive power across the entire corneal surface as it applies Snell's law of refraction instead of the basic keratometric formula, which is limited to the central corneal region. The refractive map is always presented in diopter units. The refractive map provides the clinician with appreciation for the greater refractive power of the normal cornea in the periphery than in the center, despite the fact that the normal cornea does flatten in the periphery. This is consistent with the occurrence of night myopia in a significant percentage of the normal population. Of course, in most patients there is increased curvature of the cornea in the periphery following myopic excimer laser surgery, where many of the problems of night halos and glare associated with the peripheral cornea will be even more pronounced if the area of the cornea is within the scotopic entrance pupil. Therefore, to truly understand corneal optics and its contribution to the total ocular power, the refractive map is an accurate source of data. One does not need to be concerned over posterior corneal power as a significant contributor based on the physics described earlier; therefore, once again the anterior corneal surface is the primary refractive interface for the eye. With a normal tear film consisting of a lipid monolayer on top that provides its smoothing effect, nature has provided for some ideal "polishing" of the corneal surface to enhance its optical performance.

The Z elevation map is useful in understanding the physical nature of the cornea in terms of height difference in microns from a reference sphere. The algorithms used to choose a reference sphere must be paid particular attention, as one can generate a number of different elevation measurements based solely on the reference sphere chosen. Most algorithms use a reference sphere based on the best fit to the central cornea (as is done in the case of iTrace); however, this can be highly subjective from system to system. The Z elevation map can emphasize depressions and elevations from such a best-fit sphere. The user can modify the reference sphere to get more detail in some cases. Without providing a reference sphere, the ability to discern the very subtle height differences across the cornea would be difficult. It is important to note that since the cornea is generally aspheric both in its normal and postoperative condition, there will always be some differences in the height from a sphere. Although height measurements are commonly used in topography mapping as in geographical terrain, their clinical utility is generally limited to a few instances in planning excimer laser enhancement surgeries and in studying some corneal disease progression.

The corneal wavefront map is relatively new to the scene of corneal topography, as it is an extension of wavefront

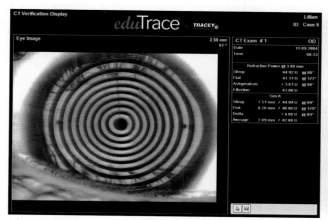

Figure 17-3. Corneal topography verification display.

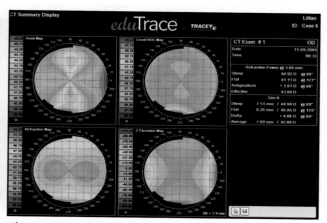

Figure 17-4. Corneal topography summary display.

analysis of the eye applied strictly to the cornea. As described later in this chapter, the corneal wavefront map is a Zernike calculation of the wavefront errors generated by the corneal surface alone. This is useful in understanding the cornea's contribution to the overall aberrations in the eye. As described later in this chapter, there are powerful diagnostic benefits to subtracting the corneal wavefront contributions from the entire ocular wavefront measurement so that one can elucidate the aberrations generated in the internal eye structures, primarily the lens. This wavefront map is described in micron units of wavefront error and must not be confused with corneal height determination. There is a direct correlation of the corneal wavefront map, which only applies to the area of the cornea within the entrance pupil, to that of the refractive map in the same corneal area.

CORNEAL TOPOGRAPHY VERIFICATION AND ANALYSIS DISPLAYS

The iTrace system uses the Vista hardware to capture the Placido image automatically upon centering and focusing of the video image as the patient fixates on a coaxial fixation point. This automatic capture occurs through triangulation of a low power laser beam reflected off of the corneal apex at a calibrated distance from the Placido. Once captured, the Placido image is displayed to the user with the ring edge detection highlighted so that the user can easily confirm correct image processing. This helps avoid artifacts and errors in processing that can sometimes be problematic in very irregular corneas, such as those following corneal transplantation. Figure 17-3 shows a typical Placido image capture verification screen with the edge detection clearly shown confirming correct analysis to the user. Also, the user can obtain the K readings and refrac-

tive power readings from this immediate display following image capture.

The corneal topography summary displays can be customized to allow for any of the color maps available to be displayed with up to four maps at once. The iTrace is generally configured to show the axial map, local radius of curvature map, refractive map, and Z elevation map. The corneal wavefront map can be added as desired. The example of corneal topography summary display in Figure 17-4 shows almost 4 D of with-the-rule astigmatism, where the steep corneal curvature is oriented vertically. As with all color maps, it is important to pay attention to scaling. With the iTrace, there is a choice to allow for auto-scaling features or user-defined fixed scaling units. Typically, 0.5-D step sizes are used to fulfill most needs and provide good corneal detail, while also providing adequate range to most corneas. User choice is available to generate practically all scaling requirements.

An example of the Z elevation map is provided in Figures 17-5 and 17-6 in a three-dimensional format that can be applied to all maps. Additionally, with this cornea, the figures demonstrate the effects of changing the best-fit sphere, so one can see how the Z elevation map can change from plus to minus elevation in certain peripheral parts of the cornea when the best-fit sphere is flattened from R0 = 7.50 mm in Figure 17-5 to R0 = 8.25 mm in Figure 17-6.

A comparison display map is also available on each of the different color map displays available with the iTrace. These maps are informative in revealing the differences that occur over time; for example, pre- and post-surgically, as well as over periods of healing or treatment. Figure 17-7 shows corneal stabilization after contact lens removal in a patient planning for excimer laser surgery. The refractive power difference between these two exams is much less than 0.25 D over most of the corneal surface, therefore indicating that the cornea has changed insignificantly between the two days examined. Overall, the difference

Figure 17-5 (left). Z elevation map with 7.50-mm reference sphere.

Figure 17-6 (right). Z elevation map with 8.25-mm reference sphere.

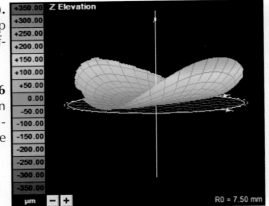

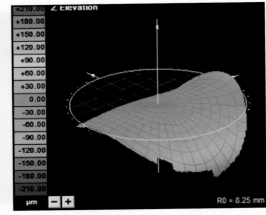

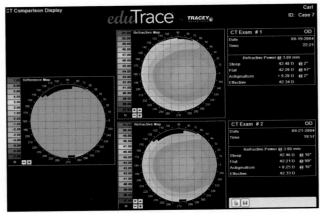

Figure 17-7. Corneal topography comparison display.

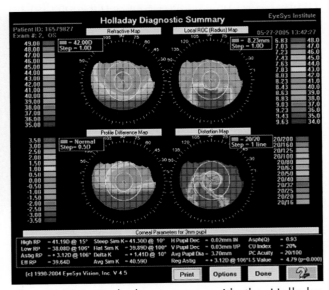

Figure 17-8. Early keratoconus with the Holladay Diagnostic Summary.

map is green, indicating little or no change in corneal topography.

The Holladay Diagnostic Summary shown in Figure 17-8 demonstrates the power of corneal topography in diagnosing an early keratoconus case. This unique display generated by EyeSys software has been widely used for over a decade in providing a single-page overview of the cornea with a number of valuable corneal indices. The cornea displayed shows the classic pattern of inferior steepening in the local radius of curvature map in the upper right and also a correlating change in the asphericity difference map in the lower left, demonstrating that the area of the keratoconus significantly alters the normal rate of flattening of the cornea from center to periphery. The potential corneal acuity map in the lower right reveals a pattern of inferior mire distortion expected in classic keratoconus as tear film break-up and irregularity over the ectasia is typical. The corneal indices at the bottom of the Holladay Diagnostic Summary are consistent with keratoconus having an I-S index greater then 1.0 (in this case 4.79) and a CUI of under 60% (in this case 20%) with a degraded PCA of 20/100. With the data presented, a clini-

cian only needs to complete the patient history to rule out contact lens warpage in making the keratoconus diagnosis with a high degree of certainty. The Holladay Diagnostic Summary demonstrates the variety of corneal topography data analysis that can be used to make the appropriate diagnosis.

ABERROMETRY/WAVEFRONT WITH THE ITRACE RAY TRACING PRINCIPLE

Historically, the optical property of the eye has been described in terms of a single group of refraction numbers: sphere, cylinder, and axis. Refraction can be measured with a variety of instruments, such as retinoscopy, refractometry, and autorefraction (Figure 17-9). However, these

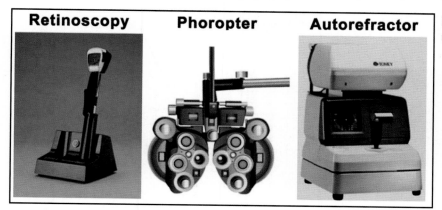

Figure 17-9. Instruments for measurement of the eye's total refraction.

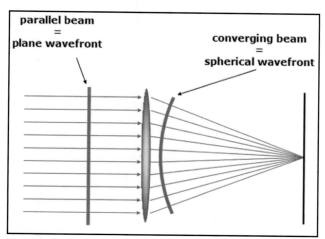

Figure 17-10. Plane and spherical wavefronts.

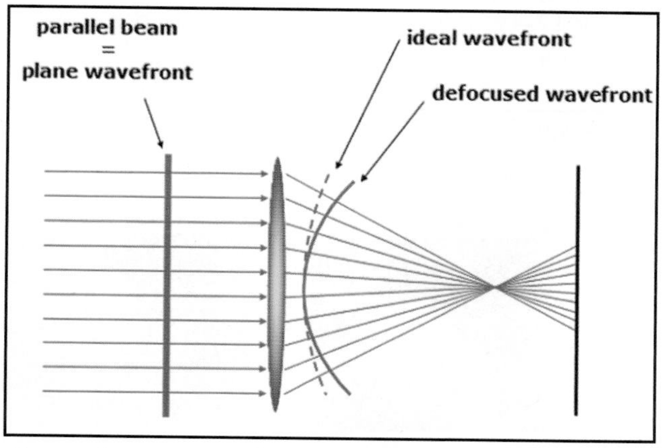

Figure 17-11. Wavefront for defocused optical system (myopia).

measurements represent only spherocylindrical measurements of the aberrations in the eye. In order to measure the spatially resolved optical properties of the eye, we must use other terminology to describe these properties. One method to describe these properties is by characterizing the wavefront or the total aberrations that the eye's optical system generate.

As used here, the wavefront is "an imaginary surface joining all points in space that are reached at the same time by a lightwave propagating through a medium." The solid, vertical red line in Figure 17-10 depicts such a wavefront. Before entering the eye, parallel light would have a flat or plane wavefront; that is, each point in the lightwave arrives at the imaginary surface in front of the eye at the same time. For an emmetropic eye, the light would have a curved wavefront because light travels different distances through different mediums at different speeds, resulting in the imaginary surface that represents the points reached at the same time being curved. For a myopic eye of the same length, the wavefront would be more curved secondary to the greater refractive power (Figure 17-11).

The difference between an ideal wavefront and the actual wavefront over the entire surface of the optical system is calculated in terms of microns of deviation. When the actual wavefront is more advanced than the ideal wavefront, the error is described as a positive deviation in microns. If the actual wavefront were retarded, the deviation would have a negative value in microns. This spatially resolved deviation of the measured wavefront from the ideal as a two-dimensional color map and a three-dimensional display is shown for the defocused wavefront in Figure 17-12.

The eye, however, is rarely described by a purely spherical or aspheric surface. Therefore, the resulting wavefront error is irregular in its deviation pattern from the ideal wavefront as depicted in cross-section in Figure 17-13. The variations in refractive power at each point over the entrance pupil can be demonstrated as irregular wavefronts in both two- and three-dimensional maps (Figure 17-14).

The deviations between the actual wavefront and ideal wavefront are referred to as aberrations, or a deviation

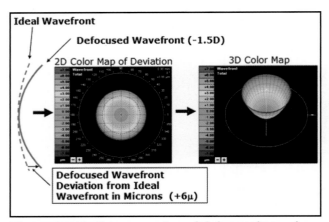

Figure 17-12. Representation of defocused wavefront from ideal.

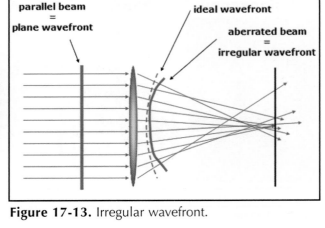

Figure 17-13. Irregular wavefront.

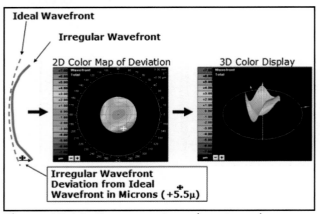

Figure 17-14. Representation of an irregular wavefront in the eye.

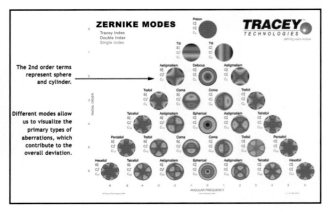

Figure 17-15. Visual representation of Zernike modes.

from the normal or expected course. In 1934, Fritz Zernike published a paper describing a set of polynomials that could be used to expand the aberration function. Each polynomial represents a particular type of optical aberration. Each wavefront can be described by coefficients (multipliers for each of the modes), which, when taken as a whole, reconstruct the wavefront map (Figure 17-15) but individually describe the relative amount of each aberration type. Figure 17-15 shows the Zernike modes (aberration type) for an expansion through 6th-order polynomials.

There are four technologies commercially available to measure aberrations in the eye. These four technologies include: Hartmann-Shack, Tscherning, differential skiascopy, and ray tracing. Tracey Technologies utilizes the ray tracing principle that projects a sequential series of thin laser beams through the entrance pupil parallel to the eye's line of sight. The location where each beam of light is focused onto the retina is measured by capturing the exiting reflected light and focusing it onto position-sensing

detectors. This principle measures the forward aberrations of light passing into the eye. This is in opposition to the Hartmann-Shack principle that assumes an ideal point source of light is generated from the retina, therefore measuring the reverse aberrations of light as it passes from the retina out the exit pupil of the eye. Measuring forward aberrations is more physiologic in analyzing vision, as it follows the natural path of light into the eye and is advantageous in measuring the optical path differences for components of the eye.

Figure 17-16 is a schematic layout of the ray tracing technique developed by Tracey Technologies. Once the position of point 1 is determined, the laser beam is moved to a new position and the location of the next point on the retina is then determined. This process continues until 256 separate points have been projected through the entrance pupil, which occurs very rapidly (approximately 100 msec). If the eye was emmetropic, then all 256 points would fall on one spot in the center of the macula (Figure 17-16).

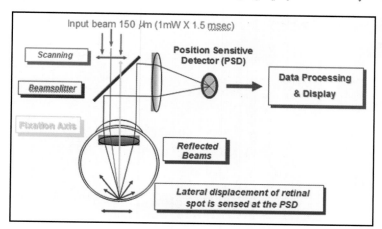

Figure 17-16. Schematic layout of ray tracing aberrometer.

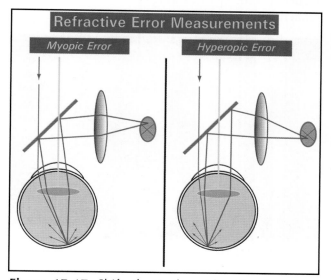

Figure 17-17. Shift of retinal spot location based on local aberrations of the eye.

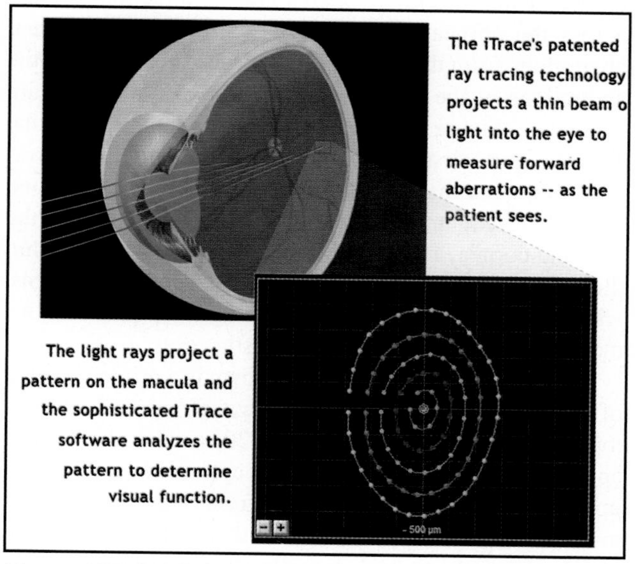

The iTrace's patented ray tracing technology projects a thin beam of light into the eye to measure forward aberrations -- as the patient sees.

The light rays project a pattern on the macula and the sophisticated *i*Trace software analyzes the pattern to determine visual function.

Figure 17-18. Schematic eye and retinal spot pattern.

Generally, local aberrations at the beam's entry point on the cornea or the lens cause a shift in the location on the retina. Figure 17-17 illustrates a single measurement point for a myopic and hyperopic eye.

When a series of points is projected sequentially through the entrance pupil, a retinal spot pattern is created (Figure 17-18). Ray tracing has several key advantages over other technologies. First, the rapid sequential capture of data means that there is no confusion in the analysis between the origin location in the entrance pupil and the reflected location from the retina, since each point is done separately and sequentially. This means that highly aberrated eyes can be measured easily with ray tracing. Second, because the pattern of laser spots projected through the entrance pupil is rapidly controlled with software, the system can track the pupil size and project all 256 points into a pupil as small as 2 mm or as large as 8 mm. Third, since each point is measured separately, the

software's task of locating the center of each spot is much easier, facilitating processing and requiring only basic computer power, which helps allow for a cost-efficient system.

ADVANTAGES OF COMBINED WAVEFRONT/CORNEAL TOPOGRAPHY DISPLAY

The iTrace system measures total ocular aberrations of the eye (aberrometry) directly through the ray tracing principle. The iTrace calculates corneal anterior surface aberrations from the corneal topography data it acquires through the EyeSys Vista Placido image. This calculation involves simply performing a Zernike polynomial computation on the data generated from the refractive map of the

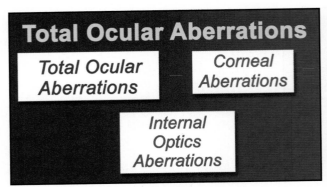

Figure 17-19. Total ocular aberrations.

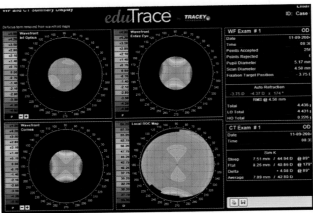

Figure 17-20. Corneal astigmatism is the source of refractive cylinder.

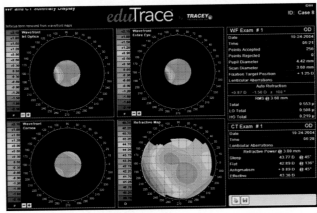

Figure 17-21. Lens aberration is a primary source of coma.

cornea, using the classic Snell's law of refraction formula across the cornea's surface. By subtracting the corneal aberrations from the total ocular aberrations of the eye, the aberrations of the internal optics (primarily the lens) are generated. Figure 17-19 illustrates this simple formula. This is a good first approximation in obtaining the aberrations of the internal optics of the eye, which provides good clinical insight into the optical relationship between the lens and cornea. The location of aberration sources within the eye is very helpful in assessing visual deficit problems, which yields great confidence in taking the ideal corrective measures for practically all diagnostic cases.

Locating the sources of astigmatism is a prime example of the power of the combined wavefront and corneal topography display. In Figure 17-20, a normal eye with approximately 4.37 D of refractive cylinder is shown. The upper right map provides the wavefront of the entire eye in microns of deviation from the ideal wavefront. This map clearly shows the typical "hourglass" shape of cylinder. To the right of this map is the autorefraction readout of the patient showing that the patient also has –3.75 D of myopia. The lower left map is noticeably larger as it represents the full corneal topography in a local ROC map. The classic vertical bowtie of corneal with-the-rule astigmatism is seen, and to the right of that map one can see that the K readings indicate corneal astigmatism of a little over 4.0 D. The map in the lower left is the corneal wavefront map calculated from the corneal topography data within the pupil. It is consistent with an "hourglass" shape almost identical to the wavefront of the entire eye. When the corneal wavefront map is subtracted from the total eye wavefront map, the map in the upper left is generated, presenting the wavefront of the internal optics of the eye, primarily from the crystalline lens. As this map is primarily green, it indicates very little source of aberrations for this patient. Obviously it is easy to conclude that most of the cylinder in this patient's refraction is due to corneal astigmatism.

Figure 17-21 shows a normal eye with a noticeable aberration in the total wavefront (upper right) that appears to be identical to the pattern in the map to the left, the aberrations of the crystalline lens. From this example, we can deduce that the source of the aberration is the lens. This type of aberration is primarily coma, which will cause double or blurred vision. Although this patient shows some corneal astigmatism, it is easy to deduce that the coma in the lens will prevent this patient from ideal correction with simple spectacles. This is particularly true at night when the pupil dilates, increasing the effect. It is important to note that if refractive laser correction was performed on the corneal surface, undergoing keratorefractive surgery for optical correction would not result in an ideal outcome. The source of the coma is behind the cornea, and all current custom LASIK algorithms assume all the eye's aberrations exist in one optical plane. The oversimplified models of custom LASIK do not discriminate between the sources of the eye's aberrations, as to which ones are from the lens or corneal plane. These algorithms will not provide an appropriate correction when the lens is a significant source of the eye's aberrations. Intraocular procedures may be better options for vision correction.

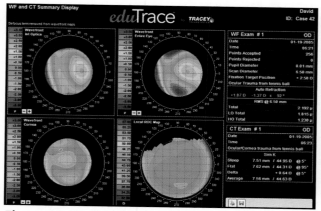

Figure 17-22. Significant coma from the lens following trauma.

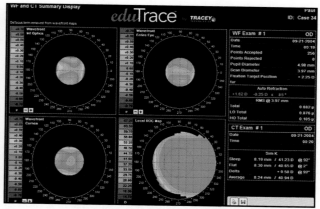

Figure 17-23. Lens and corneal aberration measures at far point of fixation.

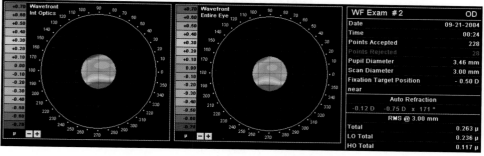

Figure 17-24. Lens aberration changes with near point of fixation.

The case in Figure 17-22 also demonstrates the existence of significant coma from the lens. This patient actually had blunt trauma to the eye from a tennis ball injury, which tore the zonules laterally leading to large lens tilt that manifested as coma. On the other hand, the corneal aberrations show a nominal amount of spherical aberration (blue ring) that is typical in normal corneas. The patient suffered a "blown" pupil and the scans measured are at the maximum of 8 mm.

The iTrace can demonstrate changes in lens aberrations with accommodation. The unit has an open field window through which the patient can see, enabling him or her to fixate on a true far target binocularly or monocularly. The measurement is then repeated while looking at a near point target, such as a reading card using an attached near point reading rod. By subtracting the wavefront measurements between near and far, a difference map represents the accommodative change of the eye. Moreover, by isolating the lens aberrations at both the near and far point measurements, we can see the actual lens aberration changes isolated at both near and far points. This information is providing new insights into how the eye achieves near point vision. Accommodation traditionally calls for a spherical change in the lens power across the pupil. But, in many cases the iTrace demonstrates that cylinder, as well as higher order aberrations, are induced by the lens, which

provides an increased depth of field (pseudo-accommodation) to assist the patient's visual processing and enhances near vision. New studies are being performed to understand mechanisms of natural accommodation and accommodating IOL technology. Figures 17-23 and 17-24 show the lens changes from far- and near-point measurements, respectively. Note the change in lenticular aberrations with primarily sphere and cylinder changes, providing almost 2 D of accommodation for this hyperopic patient. While we expect changes in lens aberrations during accommodation, the classic model of accommodation does not explain the dramatic shift of 90 degrees in the lens astigmatism observed in this patient during accommodation.

Figure 17-25 shows the difference map between the near- and far-point wavefront measurements for the same patient shown in Figure 17-23 and 17-24. It demonstrates for the first time a map of the patient's accommodative changes in refractive power across the pupil. This direct measurement of the accommodative power change of the entire eye is due to the specific lens aberration changes observed in the earlier figures. This analysis provides new diagnostic power in elucidating how a patient specifically accommodates, or does not.

The ability to reveal corneal aberrations separately from those of the lens, combined with the ability to measure a patient's ocular aberrations at true far- and near-point

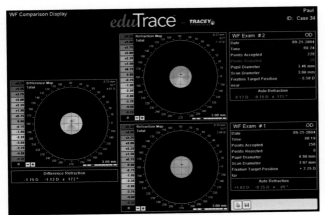

Figure 17-25. Difference map of near and far measurements showing the effects of accommodation.

fixation, are providing a new level of diagnostic information on how the eye accommodates and how well we are able to return such function through either accommodating or multifocal implants.

CONCLUSION

There is much to learn from the objective measure of corneal topography with the iTrace using the well-known Vista technology from EyeSys Vision, Inc. The cornea/tear film interface represents the majority of the eye's refractive power, but does not represent the total refraction of the eye on its own. Therefore, by integrating the iTrace refraction of the total eye through ray tracing aberrometry with the corneal aberrations derived directly from its corneal topography measurement, the device can elucidate tremendous diagnostic information to enhance vision correction and disease diagnosis. The iTrace represents a new platform of refraction to understand a patient's quality of vision and to pinpoint the source of aberrations in the eye. With this diagnostic power available in a fast, practical, and cost-efficient system, there is a tremendous added benefit to the eye care practitioner providing the best possible vision for each patient—regardless of modality.

BIBLIOGRAPHY

Holladay JT. Corneal topography using the Holladay Diagnostic Summary. *J Cataract Refract Surg.* 1997;23:209–222.

Holladay JT, Lynn MJ, Waring GO, et al. The relationship of visual acuity, refractive error, and pupil size after radial keratotomy. *Arch Ophthalmol.* 1991;109:70–76.

Gills JP, Sanders DR, Thornton SP, Martin RG, Gayton JL, Holladay JT. *Corneal Topography: The State of the Art.* Thorofare, NJ: SLACK Incorporated; 1995.

Molebny VV, Panagopoulou SI, Molebny SV, Wakil JS, Pallikaris IG. Principles of ray tracing aberrometry. *J Refract Surg.* 2000;16:S570–S575.

Zernicke F. *Physica.* 1934;1:689.

Chapter 18

Bausch & Lomb Orbscan II/IIz Anterior Segment Analysis System

Paul M. Karpecki, OD

The Bausch & Lomb (Rochester, NY) Orbscan II/IIz Anterior Segment Analysis system (Figure 18-1) performs a complete anatomical analysis of the anterior segment of the eye. The system combines two technologies: a calibrated video and slit-scanning-beam system that measures anterior segment geometry and an advanced Placido-disk system that measures the curvature of the anterior surface of the cornea.

ORBSCAN II/IIz FUNCTIONAL DESCRIPTION

During an examination, the patient fixates on a blinking light source that is coaxial with a calibrated video imaging system. The video imaging system performs 40 scans through light slits projected at a 45-degree angle. In two 0.75-second periods, 20 slits are projected sequentially on the eye from the left and right sides of the video axis. The 5-mm central zone of the cornea is sampled twice, once in each direction, through these overlapping slits (Figure 18-2). Before the slit scans, an additional image is captured using Placido rings.

The Orbscan performs noninvasive measurements of thousands of points on four surfaces of the anterior segment of the eye: the anterior cornea, posterior cornea, anterior iris, and anterior lens. An example of a raw image is shown in Figure 18-3. The system measures 9,600 points (240 from each of the 40 slits). These point measurements are used to construct mathematical representations of the true topographic surfaces of the anterior segment, including maps of elevation (z) versus horizontal and vertical (x and y) coordinates. The mathematical surface representations, which typically have continuous second-order derivatives, are used to calculate slope and cur-

vature at any point and in every direction. A tracking system measures involuntary eye movement and is used to accurately assemble the mathematical surface representation from the 40 slit images. The resulting calculations are used to describe four elements of the anterior segment: anterior corneal elevation, posterior corneal elevation, corneal power, and corneal thickness. Keratometric power is calculated using a standard keratometric index.

The Orbscan system uses a Pentium 4 computer to acquire, analyze, and present the calculated data. Displays use a color scale to show relative elevations, providing a three-dimensional view of surface topography. In all elevation maps green is the reference surface, or zero level. Red is high, positive, and anterior to the reference surface, while blue is low, negative, and posterior to the reference surface. A commonly used view of surface topography is the quad map. This presents anterior elevation, posterior elevation, corneal power, and pachymetry maps in one view. Figure 18-4 is a quad map showing typical with-the-rule astigmatism. In this figure, the anterior corneal float (elevation) appears in the upper left corner and the posterior float in the upper right corner. Keratometric topography is shown in the lower left and corneal thickness is shown in the lower right.

THEORY OF MEASUREMENT

The Orbscan system uses hybrid measurement technology. Specular reflection from a Placido disk is used to calculate the surface curvature of the cornea by measuring the specularly reflected image of a set of concentric mires. Slit scanning is used to measure the anterior segment geometry; its basic measurement is the absolute elevation of optical surfaces. These curvature and elevation measurements

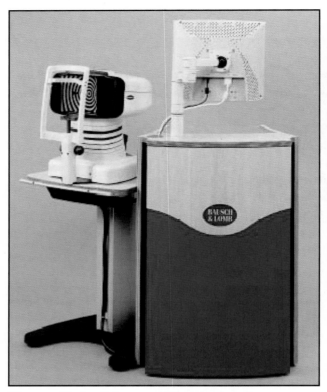

Figure 18-1. Orbscan II/IIz diagnostic systems. (Courtesy of Bausch & Lomb.)

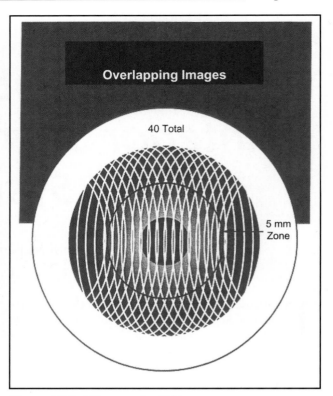

Figure 18-2. Slit scans in Orbscan.

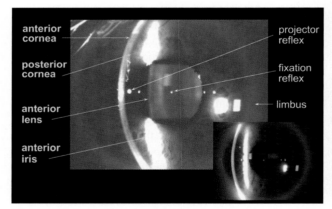

Figure 18-3. Structures of the anterior segment analyzed by Orbscan include the anterior cornea, posterior cornea, anterior lens, and anterior iris. (Courtesy of Bausch & Lomb.)

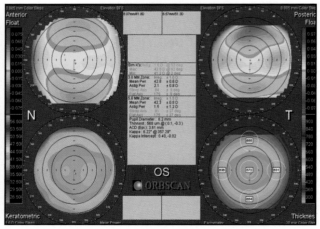

Figure 18-4. Orbscan quad map showing typical with-the-rule astigmatism. (Courtesy of John Vukich, MD.)

are combined to develop accurate maps of absolute anterior and posterior surface elevation and pachymetry. Curvature is displayed as a keratometric power.

Diffuse Reflections

When a slit beam intercepts an optically smooth surface, it is split into a specular reflection and a refracted beam that penetrates the surface and is volume scattered by internal scattering centers. Like surface diffuse reflection, volume scattering is omnidirectional. This important property allows surface points to be independently observed and triangulated, and gives Orbscan the capability to measure arbitrary surface shapes—convex or concave, aspheric or irregular. Volume (or diffuse) scattering is typically negligible from liquids such as the tear film

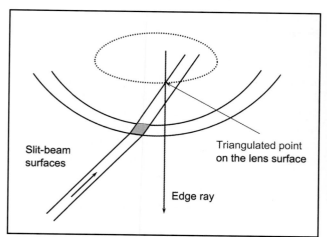

Figure 18-5. Orbscan ray trace triangulation. (Courtesy of Bausch & Lomb.)

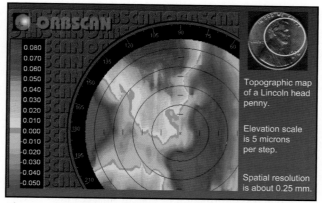

Figure 18-6. Orbscan triangulation map of a Lincoln-head penny (the area in the yellow circle is mapped). (Courtesy of Bausch & Lomb.)

and aqueous humour, because the constituent molecules are very small compared to the illuminating wavelength. In contrast, volume scattering is significant from the lens, iris, and cornea. For that reason, Orbscan sees through the tear film and captures the image of the diffusely scattered light from the corneal volume that is directly illuminated by the slit beam.

Because typical internal scatters are generally smaller than the wavelength of visible light, the magnitude of scattering is inversely proportional to the third or fourth power of the optical wavelength (Rayleigh scattering: λ^4 for spherical particles, λ^3 for cylindrical fibers). As a consequence, the diffusely scattered return consists of the shortest wavelengths found in the interrogating beam (the reason that Tyndall reflections from the cornea appear blue). Calculation of the beam and ray refraction depends on the physiologic refractive indices of the various ocular tissues and humors. Orbscan assumes that the standard physiologic refractive index of air is 1.000; aqueous, 1.336; and the cornea, 1.376.

Triangulation of Complex Surfaces

Triangulation is required to map complex surfaces, such as those of the anterior eye. Ray trace triangulation is required to accurately locate internal surface points when they lie behind an optical interface that refracts the slit beams and the conjugate image rays. The planar slit beam, diffusely reflected from the convex corneal shell, appears as an annular arc in the video image. The outer and inner edges of this arc correspond to the anterior and posterior surfaces of the diffusely reflected volume (Figure 18-5).

To locate a point on the anterior surface, an outer edge point is first detected to sub-pixel accuracy. From the video calibration, the detected edge point is then translat-

ed into its conjugate three-space ray. An example is shown in Figure 18-6. This ray is represented mathematically as:

$$y = U + Vr$$

where the (x, y, z) vector U defines the ray origin at the principal/nodal point of the camera optics; the vector V defines its direction; and the scalar r specifies the distance of a ray point from the origin.

Direct triangulation is used to locate points on the external surface of the cornea. In direct triangulation, a ray is intersected with the calibrated outer surface of the illuminating slit beam. This surface can be mathematically represented as:

$$S(x) = 0$$

where the vector x represents the (x, y, z) coordinates of any valid point on the outer beam surface. Direct triangulation finds r such that $S(U + Vr) = 0$.

Surfaces are triangulated one at a time, from front to back. Thus all the refracting surfaces in front of a desired surface point are known a priori and can be used to calculate all the necessary refractions.

FOUNDATION FOR ANALYSIS

The Measurement of Topography

The Orbscan system's analysis produces a set of data describing the true topographic surfaces of the anterior and posterior cornea, the anterior iris, and the anterior lens. All other measures and displayed maps are derived from these true three-space surfaces. This approach was taken because it avoids the pitfalls of high- and low-frequency noise generated by numerical transformation.

All numerical transformations generate noise. Mathematic extraction of curvature from elevation (differentiation) generates high-frequency noise, while the transformation required to deduce elevation from curvature or slope (integration) generates low-frequency noise. Although high frequency noise is more apparent, low-frequency noise is more difficult to deal with; in addition, *the most important optical aberrations are low-frequency.* Consequently, direct measurement of elevation and computation of curvature were the methods selected to extract the geometric information of optical surfaces in Orbscan.

Another advantage of directly measured topography is that it facilitates surface analysis and display from other points of view. Like other corneal measurement systems, Orbscan aligns with the fixation-reflex axis of the eye, which is appropriate when examining optical properties in the visual zone. However, in contact lens fitting and other procedures in which the apical shape of the cornea is important, the viewpoint should be aligned with the axis of best symmetry of the anterior surface. This alignment can be easily and accurately achieved by rotating the directly measured topographic surfaces in physical space.

Fixation-Reflex Alignment

During data acquisition with Orbscan, the eye is aligned by having the patient fixate on a blinking light source that is coaxial with the video system, while the operator aligns the fixation light reflex with the instrument axis. As slit-scan technology is relatively insensitive to misalignment of the eye, some misalignment is expected. Following data acquisition, the system determines the properly aligned fixation-reflex axis and places it at the center of the map. This fixation-reflex alignment ensures that the map center is always a point of stationary elevation with zero surface slope; for convex surfaces, this point is always a local maximum. Thus, the local surface normal at the map center is aligned with the map axis. This form of alignment is crucial for determining many relative properties that are axis-based, such as axial and tangential curvature. Because the fixation-reflex axis is very sensitive to surface inclination, refractive surgery will almost always alter this axis; for this reason, standard alignment of a postoperative eye is unlikely to coincide exactly with the preoperative alignment.

Surface Rotation

Surfaces measured by Orbscan can be rotated to any other point of view by selecting a view center, which becomes the surface point that is rotated to the map center. The view axis is automatically chosen to be coincident with the local surface normal. Because three-dimensional rotations are not commutative, the meridianal orientation of a rotated view generally depends on all the rotations that preceded it. To eliminate the ambiguity that order dependency might create and to ensure that the rotated meridians are as close as possible to the standard alignment meridians, all surface rotations are computed as simple single-axis rotations from the standard alignment position, which is always centered on the fixation-reflex axis.

Relative vs Absolute Properties

Relative properties depend on the alignment, size, and shape of a reference object; when the reference object changes, so does a relative measure. In contrast, absolute properties are intrinsic properties of the surface and are not alignment dependent; they are measured directly from the surface. Only absolute measurements can identify true ocular landmarks such as optical axes. Although absolute properties are superior, most properties are relative by their nature. In Orbscan, both relative and absolute properties are mapped, as described in Table 18-1.

GEOMETRIC ANALYSIS

Elevation

Looking at an irregular corneal surface is similar to looking at the mountains and valleys of the earth. When drawn to scale, the mean curvature of the earth overwhelms even the most significant topographic features. Hills and valleys are only apparent if elevation is shown with respect to the mean sea level. Similarly, corneal irregularities can only be seen after a reference surface is mathematically removed. Changes in the reference surface, like changes in sea level, can dramatically affect the perceived topography of the corneal landscape, while its true topography (z as a function of x and y) remains unchanged. Figure 18-7 illustrates true elevation, also known as topographic elevation. It is the perpendicular distance z of a point on the cornea from the system reference plane. True elevation data are used to determine pachymetry.

A reference sphere may be oriented with a surface in three different ways: floating, axial, or pinned (Figure 18-8). Floating alignment minimizes the surface fit error with no additional constraints. Axial and pinned alignments each add one additional constraint (indicated by the X in Figure 18-8). Axial alignment forces the sphere center to

TABLE 18-1

PREVIEW OF RELATIVE AND ABSOLUTE PROPERTIES

Geometric or Optical Property	Type	Reference Object (parameters)
Surface topography	Complete	
Normal elevation (floating alignment)	Relative	Surface (size and shape)
Normal elevation (axis alignment)	Relative	Axis + surface (size and shape)
Axial elevation	Relative	Axis + surface (size and shape)
Slope	Relative	Axis
Mean and astigmatic curvatures	Absolute	
Irregular curvature	Absolute	(Aperture size)
Axial pseudo-curvature	Relative	Axis
Tangential and sagittal curvatures	Relative	Axis
Axial thickness and depth	Relative	Axis
Normal thickness and depth	Absolute	
Optical power	Relative	Axis
Normal power	Absolute	

lie on the view axis, while pinned alignment forces the sphere surface to include the view center. Axial pinned alignment employs both constraints.

The advantage of displaying elevation with respect to a best-fitting sphere is that a sphere is rotationally symmetric, and thus it is completely described by its radius and center. Unfortunately, corneal surfaces are not spherical (Figure 18-9). To view elevation asymmetries with respect to the axisymmetric surface that fits the cornea no matter what its shape, it is necessary to select a rotor reference surface. The name rotor is derived from its method of construction, which is to find a surface of revolution by spinning the data surface around the view axis. A rotor (without modifiers) is the mean surface of revolution. The high rotor (or low rotor) is the surface of revolution lying just above (or below) the data surface. Orbscan setup options and parameters that affect the relative elevation of a single topographic surface include surface rotation from the instrument axis; reference surface type (plane, sphere, cone, or rotor); reference surface size, shape, and alignment (floating, axial, or pinned); and elevation direction (normal to the reference surface or axially directed).

Corneal Thickness (Pachymetry)

Corneal thickness is calculated as the distance from the anterior to the posterior surface, in the direction perpendicular to the anterior surface. A typical cornea has a single minimum thickness point, located temporally and inferiorly to the fixation-reflex axis. However, the cornea is not uniformly thick and is not always thinnest at the center. Orbscan pachymetry calculations have been correlated with manual ultrasound pachymetry; in general, Orbscan determinations of corneal thickness are several percent thicker than ultrasound measurements of the same corneas. Orbscan pachymetry measurements can be automatically converted to their acoustic equivalent values, and the correlation factor can be set individually for each Orbscan system. The refractive surgeon can overlay the intended radial and astigmatic keratotomy (RK and AK) cuts on any Orbscan anterior corneal map. The values of minimum corneal thickness are shown on each incision.

Anterior Segment and Chamber Depths

The anterior chamber depth from the posterior cornea to the anterior lens or iris is calculated differently, as the straight-line axial distance between anterior chamber surfaces. Anterior chamber volume is easily determined by integrating this distance across the cornea. In addition, the rate of change of this distance in radial directions can be used to estimate the anterior angle.

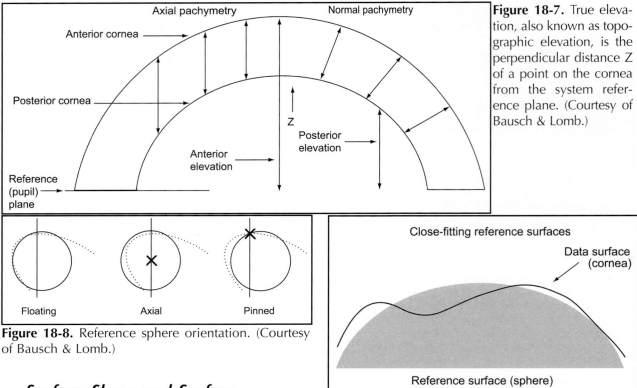

Figure 18-7. True elevation, also known as topographic elevation, is the perpendicular distance Z of a point on the cornea from the system reference plane. (Courtesy of Bausch & Lomb.)

Figure 18-8. Reference sphere orientation. (Courtesy of Bausch & Lomb.)

Figure 18-9. Close-fitting reference surfaces. (Courtesy of Bausch & Lomb.)

Surface Slope and Surface Curvature

Surface slope measures the rate of change of surface elevation in a particular direction. Determination of the radially directed slope of the corneal surfaces is important in contact lens fitting and in the implantation of intracorneal rings for refractive correction. Surface curvature measures the bending (or rate of change of slope, or second derivative) intrinsic to a curve or a surface. Because curvature is inversely related to radius of curvature, a small radius sphere has a large curvature.

Surface curvature can be described as cutting the surface of an object with a plane and then fitting a circle to the plane intersection. The inverse radius of the circle gives the surface curvature in the direction of the plane. Obviously, the value measured is highly dependent on the orientation of the cutting plane. Every surface point has an infinite number of surface normal planes—each containing the local surface normal, but each cutting the surface in a different direction. Thus every point on a smooth surface has a direction-dependent curvature, whose complete description is captured by a mathematical object known as a tensor. Orbscan calculates the complete curvature tensor field from the derivatives of the fitted topographic surfaces. From this tensor field, the curvature at any surface point and in any direction can be directly calculated.

A theorem of differential geometry states that every point on a smooth surface has a minimum and a maximum

curvature (called principal curvatures) that lie in perpendicular surface normal planes. Thus the curvature at any smooth surface point can be completely specified by three independent quantities: the minimum and maximum (principal) curvatures and their directions. Two curvatures at a point in nonprincipal directions do not contain sufficient information to construct the complete curvature tensor.

Curvature of an optical surface is directly related to the focusing power of a normally incident bundle of light rays. Because of this property, curvature is often expressed in diopters (the unit of optical power) and is often referred to as power, which is a potential cause of confusion. Orbscan emphasizes the distinction between curvature and power by exclusively reserving the name power for optical properties. Curvature, whether expressed in standard geometric units (inverse meters, 1/m), radius of curvature units (millimeters, mm), or scaled by diopters, is always called curvature by Orbscan.

Three concepts are important in understanding Orbscan's mapping of surface curvature. First, curvature applies only to a single surface. In contrast, optical power is generally calculated for a sequence of surfaces (always beginning with the anterior cornea). Second, surface curvature is not single-valued, but direction dependent. A

TABLE 18-2 ASSUMED REFRACTIVE INDICES AND TYPICAL SPHERICAL CURVATURES				
Ocular Surface	Index Type	Posterior Index	Curvature (Geometric)	Curvature (Diopters)
Keratometric cornea	Standard keratometric	1.3375	128 1/mm	43.2 D
Anterior cornea	Physiologic	1.376	128 1/mm	48.1 D
Posterior cornea	Physiologic	1.336	149 1/mm	–6.0 D
Anterior lens	Physiologic	1.425	98 1/mm	8.7 D

complete specification of curvature requires three values: the two principal curvatures and their orientation. As a color contour map (without overlays) can only show the variation of one value, many different curvature maps are used to display combinations of the three principal values in useful ways. These maps are grouped into two families: absolute local curvatures (mean, astigmatic, and irregular), and relative axis-based curvatures (axial, tangential, and sagittal). The third concept important in understanding Orbscan maps is that curvature expressed in diopters is proportional to an assumed refractive index difference. The assumed index difference may be physiologic (the real value averaged over the population) or it may be invented (eg, the standard keratometric index). Table 18-2 lists the assumed posterior indices (air = 1) for each optical surface in the anterior segment, together with their typical curvatures, expressed in both geometric and diopter units. Note that the curvature (in diopters) of the posterior cornea is negative, not because the geometric curvature is negative but because the interfacial index difference is negative ($\Delta n = -0.040 = 1.336 - 1.376$). The standard keratometric index is applicable only to the anterior cornea. When so applied, the anterior cornea is referred to as the keratometric cornea.

Mean and Astigmatic Curvature

Mean curvature is a measure of absolute local sphericity. A local sphere is the one that best fits a point and its surface derivatives. The inverse radius of this sphere is an absolute measure of the local spherical component of curvature. Because it is absolute, mean curvature is intrinsic to the surface and is independent of surface alignment. Absoluteness is important in the diagnosis of certain corneal diseases like keratoconus, as it ensures that any geometric abnormality will appear as it exists. Hence, keratoconus appears as a symmetric local maximum, because the mean curvature of a cone increases toward its apex.

Maps of mean curvature display the variation of local sphericity. Thus, the mean curvature of a normal cornea is typically very uniform, even when its astigmatism is significant. Mean curvature typically filters out global astigmatism in favor of the local spherical component. As a rule, any residual astigmatism seen in a mean curvature map is greatly reduced and rotated 90 degrees from the real astigmatism. To see the local axes of astigmatism, the principal direction's overlay is used.

Astigmatic curvature is a measure of absolute local cylinder. Astigmatic curvature typically filters out the global spherical component in favor of astigmatism or local cylinder. As maps of astigmatic curvature display the variation of local cylinder, an eye with regular astigmatism will have a fairly uniform astigmatic map. The bowtie pattern typically associated with astigmatism and seen in axis-based maps (eg, axial, tangential, and sagittal curvatures) is not physical, but is really an artifact of the measurement.

Irregular Curvature

A normal but ametropic eye with regular astigmatism is correctable with spherocylindrical spectacles. Surface irregularity includes the curvature variation of an optical surface that cannot be corrected with a spherocylindrical lens, thereby producing an uncorrectable loss in visual acuity.

As the mean and astigmatic curvature maps of a normal eye are fairly uniform, the variation of these curvatures is a measure of surface irregularity. Irregular curvature is the statistical combination of the standard deviations of the mean and astigmatic curvatures, measured over a local aperture (typically 1 mm in diameter). Surface irregularity caused by incisional keratotomy, such as the RK artifact, is recognizable in maps of irregular curvature.

Axial, Tangential, and Sagittal Curvatures

Axial, tangential, and sagittal curvatures are relative properties measured with respect to the arbitrary view axis. Because the measurement directions radiate from or encircle this axis, these axis-based maps always contain a conspicuous axial artifact, the familiar bowtie pattern seen in Figure 18-10. The direction of this artifact effectively locates the meridians of astigmatism, but only with respect to the view axis.

Unlike absolute curvature, which is a property of the surface and requires no reference object, axis-based curvature maps change dramatically when their axes are repositioned. Axis-based maps also distort corneal abnormalities, like keratoconus, making it impossible to locate the true conical apex.

The curvature of an aligned sphere is correctly determined by any of the axis-based curvatures and the mean curvature (which gives the correct value even when the sphere is off center). Axial curvature, however, is not a true measure of curvature, but is a spherical equivalent not applicable to aspheres or to asymmetric surfaces. Tangential and sagittal maps, although true measures of curvature, do not contain sufficient information to construct the complete curvature tensor, except for the special case of aligned axisymmetric surfaces.

THEORY OF OPTICAL ANALYSIS

Optical Power

Optical power is defined as the posterior refractive index divided by the posterior focal length:

$$P = n_2/f_2$$

(Figure 18-11, left panel). Light rays, originally parallel to an arbitrary power axis, are refracted by both surfaces of the cornea and are brought to focus on the power axis, which is also refracted. The refractive index is included in the definition so that power measured in either direction is the same. Optical performance can be calculated from topographic surface data when the material refractive indices are known (see Table 18-2).

Peripheral rays are brought to a shorter focus than central paraxial rays. This is illustrated in Figure 18-11. This spherical aberration is apparent in optical power maps of the cornea, which show increasing power peripherally. When astigmatism is present, the familiar bowtie pattern will also be seen. This pattern arises from the interaction of light, collimated along the line of sight, with a smooth optical surface or sequence of surfaces. Optically, the bowtie pattern is real, while geometrically it is an artifact.

Normal Power

Normal power is a measure of the normally incident mean focusing power of a sequence of surfaces, beginning

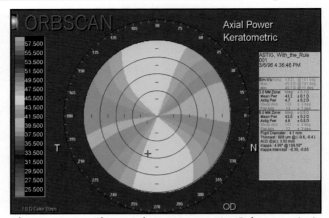

Figure 18-10. The axial power map in Orbscan, similar to the sagittal map from Placido systems, produces its image using only the Placido rings. (Courtesy of Bausch & Lomb.)

with the anterior cornea (Figure 18-11, right panel). Unlike optical power, which is a relative property defined with respect to some arbitrary power axis, normal power is an attempt to define an optically relevant absolute measure.

Normal power can be calculated locally for any point on the anterior corneal surface by orienting a ray pencil (a tight bundle of paraxial rays) initially perpendicular to the point of interest. The ray pencil is mathematically propagated through the specified surface sequence and the mean paraxial focus calculated. The normal power is calculated from the mean focal length.

Because the normal power of an anterior surface point is independently calculated, neither a common focal point nor power axis exists. However, when the optical power axis is aligned to the local surface normal, normal power and paraxial optical power are equivalent. Hence, normal power is the paraxial portion of optical power as seen from any point on the cornea.

Optical Axes

An optical axis can be defined for any two surfaces by the alignment of a point source and its two catoptric images. Thus, an optical axis is the refracted light ray oriented perpendicularly to both surfaces. In tilted optical systems, like the human eye, the optical axis is not a straight line, but is bent or curved by refraction occurring between the two defining surfaces.

Normal pachymetry and normal anterior segment depth are both distances measured along the refracted light ray that is initially perpendicular to the anterior corneal surface. Maps of these quantities each show a local extreme, which locates a two-surface optical axis. The local minimum in corneal thickness is the origin of the corneal optical axis, as defined by its anterior and posterior surfaces. Similarly, the local maximum in anterior segment depth is

Figure 18-11. Optical power and normal power. (Courtesy of Bausch & Lomb.)

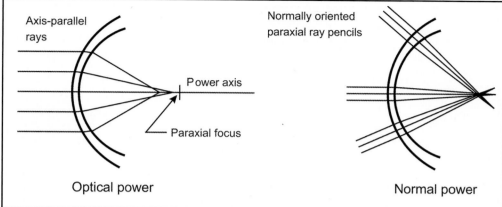

the origin of the anterior optical axis, as defined by the anterior cornea and lens.

Both of these optical axes lie close to the traditional optical axis of the eye, which is defined by the confluence of the four Purkinje images. However, because four images can not generally be brought into alignment, the traditional axis is undefined for many eyes. When the traditional axis exists, it is coincident with both the corneal and anterior segment optical axes, which always exist.

OCULAR LANDMARKS USED BY ORBSCAN (SURFACE CENTERS)

In general, a surface center is any well-defined point on a surface, usually the anterior cornea. A landmark center is any uniquely defined physical or optical point of the eye, whereas a reference center is defined by the arbitrary reference object employed. Fixed centers are points on ocular surfaces that rotate with the eye and any reference objects, whereas movable centers are dependent on the rotational point of view (eg, entrance pupil center). Nine centers used by Orbscan are defined in Table 18-3. The tabulated accuracy reflects the theoretical precision with which these centers can be calculated from a set of topographic surfaces.

OPTICAL SURFACE IRREGULARITY

Irregularity is a statistical term that describes the variation of values in a data set. Optical surface irregularity is proportional to the standard deviation of surface curvature. As applied to the Orbscan, it is a spatial variation in curvature and quantified as the statistical combination of the standard deviations of the mean and toric curvatures. Irregularity is calculated for a specific area using the following formula:

$$Irregularity = I = [(\sigma(\kappa))^2 + (\sigma(\Delta\kappa))^2]^{1/2}$$
$$where$$
$$\sigma = standard\ deviation$$
$$\kappa = mean\ curvature\ \frac{\kappa_1 + \kappa_2}{2}$$
$$\Delta\kappa = toric\ curvature\ |\kappa_1 - \kappa_2|$$
$$\kappa_1\ and\ \kappa_2\ represent\ the\ principal\ curvatures$$

The Orbscan system calculates irregularity using the following method. First, initial parameters are set using default values that can be changed in an initialization file. The beginning default pupil diameter is 3 mm, and the increment for increasing the diameter is 2 mm. With these settings, there are four possible irregularity zones on the pupil (3, 5, 7, and 9 mm). Next, the algorithm defines the sampling rules for each zone. Nine concentric rings are defined in the 3-mm zone; each ring is divided into segments using a formula to ensure uniform sampling density. (For example, the center ring has three segments, the second ring has nine segments, the third has 15 segments, etc.) The center point of each segment is defined. In the third step, the algorithm calculates all the map zone statistics at each center point, including the principal and mean, toric curvatures, etc. Then, the algorithm calculates the standard deviation of these values for the first zone and applies the formula for calculating irregularity. These calculations are repeated for each zone.

Optical surface irregularity is proportional to the standard deviation of surface curvature. Consequently, only axis-independent surface curvatures are used in the calculation, as only they are true surface properties. These include the mean curvature, which is a measure of local surface sphericity, and astigmatic curvature, which is a measure of local cylinder. As both curvature variations are important, the standard deviations of the mean and astigmatic curvature are statistically combined (their variances are added) to yield the irregularity in standard curvature units (reciprocal meters). Curvature in reciprocal meters can be converted to diopters by multiplying it by the surface refractive index

TABLE 18-3

OCULAR LANDMARKS (SURFACE CENTERS) USED BY ORBSCAN

Surface Center	Definition	Type	Accuracy	Map mark (typically white)
Fixation reflex	Corneal reflex point of a fixating patient, measured by a coaxial optical system and corrected for acquisition misalignment	Fixed landmark	High	Oblique cross, x
Pachymetry minimum	Anterior corneal point with minimum normal thickness; defines the 2-surface optical axis of the cornea	Fixed landmark	Low	C
Anterior segment maximum	Anterior corneal point with maximum normal anterior segment depth; defines the 2-surface optical axis of the anterior cornea and lens combination	Fixed landmark	Low	S
Anterior corneal apex	Geometric center of the cornea, or the location where the axis of best anterior symmetry intersects the anterior surface	Fixed landmark	Low	Triangle
Entrance pupil	Physical pupil of the eye imaged through the cornea. Its center is taken to be the geometric centroid of the pupil image.	Movable landmark	Medium	Dot
Sphere center (of an axisymmetric reference object)	View axis projection of its apical center of curvature	Movable reference	Exact	Circle
View center	Point at which the view axis pierces the surface; placed at the map center in standard alignment	Movable reference	Exact	Black cross (map center)
Summit	Highest surface point measured with respect to the current view axis; placed on the view center (and therefore at map center) in standard alignment of a convex surface	Movable reference	High	
Instrument or system center	Point at which the instrument axis (defined by the video camera) pierces the data surface; if located on the unrotated anterior cornea, is a measure of acquisition misalignment	Fixed reference	High	

difference, which is 0.3375 for the keratometric surface. Thus, the diopter equivalent of irregularity is about one-third the curvature measure in reciprocal meters.

Clinical Implications of Irregularity Calculations

Optical surface irregularity is important to the refractive surgeon, because it often represents a loss in BCVA. A regular astigmatism has a low irregularity, while an irregular astigmatism has a high degree of irregularity. Higher-order aberrations may also have a high degree of irregularity. Measures of irregularity may also be useful as a supporting indicator (but not the sole indicator) in evaluating keratoconus. A 3-mm irregularity greater than 1.5 or a 5-mm irregularity greater than 2.0 may be an early sign of keratoconus, while a 3-mm irregularity greater than 2.0 or a 5-mm irregularity greater than 2.5 may indicate full keratoconus. Irregularity cannot be corrected with spherocylindrical lenses.

CLINICAL EXAMPLES

Risk of Ectasia

One of the most frequent uses of Orbscan is in the screening of patients for LASIK surgery. The risk of ectasia can be accurately assessed using six indices: the number of abnormal maps using the normal band scale, a variance of more than 1.00 D in astigmatism between the eyes, keratometric or corneal steepness on the mean power map, a posterior surface float greater than 0.050 mm (the difference between the highest and lowest spots) (Figure 18-12), 3-mm and 5-mm irregularity (Figure 18-13), and a minimum peripheral corneal thickness that is not at least 20 microns greater than the thickness of the central cornea (Figure 18-14). Although the 0.050 mm dimension is critical to diagnosing an ectatic disease such as keratoconus of PMD, a reading over 0.040 with other suspicious maps is also a potential indicator.

Figure 18-12 shows a posterior float of approximately 0.063 mm, indicated by the dark reddish color near the center of the posterior elevation map (upper right). A posterior float greater than 0.050 raises a strong red flag for forme fruste keratoconus or PMD, and confirms the diagnosis if supported by other maps and measurements. Note that when the posterior float is greater than 0.050, posterior elevation is rarely the only abnormal map. In this example, the pachymetry map shows a significant irregularity in corneal thickness, with a central area whose thickness is

only approximately 0.050 mm—two indices suggesting that LASIK may not be appropriate for this patient.

Figure 18-13 shows surface irregularity of 2.1 D in the 3-mm zone and 2.2 D in the 5-mm zone. It does not indicate forme fruste keratoconus in and of itself, but raises suspicion to look for other signs, such as the number of abnormal maps or a posterior float greater than 0.050 mm (50 microns). Irregularity at 3.00 mm and 5.00 mm may simply indicate the presence of higher-order aberrations without pathology, so this index should only be used in conjunction with other findings to diagnose keratoconus.

In the lower left corner of the pachymetry map (Figure 18-14), the thinnest area is more than 30 microns thinner than the central cornea (marked in red). Peripheral pachymetry measurements in which the peripheral cornea is not at least 20 microns thicker than the central cornea may be a sign of keratoconus, which should be corroborated with other observations. Another potential source of concern is a cornea in which the thinnest point is outside the central 5 mm of the cornea.[1]

One abnormal map on the Orbscan normal band scale does not usually indicate forme fruste keratoconus, but requires patient education or having the patient return for monitoring of changes in 6 to 12 months. Two abnormal maps may indicate early keratoconus; or, if the posterior float is abnormal with a slightly thinner cornea (less than 500 microns), two abnormal maps may still indicate keratoconus depending on other variables described in this chapter. If a patient has two abnormal maps but no indication of forme fruste keratoconus, surface ablation would likely be a better procedure than LASIK for this patient. Three or more abnormal maps is a contraindication to corneal surgery and often indicates a high risk of post-LASIK ectasia.[2]

A difference of more than 1.00 D cylinder between the eyes, increasing cylinder over time, a bending of the bowtie in the axial topography map, or against-the-rule astigmatism are also potential indicators of keratoconus that can be detected with the Orbscan.[3] Since keratoconus is known to be an asymmetric condition, one eye usually progresses faster than the other.[4] A higher risk of keratoectasia is also suggested by a K reading of more than 46.00 D at the steepest point on the Orbscan keratometric mean power map.

Anterior Chamber Map

The anterior chamber map, which shows the depth of the anterior chamber, can be useful in surgical planning for phakic IOLs. The endothelial anterior map (Figure 18-15) shows the true available space. This map is likely to grow in its usefulness in the future as the use of phakic IOLs increases.

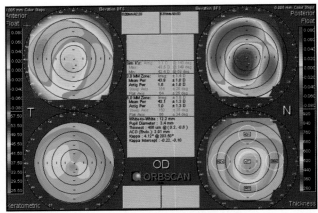

Figure 18-12. This Orbscan quad map shows a posterior float of approximately 0.063 mm, a strong red flag for forme fruste keratoconus or PMD. (Courtesy of John Vukich, MD.)

Post-LASIK Follow-Up

After approximately 1 month following LASIK, the Orbscan system may be used to assess problems such as dry eye and corneal edema and to map the change in corneal shape as a reference for an enhancement procedure. Earlier than 1 month, reflections from the recovering tear film or corneal edema may produce an Orbscan reading that incorrectly suggests ectasia.

Dry Eye and Corneal Edema

Dry eye that continues for more than 1 month after LASIK can be evaluated in a distinctive Orbscan map, shown in Figure 18-16. Note the irregularity on the keratometric mean power map, as well as the significant missing data points. These anomalies confirm that the maps are not reliable. After artificial tears were instilled, the images were normal. An Orbscan map with irregularity on the anterior elevation map and with thinning present on pachymetry is an indicator of dry eye.[5]

Corneal edema also produces a distinctive Orbscan map (Figure 18-17). The specular reflection from corneal edema might be interpreted as Descemet's layer, and therefore the edema will often look similar to a case of ectasia.

Post-LASIK Enhancement Planning

LASIK surgery results in significant changes to the corneal surface geometry (Figure 18-18). The blue areas in the center and at the edges of the Orbscan map show the changes in the cornea that result from LASIK, including a flattening of the center and sides of the cornea with respect to the reference sphere. Although the map appears to show

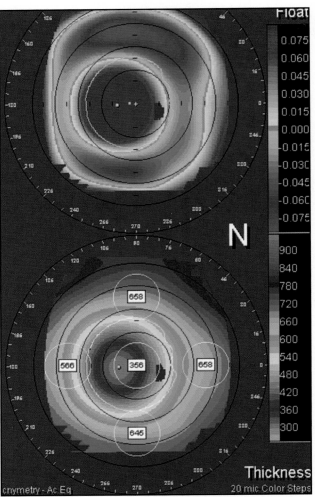

Figure 18-13. This Orbscan quad map shows surface irregularity of 2.1 D in the 3-mm zone and of 2.2 D in the 5-mm zone. This suggests that the clinician should look for other signs, such as the number of abnormal maps or a posterior float greater than 0.050 mm (50 microns).

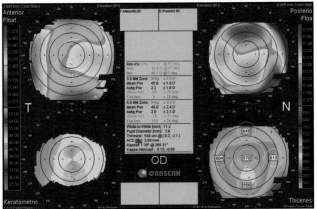

Figure 18-14. In the pachymetry map at the lower left corner of this quad map, the thinnest area is more than 30 microns thinner than the central cornea.

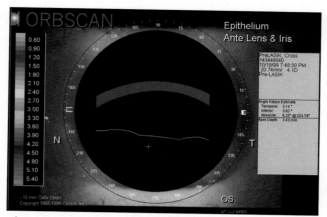

Figure 18-15. The endothelial anterior chamber map shows the depth of the anterior chamber.

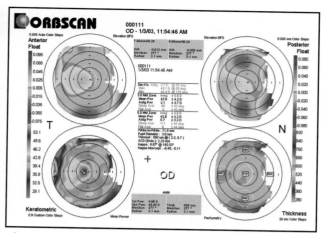

Figure 18-16. Post-LASIK dry eye.

that the cornea is concave, this is not the case; the depression in the center of the cornea is lower than the reference sphere but not lower than the outer corneal edges. A three-dimensional Orbscan map of the post-LASIK cornea provides the surgeon with a means to visualize the cornea and determine an enhancement strategy when an enhancement procedure is desired.

NONREFRACTIVE USES OF ORBSCAN TECHNOLOGY

Pellucid Marginal Degeneration

Pellucid marginal degeneration (PMD) is a rare form of corneal ectasia, with an arcuate band of corneal thinning in the inferior cornea. The Orbscan system can be used in the diagnosis of patients with this disorder. PMD typically presents with topography similar to Figure 18-19. Note the classic kissing bird appearance in the bottom left keratometric axial map, as well as the extreme peripheral elevation on the anterior and posterior floats (upper right and left maps). Note also that the steepest part of the cornea is located more inferiorly in PMD, and the axial topography shows a bending of the bowtie pattern. The keratometric mean map shows a localized inferior corneal steepening, especially in the peripheral areas.

Keratoconus

Diagnosis of keratoconus is facilitated by the use of Orbscan maps, which show the magnitude and location of corneal thinning and protrusion (Figure 18-20). Orbscan

maps can also be used to detect early keratoconus (which always appears initially on the posterior surface) and document the progression of the disorder. Note the normal pachymetry map and the irregularity in the 3- and 5-mm zones, and the deeper cone on the posterior surface. The mean power map shows Ks in the inferior cornea greater than 54 D. Indices for the detection of keratoconus are described above, in the discussion of the risk of post-LASIK ectasia.

RAY TRACE ANALYSIS AS A DIAGNOSTIC TOOL

Ray trace analysis can calculate optical properties even more informative than power. The retinal point spread function (PSF) is the retinal image of a point of light. It contains all the information needed to reconstruct what the patient sees. The PSF describes how an object point is aberrated (spread out) in the retinal image. PSF size and shape indicate the ocular aberration. In an emmetropic, unaberrated eye, the image is concentrated at one point. In an astigmatic eye, the image takes on an elongated shape, while in monocular diplopia the image is double peaked. Figure 18-21 shows an original picture and a simulated retinal image, produced with the retinal PSF, in a patient with monocular diplopia.

The patient complained of double vision, halos, and night driving difficulties—but only for the left eye. Ray trace analysis through the anterior corneal surface did not reveal any visual impairment. When both corneal surfaces were ray-traced, the left eye showed several ghost images that are associated with the posterior corneal surface. An analysis of posterior elevation maps showed that each eye

Figure 18-17. Post-LASIK corneal edema. (Courtesy of Dan Durrie, MD.)

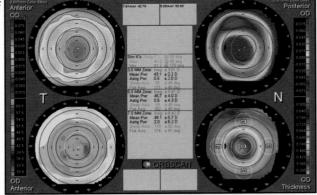

Figure 18-18. Corneal topography S/P myopic LASIK. (Courtesy of John Vukich, MD.)

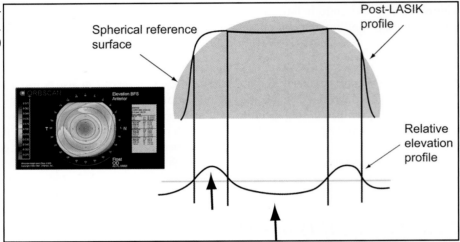

had a posterior cone, but the off-axis eccentricity of the OS cone resulted in the optical aberrations reported by the patient. Retreatment was not undertaken, because of concern that it would increase the posterior ectasia and the associated visual impairment.

ORBSCAN DIAGNOSTICS AND WAVEFRONT TECHNOLOGY

A unique aspect of the Bausch & Lomb Zyoptix Diagnostic Workstation is that it combines wavefront aberrometry information with data from the Orbscan system. This allows for potentially greater data capture and optimal results based on that data. Functions such as pachymetry and the new 2-mm to 1-mm laser flying spot placement allow the Zyoptix system to be one of the few systems that is tissue sparing when moving from conventional to wavefront LASIK procedures. Furthermore, it is becoming apparent that wavefront data can also enhance topography diagnostic capabilities. In a study reported by Pepose and Applegate,[6] posterior float signs of ectasia noted on the Orbscan Diagnostic System were differenti-

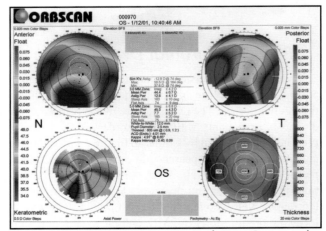

Figure 18-19. PMD. (Courtesy of Tim Cavanaugh, MD.)

ated from PMD and keratoconus based on wavefront data. Patients with PMD tended to have higher degrees of peripheral aberrations on the Zywave system, including trefoil, whereas patients with keratoconus tended to have

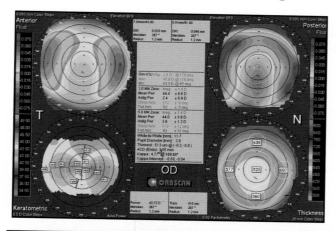

Figure 18-20. Keratoconus.

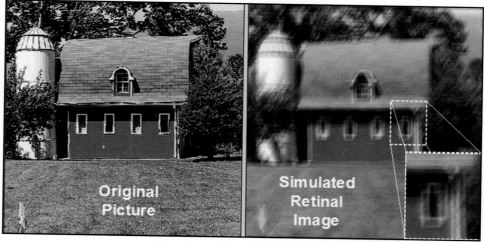

Figure 18-21. Reconstruction of the patient's view of an object using retinal point spread function in ray trace analysis. (Courtesy of Bausch & Lomb.)

higher degrees of coma. Combining the wavefront data with the Orbscan data will enhance diagnostic capabilities and wavefront data, potentially improving outcomes.

SUMMARY

This chapter has described the Bausch & Lomb Orbscan Anterior Segment Analysis System, focusing on the principles underlying its measurement and analysis technology. The Orbscan system provides unique tools for the refractive surgeon to use in the evaluation and diagnosis of visual disorders of the anterior segment.

ACKNOWLEDGMENT

The author thanks Barry Eagan, Director of Optical Systems Design & Numerical Analysis for Bausch & Lomb, Rochester, NY, for his assistance in the development of this chapter.

REFERENCES

1. Pflugfelder SC, Liu Z, Feuer W, Verm A. Corneal thickness indices discriminate between keratoconus and contact lens-induced corneal thinning. *Ophthalmology.* 2002;109(12):2336–2341.

2. Tanabe T, Oshika T, Tomodokoro A, Amano S, Tanaka S, Kuroda T, Maeda N, Tokunaga T, Miyata K. Standardized color-coded scales for anterior and posterior elevation maps of scanning slit corneal topography. *Ophthalmology.* 2002;109(7):1298–1302.

3. Davis LJ, Schechtman KB, Begley CG, Shin JA, Zadnik K. Repeatability of refraction and corrected visual acuity in keratoconus. The CLEK study group: collaborative longitudinal evaluation of keratoconus. *Optom Vis Sci.* 1998;75(12):887–896.

4. Zadnik K, Steger-May MA, Fink BA, et al for the CLEK study group. Between-eye asymmetry in keratoconus. *Cornea.* 2002;21:671–679.

5. Liu Z, Pflugfelder SC. Corneal thickness is reduced in dry eye. *Cornea.* 1999;18(4):403–407.

6. Pepose JS, Applegate RA. Making sense out of wavefront sensing. *Am J Ophthalmol.* 2005;139(2):335–343.

Chapter 19

Artemis VHF Digital Ultrasound Technology

Dan Z. Reinstein, MD and Ronald H. Silverman, PhD

Digital signal processing of ultrasound backscatter was pioneered by Coleman and coworkers at the Bio-Acoustic Research Facility in the Department of Ophthalmology of the Weill Medical College, Cornell University (New York) in the 1980s. In the early 1990s we began the integration of very high-frequency (VHF) probes originally designed for quality control in the metallurgical industry into the Cornell University three-dimensional ultrasound scanning prototype. Pavlin, Sherar, and Foster at the University of Toronto also produced a VHF ultrasound scanner, but it was based only on conventional analog signal processing.[1] The Toronto prototype became a commercial unit called the Ultrasound Biomicroscope (UBM) manufactured by Humphrey Zeiss (Dublin, CA). The Cornell prototype and patents were assigned to Ultralink, LLC (St. Petersburg, Fla). They have subsequently developed and commercialized the first Artemis VHF digital ultrasound arc B-scanner.

The Artemis (Figure 19-1) was created in conjunction with Cornell University researchers Reinstein, Silverman, Raevsky, Coleman, and colleagues,[2] and is based on their intellectual property and patents from the Bio-Acoustic Research Facility in the Department of Ophthalmology of the Weill Medical College of Cornell University.

The Artemis was designed to help ophthalmologists in all disciplines, but particularly in refractive, cataract, and presbyopic surgery to improve anatomical diagnosis for surgical planning and postoperative diagnostic monitoring. The Artemis' primary functions are to provide very high resolution ultrasound B-scan imaging of the anterior and posterior segment, high-precision three-dimensional mapping of individual corneal layers, and three-dimensional mapping of anterior segment dimensions and axial length by a combined additional immersion A-scan probe. The Artemis is designed to scan in an arc of adjustable radius, thus following the curved surfaces of either the cornea, the iris plane, or the globe, and enabling wide segments (up to 15 mm) to be imaged within one scan sweep.

The resolution of the Artemis, when set to scan cornea, is sufficient to distinguish individual corneal layers such as the epithelium, stromal component of the flap, residual stromal bed, and others in three-dimensions thanks to multi-meridional scanning. The Artemis VHF digital ultrasound technology is able to consistently detect internal corneal lamellar interfaces (such as the keratectomy track) because of the permanent "mechanical" interface present even years after surgery, and despite total optical transparency. Analog UBM is not able to image the interface consistently because analog processing does not produce a high enough signal-to-noise ratio between interface echo complex and the surrounding tissue. OCT has been shown to be capable of detecting the interface in LASIK in the early postoperative period, but this ability diminishes with time as edema subsides in the cornea and the optical properties of the corneal lamellar interface homogenize. We have scanned former non-freeze keratomileusis patients more than 10 years after surgery and have been able to clearly delineate, end-to-end, the stromal lamellar interface.

In 1993, we reported the first confirmed measurement of the epithelium of the cornea in vivo using VHF ultrasound, demonstrating that the acoustic interfaces that were being detected were indeed located spatially at the epithelial surface and at the interface between epithelial cells and the surface of Bowman's layer.[3] We also reported the first high-precision three-dimensional thickness mapping of the corneal epithelium and flap.[4] This system, by acquiring a series of parallel, rectilinear B-scans, was capable of mapping the epithelial layer thickness within the central 3- to 4-mm area. By using digital signal processing techniques (eg, the I-scan), a 2.0-micron reproducibility for epithelial thickness measurements was obtained.[5] The I-scan is an A-scan-like trace produced by digital processing of the stored radiofrequency ultrasonic data. The trace represents the instantaneous energy intensity with time, as opposed to the average amplitude as is represented by the conventionally employed A-scan. Previous studies demonstrated that the I-scan more than doubles the measurement precision afforded by the analog A-scan process.[5] We further improved epithelial thickness measurement precision to 1.3 microns by increasing the fidelity of the digitized signal.[6] Measurement precision within the cornea in LASIK has been formally tested and published. The axial measurement precision within 9-mm wide corneal scans is approximately 1 µm.[2] When scans are expanded to include the entire anterior segment (15-mm width), the axial precision remains similar, while the lateral precision for measuring angle-to-angle is 0.15 mm, and sulcus-to-sulcus is 0.20 mm.[7] Axial measurement precision will be higher than lateral measurement precision because axial measurements are made from analysis of data within scan lines (pulse-echo axis), while lateral measurements are made from analysis of data between adjacent scan lines.

This Artemis VHF digital ultrasound system has been used to characterize central epithelial lenticular anatomy and to demonstrate that the power of the epithelium is not constant from eye to eye.[8] We have also examined the shape of Bowman's layer,[9] the measurement of anterior corneal scars for planning therapeutic keratectomy,[10–12] the quantitative analysis of corneal scarring (haze) after PRK,[13] and the measurement of the depth of radial keratotomy incisions.[14] In 1999, we were the first to publish on the analysis of epithelial and stromal changes after lamellar corneal surgery, demonstrating significant epithelial changes after uncomplicated LASIK and the masking of stromal surface irregularities that were producing optical complications.[6] This chapter will focus on this application.

ARTEMIS TECHNOLOGY

Details of the scanning and signal processing technology have been described comprehensively elsewhere.[2,3,10,15] Briefly, a broadband 50 MHz VHF ultrasound transducer (bandwidth approximately 10 to 60 MHz) is swept by a reverse arc high-precision mechanism to acquire B-scans as arcs that follow the surface contour of anterior or posterior segment structures of interest. The Artemis possesses a unique scan-arc adjustment mechanism to enable maximum perpendicularity (and signal to noise ratio) to be obtained for scanning any of the different curvatures within the globe (cornea, iris plane, retina). Ultrasound data is first digitized and stored. The digitized ultrasound data is then transformed, using Cornell digital signal processing technology. Digital signal processing significantly reduces noise and enhances signal-to-noise ratio. We have

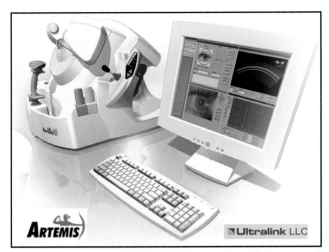

Figure 19-1. Artemis 2: Artemis VHF digital ultrasound 50 MHz 3D arc B-scan (Ultralink, LLC).

demonstrated that using digital signal processing on 50 MHz ultrasound data doubles resolution and increases measurement precision by a factor of three when compared to conventional analog processing of the same very high-frequency data.[5] Scanners produced by Paradigm Medical (Salt Lake City, Utah) (UBM), OTI (35 MHz), and others employ only analog ultrasound processing. As a result of a unique, coaxial, simultaneous video image capture at each scan position (Figure 19-2), a correlation of measurements made from the ultrasound scans can be formed into visible ocular landmarks, such as the corneal reflex. This enables accurate three-dimensional reconstructions made from multiple meridional scans and the production of corneal mapping. Simultaneous optical and ultrasound imaging also enables the anterior segment sulcus-to-sulcus distance to be determined in a verified plane, such as the visual axis for surgical planning in phakic IOL surgery.

For the first time, it also enables localization of the optimum implantation site for devices, such as scleral expansion bands, that need to be positioned based on internal (invisible) landmarks. The Artemis possesses a software application that will give the surgeon external landmarks, identifiable under the operating microscope, that locate the lens equator based on a caliper measurement from the corneal reflex (Figure 19-3). The intersection of the cornea with the line-of-sight is indicated by an arrow and the letter C. The lens equator plane is localized based on the ultrasound image, and the eternal intersection of this plane at the scleral surface is localized. The distance from C to the equatorial plane is identified for exact localization of the scleral implant to achieve maximum effect. The thickness of the sclera is provided in order to maximize depth without intraoperative exposure of the choroid.

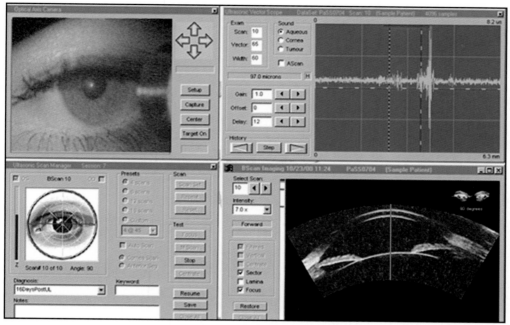

Figure 19-2. Artemis advanced control display panel.

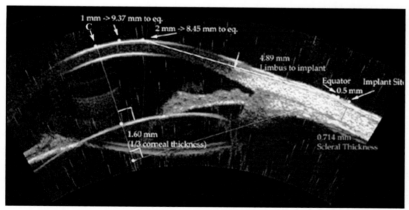

Figure 19-3. Annotated arc B-scan ultrasound image showing all measurements required for the accurate implantation of a scleral expansion band.

While Artemis scanning is a noncontact test, it does require an ultrasonic standoff medium, and thus provides the advantages of immersion scanning. The Artemis 2 was designed specifically to enable quick set-up of this immersion scanning by a novel (patented) reverse-immersion technique. The patient sits and positions his or her chin on a three-point forehead and chin rest, while placing the eye into a soft rimmed eye-cup akin to a swimming goggle (Figure 19-4). The sterile coupling fluid fills the compartment in front of the eye and the scanning is performed via an ultrasonically transparent (sterile) membrane, without the need for a speculum. Thus, there is no contact by the scanner probe with the eye. Performing a three-dimensional scan set with the Artemis requires 2 to 3 minutes for each eye.

CLINICAL UTILITY

Figure 19-5 demonstrates an arc B-scan taken along the horizontal plane of the cornea of a patient 4 months after LASIK. The interfaces of saline-epithelium (E), epithelium-Bowman's (B), the keratectomy interface (K), and the posterior surface (endothelial-aqueous) (P) are clearly visualized along the 9-mm chord-length of the preoperative B-scan. The keratectomy interface can be seen with an entrance track nasally (S), coursing temporally to a stop at the hinge (H). Magnification of the keratome entrance position shows that the flap was not fully distended and Bowman's was not fully apposed, potentially inducing astigmatism and/or increasing the risk of epithelial ingrowth. The interface track has a small irregularity (I)

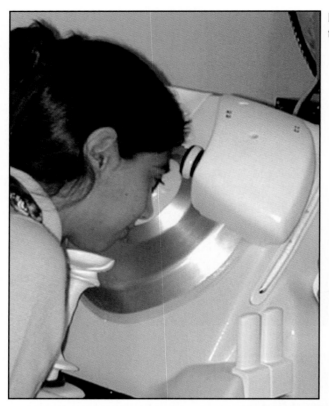

Figure 19-4. Patient demonstrating the simple set-up of the reverse immersion scanning system.

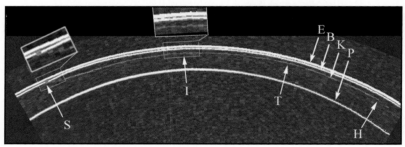

Figure 19-5. Horizontal B-scan through the visual axis of a cornea 4 months post-LASIK.

(magnified insert), perhaps caused by a patient squeeze during passage of the keratome. The flap can be seen to be thicker temporally and thinner (T) nasally.

This C12 display configuration shown in Figure 19-6 forms the mainstay, and state-of-the-art, in anatomical diagnosis after LASIK. Figure 19-6 shows such a display created from scans of the right cornea of a patient scanned before and 6 months after LASIK for myopia of –4.75 –0.25 x 55. Uncorrected visual acuity was 20/16 with a residual subjective manifest refraction of plano. Videokeratographic examination showed the customary central flattening with a small surface with-the-rule astigmatism. The lamellar interface was only faintly detectable in places by slit lamp examination.

This display of twelve pachymetric maps was designed as a standardized layered pachymetric summary of corneal anatomical changes following LASIK. We have chosen to name this presentation a Reinstein C12 diagnostic display,

for it consists of twelve corneal pachymetric topographical maps of the same cornea before and after LASIK. Each map depicts the local thickness of a given corneal layer represented on a color scale in μm. The Reinstein C12 display was designed as a layout of map groupings by time, anatomic depth, and calculation. Columns 1 and 2 depict maps pre- and postoperatively. Within these columns, the rows represent depth within the cornea. Thus the first column depicts the thickness profiles of the preoperative corneal epithelium (Figure 19-6, map 1), full stroma (Figure 19-6, map 2), and full cornea (Figure 19-6, map 3), respectively. The second column demonstrates the postoperative thickness profiles of the corneal epithelium (Figure 19-6, map 4), stroma (Figure 19-6, map 5), and full cornea (Figure 19-6, map 6). Epithelium, full stroma, and full cornea color scales are identical for pre- and postoperative stages to allow direct comparison. The third column consists of calculated maps representing topographical

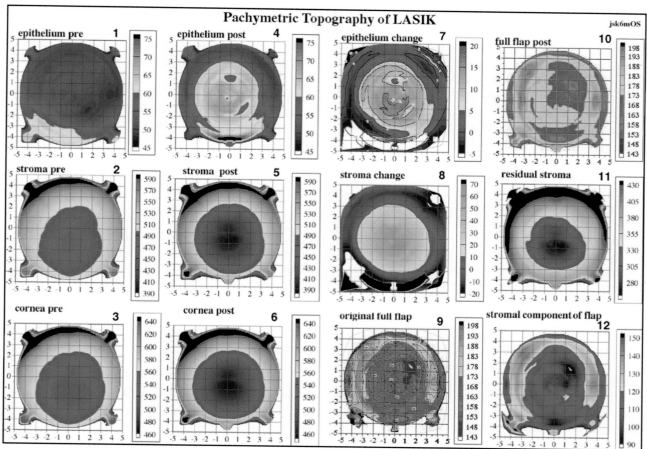

Figure 19-6. Reinstein "C12" display of the cornea of a patient pre- and six months post-LASIK OS. All 12 maps are pachymetric representations of particular corneal layers depicted on a color scale in microns. The preoperative epithelial (1), stromal (2), and full corneal (3) thickness maps appear in the first column. To the right of each of these maps (column two) is the post-LASIK pachymetric maps of epithelium (4), stroma (5), and full cornea (6) on identical color scales for direct comparison to preoperative measurements. The third column depicts calculated maps only. The calculated epithelial change map (map 7, 3rd column, 1st row) is derived in point-by-point subtraction of the preoperative from the postoperative epithelial pachymetric map. Thus the epithelial change map shows on a color scale the number of microns increased due to surgery. Note that the pattern of epithelial thickness change is such that it is greatest centrally, with a decrease in a symmetrical centrifugal fashion; thus producing an increase in outer curvature of the postoperative cornea. Note that the area of epithelial thickening is confined to the ablation zone or the zone of surgical corneal flattening. The calculated stromal change map (map 8, 3rd column, 2nd row) is derived in point-by-point subtraction of the postoperative from the preoperative stromal pachymetric map. Thus the stromal change map shows on a color scale the number of stromal microns decreased due to surgery in a topographic fashion and hence represents the ablation volume of tissue. The calculated map of the "original flap" (map 9, 3rd column, 3rd row) is derived by addition of the preoperative epithelial thickness profile (1) to the postoperative "stromal component of the flap" (map 12, 3rd column, 3rd row). It is necessary to perform a temporally displaced addition of epithelial and stromal components of the flap separately because of the epithelial changes present post-LASIK, leading to a flap anatomy post-LASIK (map 10, 3rd column, 1st row) that is different from that at the time of creation by the keratome. Finally, the pachymetric topography of the "residual stromal layer" comprising all stroma beneath and around the flap is shown in map 11 (3rd column, 2nd row). This map can be critically important in determining the adequacy of the stromal bed for further LASIK enhancement surgery under the flap in that the thinnest point is not always located centrally and may be missed by any form of intraoperative single-point measurement of the bed. Thus the C12 display is set out to be read by temporal grouping (columns) or anatomical grouping (rows). See text for further descriptive analysis.

epithelial change (Figure 19-6, map 7) (derived by subtraction of the preoperative from the postoperative epithelial map), the stromal change (Figure 19-6, map 8) (derived by subtraction of the postoperative from the preoperative stromal map), and the (calculated) original flap produced at the time of surgery, or "Reinstein Flap Profile"[16] (Figure 19-6, map 9). The Reinstein Flap Profile is calculated by adding the stromal component of the flap (Figure 19-6, map 12) to the preoperative epithelial thickness. The fourth column represents postoperative corneal layers: the thickness profile of the flap at 6 months (including epithelial changes) (Figure 19-6, map 10), the three-dimensional thickness profile of the residual stromal layer (stroma excluding the flap), and the postoperative stromal component of the flap (Figure 19-6, map 12).

The profile map of the preoperative epithelium OS was approximately 9.25 mm in diameter (Figure 19-6, map 1). The epithelial change map (Figure 19-6, map 7) shows the pattern of epithelial thickening and thinning. The epithelium thickened between 15 and 20 µm centrally, with a concentric decrease in thickening progressing toward the 7.5-mm diameter zone. It is interesting to note that within a 1-mm annulus at the 8-mm diameter zone, there was circumferential epithelial thinning after LASIK. We also note in this case that the pattern of epithelial change increased anterior corneal power (greater tissue addition centrally), but the patient had a plano refraction postoperatively. This indicates that the optical power shift produced by the epithelium in this case was exactly as expected by the nomogram setting used.

The stromal change map (Figure 19-6, map 8) shows a well-centered difference about the center (0,0 coordinate) of the cornea. The difference in stromal thickness prior to surgery is 70 µm centrally, decreasing to zero at the 7.5-mm diameter zone. Thus, the zone depicted on the color scale from green to red represents the effective volume of tissue change in the cornea (the predicted central ablation depth by the Nidek EC5000 readout was 73 µm for a 6.5-mm optical zone, transition to 7.5 mm). Within the peripheral 8- to 9-mm zone there is annular stromal thickening of between 10 and 20 µm. We were the first to publish this finding,[2] and Roberts has proposed a mechanism to account for it.[17] It is also interesting to note that this annulus of stromal thickening coincides with the annulus of epithelial thinning described previously, consistent with the Reinstein's law of epithelial compensation (see following).

Examination of the anatomy of the calculated original flap (Figure 19-6, map 9) by the Moria LSK-One keratome (predicted mean 160 µm) reveals a central thickness of 158 µm. Within the 4-mm diameter zone, the flap thickness was generally homogeneous between 160 and 165 µm although irregularity is evident. Note that direct measurement of the flap thickness at 6 months (Figure 19-6,

map 10) would not provide an accurate description of the flap anatomy at the time of creation due to the epithelial thickness changes present after LASIK. The stromal component of the flap (Figure 19-6, map 12) can be seen to possess a thickness profile of approximately 110 to 120 µm within the central 6-mm diameter zone, except for the quadrant superotemporally within the 4-mm diameter zone, where this is decreased to approximately 95 µm. This area may have been thinner due to the presence of thicker epithelium preoperatively in the corresponding quadrant and the passage of the keratome parallel to the surface of the cornea during applanation by the keratome head.

The three-dimensional thickness profile of the residual stromal layer (Figure 19-6, map 11) shows a thinnest point of 280 µm approximately 1 mm inferior to the center of the cornea. This is an example of why intraoperative handheld ultrasound residual stromal pachymetry can be unsafe. Lateral position variations of only a few hundred microns could completely alter the course of an ablation by providing a residual stromal thickness (RST) that is not the minimum.

Preoperative Assessment

The importance of accurate preoperative corneal thickness profile determination is now generally accepted, as an aid in the determination of candidacy for safe LASIK with avoidance of ectasia.[18] Concentric patterns of thickness about the corneal center is also a contributor in screening for keratoconus. Because of the significant added expense to the patient for Artemis scanning, at present we offer this but do not routinely use it preoperatively in every patient. Current indications for Artemis scanning in our practice include a greater than 15 µm discrepancy between Orbscan and handheld ultrasound pachymetry, and a predicted RST of less than 300 µm based on whichever is the thinnest, Orbscan or handheld ultrasound pachymetry.

The accuracy of measurement is defined as the concordance between the measured and the true value. A theoretical error analysis to estimate the accuracy of Artemis pachymetry has been published.[2] The accuracy of Artemis thickness measurements within the cornea was found to be at worst ±1.8%. This means that the 95% confidence interval for concordance between the measured and the true value is expected to be within ±5 µm for corneal thickness measurements (mean thickness 515 µm by Artemis VHF digital ultrasound[5]).

Optical methodology for the determination of corneal back surface shape and hence three-dimensional corneal thickness mapping, although possessing the convenience of in-air data acquisition, suffers from variable accuracy,[19–21] almost certainly due to a large extent to the variable optical properties of the cornea before and after corneal refractive surgery.[22] But variations in the refractive index of the cornea probably also exist between normal, unoperated individuals. We conducted a central corneal thickness study in which we compared measurements in 52 unoperated eyes obtained by Orbscan with those from Artemis VHF digital ultrasound scanning. Orbscan was found to be approximately four times less accurate; the variance was ±25 μm (SD) greater in the Orbscan group compared to the Artemis VHF digital ultrasound group (with a 95% confidence interval ±35 μm).

POSTOPERATIVE ASSESSMENT WITH ARTEMIS TECHNOLOGY: TRUE DIAGNOSIS AFTER LASIK AND OPTIMAL TREATMENT PLANNING

While LASIK and PRK are already relatively safe procedures today, we are constantly striving to make them safer. We need to prevent complications, and when these do occur, we need methods for correcting them and restoring visual function. In keeping with basic principles of surgery, accurate imaging and biometry will be the cornerstone of these goals, since accurate diagnosis enables optimal treatment planning.

Surface topography has been the mainstay of diagnostic testing in complicated LASIK cases. Recently, the introduction of aberrometry has greatly enhanced our diagnostic capabilities in being able to understand in a quantitative way how irregular astigmatism and other shape irregularities produce visual complaints. However, neither the understanding of the optical defect nor the surface shape of the cornea will necessarily provide a diagnosis for the cause of the problem.[6] The anatomical cause of a surface abnormality may only be understood at an internal corneal level, eg, irregularities in the flap versus the stromal bed. With burgeoning surgical rates of PRK and LASIK worldwide, it is becoming increasingly evident that there is a distinct need for a method of determining the layered anatomy of the changes induced. Without an accurate anatomical diagnosis, topography- or wavefront-guided treatments may lead to a suboptimal treatment plan.

The development of digital VHF ultrasound corneal scanning technology was first reported in 1991, where digital signal processing was used to identify and analyze the epithelium and scar layers formed in an experimental rabbit model.[10] In 1993, we reported the first confirmed measurement of the epithelium of the cornea in vivo, demonstrating that the acoustic interface detected within the intact cornea was localized spatially at the interface between epithelial cells and the surface of Bowman's layer.[3] This system, acquiring a series of parallel, rectilinear B-scans, was further developed to enable mapping of the thickness profile of the epithelium[4] as well as the lamellar flap within the central 3- to 4-mm area. By using digital signal processing techniques (the I-scan5), a 2.0 μm reproducibility for epithelial thickness measurements was obtained.[5] Subsequently, by increasing the fidelity of the digitized signal, flap thickness measurement precision was further improved to 1.3 μm, with epithelial and corneal measurements attaining a reproducibility of under 1 μm.[2] In clinical application, analysis of epithelial and stromal changes after lamellar corneal surgery has demonstrated significant epithelial changes after uncomplicated LASIK and the masking of stromal surface irregularities that were producing optical complications.[6]

The importance of epithelial changes in corneal refractive surgery has probably been underestimated. Significant changes in epithelial thickness profiles in both PRK[23,24] and LASIK[25,26] have been demonstrated and implicated in regression as well as the inaccuracy of topographically guided excimer laser ablation.[6] The curvature of Bowman's layer in the center of the normal cornea is on average greater than that of the epithelial surface.[9] As the refractive index of the epithelium and the stroma are sufficiently different (1.401 vs 1.377),[27] the epithelial-stromal interface constitutes an important refractive interface within the cornea, with a mean power contribution estimated at approximately 3.60 D.[9] Thus, unpredicted changes in the epithelial lenticule after surgery will result in unplanned refractive shifts. This is one of the reasons why current ablation depths and profiles ("nomograms") differ from theoretical ablation profiles. They incorporate the average change of epithelial power for a given level of stromal surface flattening (level of myopia treated). Thus the understanding of epithelial dynamics and their patterns begins to unfold,[26] and these factors potentially may be used to improve the accuracy of corneal refractive outcomes.

Artemis scanning will significantly contribute to LASIK accuracy and safety. Accuracy in LASIK translates to the chances of an eye achieving target refraction. Safety relates to achieving this target without loss of BSCVA or other visual disturbance.

Ectasia is one of the most devastating potential consequences of LASIK, and it behooves us to prevent it from happening in every possible way. The thickness of the flap determines at what level stromal tissue removal commences, and hence is directly related to the amount of stromal tissue remaining in the posterior cornea under the flap after surgery. The thinner the flap, the more difficult it is to handle surgically; however the thicker the flap, the less tissue remains for the correction of ametropia by LASIK.

TABLE 19-1
REINSTEIN CLASSIFICATION FOR MICROFOLDS

Type	Anatomic Location	Loss of BSCVA	Flourescine Pooling	Clinical Findings	Anatomical Basis	Management
Corrugation	Stroma	√	√	Gross folds, differential pooling of gutters, mixed-cylinder	Flap slip	Flap repositioning
True Microfolds	Bowman's	√	√	Grooves in Bowman's	Grooves in Bowman's	Flap repositioning and microfold distension
Bowman's Cracks	Bowman's	√	Ø	Gray lines, no groove	Fractures in Bowman's	Observe only

Following are some clinical examples demonstrating the importance of distinguishing biomechanical from epithelial components of ametropia after an initial treatment.

Despite all the advances in corneal topography and ocular wavefront measurement, it is not always possible to diagnose the cause of subjective visual complaints by these means alone.[6] This is due to the fact that internal corneal refractive interfaces (such as the epithelial–stromal interface) are not being measured independently. In fact, topography is often not, strictly speaking, a diagnostic test but rather a descriptive one. For the diagnosis and correction of complications, identifying the anatomical cause of a corneal surface abnormality—front or back—may only be possible by understanding the layered internal corneal anatomy. For example, the distinction between irregularities in the flap profile (keratome), flap positioning (surgeon), and the stromal bed (laser) will aid in planning further surgical correction. In addition, further surgery on the cornea should always be based on a full knowledge of the remaining tissue available.

Below are several examples of cases within, and commonly referred to, our practice for Artemis anatomical evaluation after complicated LASIK in which Artemis provided essential information for further treatment planning.

Microfolds

The occurrence of microfolds in the LASIK flap is often a visually compromising complication. There have been numerous suggestions as to how to treat microfolds, but not all have been based on an anatomical diagnostic classification.

We have studied the anatomical morphology of microfolds, while correlating the Artemis VHF digital ultrasound scans to clinical slit lamp examination and functional impact on vision. We have devised a classification system founded on these studies that is based on clinical

management options. The Reinstein classification is shown in Table 19-1. Folds are initially classified as either involving the stromal component of the flap or Bowman's layer alone. If involving the stromal component of the flap, these are classified as flap corrugations that represent gross flap malposition that in effect leads to undulation and waviness of stromal lamellae within the entire flap substance. Flap corrugations must clearly be managed by flap lifting and repositioning. If the folds involve Bowman's layer, a distinction must be made between true microfolds and Bowman's cracks because their management is completely different. True microfolds are literally grooves in Bowman's layer (Figure 19-7) produced by redundancy due to flap malposition or incomplete distension. Bowman's cracks are fractures in Bowman's layer with no grooving (Figure 19-8). Bowman's cracks are caused by trauma to the flap that may result either from the stretching of Bowman's on dragging the flap from the hinge with a spatula, or from folding or bending of Bowman's on returning the flap to the bed (especially if the flap has dried during the period of ablation). The distinction between true microfolds and Bowman's cracks is very important because while it may be warranted to relift a flap with true microfolds to adequately reposition the flap and distend the grooves to improve refraction and BSCVA, lifting a flap with Bowman's cracks will further traumatize the flap and cause additional damage as well as potentially delaying the return of BSCVA.

Flap Complications

The postoperative assessment of flap complications is greatly aided by Artemis VHF digital ultrasound scanning. Determination of the exact anatomy of the faulty lamellar dissection will show at what depth the flap was created and whether the flap repositioning was optimal. This information is important in the planning of a subsequent

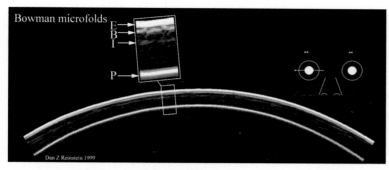

Figure 19-7. True Bowman's microfold. Horizontal Artemis VHF digital ultrasound corneal B-scan through the visual axis of a patient 6 months after LASIK. The surface of epithelium (E), Bowman's (B), the keratectomy interface (K), and the endothelium (P) are labeled. Inspection of the surface of Bowman's demonstrates a true microfold, with Bowman's showing a groove approximately 25 μm in depth and 100 μm in width.

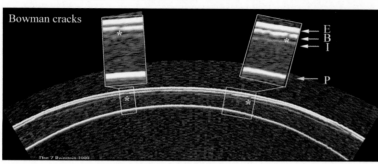

Figure 19-8. Bowman's cracks. Horizontal Artemis VHF digital ultrasound corneal B-scan through the visual axis of a patient 9 months after LASIK. The surface of epithelium (E), Bowman's (B), the keratectomy interface (K), and the endothelium (P) are labeled. Inspection of the Bowman's interface demonstrates fractures or discontinuities (*) that do not involve grooving or puckering of Bowman's.

recutting of another flap. In addition, for cases with central flap dissections or irregularities, Artemis VHF digital ultrasound can determine if the edges of Bowman's layer were properly and adequately apposed in order to help avert epithelial ingrowth.

In the following example, a 33-year-old nurse underwent LASIK in 1998 with the Moria LSK-One and the Nidek EC5000 for a –5.50 sphere. The preoperative corneal thickness was 509 μm and the predicted RST was 280 μm (based on a 160-μm flap). She lived far away, and eventually presented in 1999, almost 2 years later, requesting that one of the eyes, which had regressed in the first 3 months after surgery, be enhanced. General opinion at the time dictated recutting flaps rather than lifting, ostensibly because flap lifting after 6 months was assumed to be difficult and recutting was assumed to lead to less chance of epithelial ingrowth due to the sharp edges of the new flap. The patient underwent recutting with the Hansatome using the 160-μm head and the 9.5-mm ring (aiming to go outside, but superficial to the original flap to save residual stromal tissue). The result was a central buttonhole within a double flap dissection that was replaced without performing laser ablation. Figure 19-9, shows the exact anatomical result 1 day after flap replacement. From the ultrasound scans it was clear that the Hansatome flap had managed to stay superficial and within the original flap, only to then exit (Figure 19-9, X_1) through Bowman's layer and the epithelium and then re-enter (Figure 19-9, X_2) the cornea to regain the plane superficial to the original flap interface. The scan reassured us that Bowman's was properly apposed and that anatomical restoration had

been achieved for a good prognosis. At 2 years thereafter, she had not developed epithelial ingrowth and remained without loss of BSCVA.

In 1994, we coined Reinstein's Law of Epithelial Compensation for irregular astigmatism[28]: "irregular astigmatism results in irregular epithelium." The epithelium often compensates fully for stromal surface irregularities, keratoconus being an excellent example of this. Everyone knows that as cone formation in keratoconus progresses, the epithelium overlying the cone becomes progressively thinner. This is because the epithelium becomes invaginated by the underlying bulging stromal surface while its outer surface is kept as regular as possible by the action of 10,000 blinking events a day. In fact, this is why keratoconus can be detected earlier by looking at the back surface topography of the cornea rather than the front surface. We are investigating whether examination of epithelial thickness profiles may provide an even earlier and therefore more sensitive screening tool for keratoconus. According to Reinstein's Law of Epithelial Compensation, if a patient presents with stable irregular astigmatism, by definition the epithelium has reached the maximum compensatory function.

In the following example, a 23-year-old patient underwent LASIK in 1998 in the left eye, using the Moria LSK-One microkeratome in which a short, nasal hinged flap was obtained and the laser ablation was performed. Artemis VHF digital ultrasound scanning is shown in Figure 19-10. A large amount of epithelial compensation takes place in cases like this, in which there are large steps in the shape of the stromal surface. This is why neither

Figure 19-9. Geometrically corrected horizontal Artemis VHF digital ultrasound corneal B-scan of a cornea 1 day after recutting a second flap and obtaining a simultaneous separation of the original flap from the bed and a buttonhole (A). An axially zoomed image in a different horizontal plane is shown below (B). The surface of epithelium (E), Bowman's (B), the keratectomy produced by the second-cut Hansatome 160-head (H), and the original Moria keratectomy interface (M) are labeled. The Hansatome interface is seen to course superficially to the original keratectomy as intended

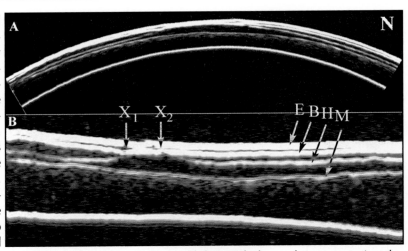

from left to right; but move superficially, exiting through Bowman's (X_1) and the epithelium, then re-entering the epithelium and crossing Bowman's (X_2) to again find a plane superficial to the original keratectomy. Exact anatomical apposition of Bowman's is confirmed by the scan, thus confirming perfect flap repositioning and minimizing the probability of epithelial ingrowth in the visual axis.

Figure 19-10. Horizontal Artemis VHF digital ultrasound corneal B-scan through the visual axis of the left cornea of a patient in whom a slightly short flap was created and the ablation was carried out. The surface of epithelium (E), Bowman's (B), the keratectomy interface (I), and the endothelium (P) are labeled. The abrupt termination of the keratectomy producing a short hinge is shown (SH). Lack of ablation nasal to this has produced a

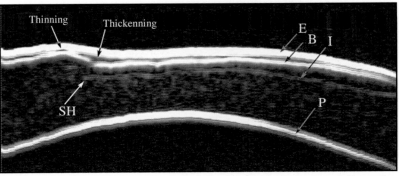

large step in the cornea. The stromal surface step is partially compensated for by epithelial remodeling; the epithelium characteristically thins over the "bump" while thickening in the crevice is produced. This cross-section clearly demonstrates why topography-guided ablations (or even wavefront-guided ablations, which are 70% biased to the front surface) will not be fully successful in correcting the stromal irregularity.

topography- nor wavefront-guided ablations will be sufficient to correct such complications. In this case, the stromal surface is asymmetric. The epithelium has compensated as much as it can, but is still leaving asymmetry. The patient presents with topographic asymmetric astigmatism. If one were to base the corrective ablation profile on the topography or ocular wavefront now (70% epithelial surface shape-dependent), there would clearly be ineffective correction of the stromal surface shape. Following such a case, the epithelium may or may not compensate fully for the remaining stromal surface asymmetry. If it does, the topography would become regular but the patient may still have symptoms, due to the significant refractive index difference between epithelium and stroma.[9]

Decentration is a diagnosis made postoperatively by inspection of topography. Decentration denotes off-center

ablation. We have found that what appears to be decentration by topography is not always due to off-center ablation. In the following example, a patient presented to us complaining of monocular double vision after LASIK. The initial refraction was –6.50 D. Treatment was carried out with the Moria LSK-One microkeratome and the Nidek EC5000. Preoperative corneal thickness by Orbscan was measured as 516 µm. With an ablation depth of 90 µm, the predicted postoperative RST was 266 µm. On examination, his UCVA was 20/70 and manifest refraction was +3.00 –3.75 x 96, yielding a BSCVA of 20/40+2. Slit lamp examination showed a clear cornea with an unremarkable flap possessing a few very faint, faded shallow-appearing vertical microfolds. Orbscan anterior best-fit sphere mapping is shown in Figure 19-11, providing a differential diagnosis of decentration of the ablation zone or ectasia.

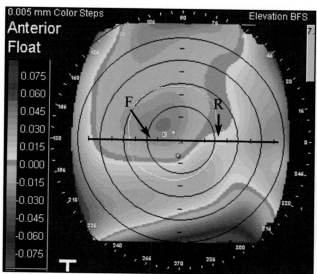

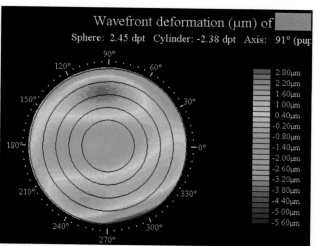

Figure 19-11. Orbscan anterior best-fit sphere (default 10-mm zone fit) plot of the cornea in a patient presenting with monocular diplopia and a topographic diagnosis of "decentered ablation," proved incorrect by B-scan imaging in the plane represented by the horizontal black line.

Figure 19-12. Zywave aberrometry displaying the higher-order wavefront plot of the eye represented in Figure 19-11 There is marked coma.

Figure 19-12 shows Zywave (Bausch & Lomb, St. Louis, MO) aberrometry of the same eye, demonstrating coma-like higher-order aberrations.

Horizontal three-dimensional Artemis VHF digital ultrasound B-scan cross-section of the cornea revealed anatomical features that provided further diagnostic information. Figure 19-13 shows the B-scan demonstrating a flatter (F) nasal side of the cornea, with a raised (R) surface temporally as found also on the Orbscan best-fit sphere surface shape map. Beneath the raised (R) area the epithelial thickness is seen to be reduced, due to invagination by the underlying Bowman's layer (B). Bowman's (B) is highly irregular, showing three major ultrasonic discontinuities (*) representing either cracks or microfolds in the flap surface. Three-dimensional pachymetric topography of this cornea is shown in Figure 19-14. The epithelial thickness profile is seen to vary continuously, filling in and smoothing out the surface of Bowman's layer. The thinnest point within the residual stromal bed, as determined by three-dimensional thickness mapping in a Reinstein C6 display (post-LASIK with no preoperative data for subtraction maps), shown in Figure 19-14 is 223 µm. The residual stromal layer thickness profile appears slightly asymmetric or decentered in the nasal direction. Inspection of the stromal component of the flap map (Figure 19-14; second column, second row) shows the reason for this: the stromal component of the flap was thicker temporally than nasally. The central stromal component of the flap was 8 µm, thus implying that the central flap

thickness was originally approximately 130 µm (80 + 50). The original surgeon had calculated that the patient would still have 266 µm under the flap after treatment. Given that this is 43 µm less than observed, and that the flap was 30 µm thinner than intended, it is probable that his preoperative pachymetry (by Orbscan) was underestimated by approximately 43 µm, and the original corneal thickness must have been closer to 473 µm.

A diagnosis was made of flap malposition and possible asymmetric biomechanical shift. In addition, the RST was noted to be too thin for further under-the-flap ablation, despite the fact that the preoperative parameters would have implied that there was room for further treatment.

This case clearly illustrates the importance of anatomical diagnosis in contrast to a topographical description in planning the management of the complications of LASIK. By topography alone, this case may well have been diagnosed as a decentration. The eye may well have then undergone a topographically guided treatment under the flap. Given the low RST, it is conceivable that further tissue removal would have led to further mechanical shifts and an unpredictable result, with a high possibility of inducing progressive ectasia.[29]

Flap profile irregularities can lead to irregular biomechanical shifts in refraction. A patient was able to undergo LASIK for the correction of −10.00 D OD because she had 5.5 mm scotopic pupils, and adequate corneal thickness to leave 250 µm in under an assumed 160 µm flap. The Moria CB microkeratome employing the 110 head, which is

Figure 19-13. Horizontal Artemis VHF digital ultrasound corneal B-scan through the visual axis of the right cornea of a patient presenting with monocular diplopia and a topographic and wavefront diagnosis consistent with "decentered ablation." The upper image (1) shows the geometrically corrected image, while the lower image (2) shows the raw ultrasound data with axial zoom to better appreciate the interfaces. The surface of epithelium (E), Bowman's (B), and the keratectomy interface (I) are labeled. It is clearly noted that Bowman's surface is highly irregular, with numerous true microfolds (*) that were only very faintly visible on slit lamp examination due to the impressive epithelial compensation producing excellent smoothing of the corneal surface. The diagnosis of "decentered ablation" is clearly less likely than that of an inadequately distended flap, producing surface asymmetry.

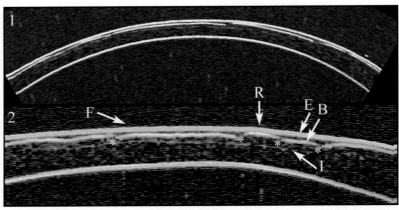

designed to cut an average of 140 µm, was used in manual mode with a deliberate "fast pass" of about 1 second in order to attempt to obtain a thinner flap. It was proposed that Artemis VHF digital ultrasound scanning would be used postoperatively to measure flap and RST to decide if it would be possible to perform further enhancement if required. The procedure was uneventful, and the flap intraoperatively was noted to "feel" thin, and was noted to be of "good quality for a future flap lift." Day 1 postoperatively the refraction was +5.00 D with no loss of BSCVA. This only regressed to +4.00 D by 3 months. Figure 19-15 shows a horizontal cross-section of the flap 3 months after LASIK. It can be seen that the flap centrally was indeed thin, the stromal component of the flap was in the region of 90 to 100 µm thick. However, peripherally the stromal component of the flap reached over 200 microns (equating to an original flap thickness of over 250 µm). It is conceivable that this patient's gross overcorrection was partly due to a biomechanical cause: deep keratectomy peripherally may have produced excess flattening centrally through a mechanism of peripheral thickening as proposed by Roberts[17] combined with an effect similar to radial keratotomy and mid-peripheral bulging due to localized deep keratectomy causing central flattening. Clearly in this case knowledge of the flap anatomy created will be essential in planning further treatment. The relifting of the apparently good quality flap (as assessed intraoperatively) for hyperopic ablation to be performed would deepen the midperipheral keratectomy further, and would probably not be ideal given the apparent mechanisms producing this excessive overcorrection.

Elastic changes in the cornea are composed of forward or backward bending of the central cornea due to surgically induced lamellar structural changes, the influence of intraocular pressure, and other external forces to the cornea, but by definition should not be described as ectasia. Ectasia, as it relates to lamellar refractive surgery (and keratoconus, actually), should be defined according to the way it was done by the father of lamellar corneal refractive surgery, Jose Ignacio Barraquer-Moner. Barraquer defined ectasia as a progressive deformation of the cornea in which there is progressive corneal steepening and thinning.[30] As such, it describes a plastic and/or viscoelastic deformation.

In LASIK, it is important to determine the true anatomical diagnosis for secondary ametropia (ie, epithelial or biomechanical corneal changes), so that accurate cognitive surgical planning for enhancement surgery can be accomplished. Given the lack of consistency in flap thickness, when considering correction of secondary ametropia (enhancement surgery), knowledge of the whole RST bed is paramount for maximum safety. Currently, only the central RST is determined either from the assumed presurgical parameters, or it is measured manually intraoperatively using a handheld ultrasonic pachymeter.

In the following example, a 30-year-old woman underwent LASIK OS with the Nidek EC5000 and the Moria LSK-One 130 head microkeratome in June of 1998. The preoperative corneal thickness by Orbscan was 555 µm. The predicted ablation depth for correction of –6.25 –1.25 x 175 (BSCVA 20/20) in a 6.5-mm zone was 101 µm, and the flap thickness used for predicting the RST was 160 µm. Therefore, the predicted RST was 293 µm (555 – 101 – 160 = 293). One week after treatment, the refraction was –1.00 –1.00 x 170, and at 3 months the refraction was –0.50 –1.75 x 175 (BSCVA 20/20). Note that there was *no* correction of the original on-axis cylinder, and an undercorrection of myopia. Given that there were 43 µm of

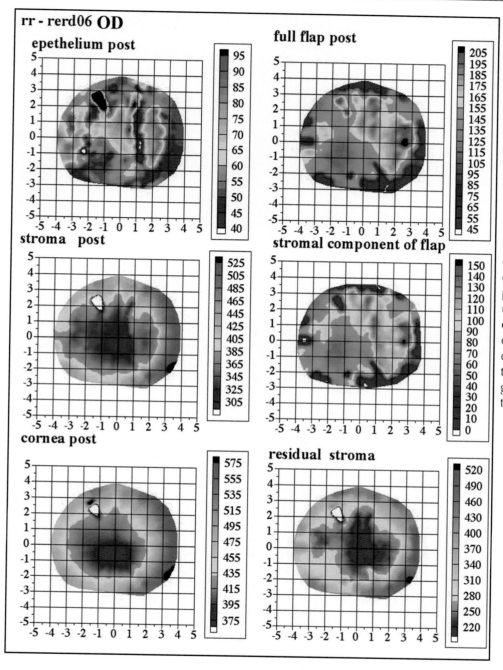

rr - rerd06 OD

epethelium post

stroma post

cornea post

full flap post

stromal component of flap

residual stroma

Figure 19-14. Reinstein "C6" corneal pachymetric map display of the thickness in microns (color scale) of the epithelium, stroma, full cornea, stromal component of the flap, and residual stromal bed in the case of monocular diplopia with a topographic diagnosis of "decentered ablation." The residual stromal thickness minimum is 223 microns (third row, second column). Inspection of the epithelial thickness profile (first row, first column) demonstrates the error introduced by epithelial compensation if one were to attempt topography- or wavefront-guided ablation to correct the optical defect.

residual stroma predicted still left over the 250 μm limit, an enhancement was performed lifting the original flap in September 1998 using the Bausch & Lomb 217C (predicting a removal of a further 42 μm, bringing the predicted RST to a level of 251 μm). Intraoperative bed pachymetry (Sonogage II handheld ultrasound pachymeter) measured 305 μm in the central bed under the flap before ablation of 42 μm as predicted by the laser. Six months following this enhancement, refraction was +2.75 –2.50 x 90 (BSCVA 20/20) and the patient was complaining of double vision in that eye (even with best spectacle correction). There was a

greater than 100% overcorrection of on-axis cylinder. Given the fact that no further tissue was left under the flap for further treatment, it was decided to enhance as a photorefractive keratectomy (PRK) over the original flap in April of 1999, by what is now termed advanced *surface ablation*—removal of the epithelium using 20% ethanol and ablation with the Bausch & Lomb 217C. The treatment performed was a positive cylinder ablation of plano +2.50 x 180. Although the cornea remained clear and no haze developed, the refraction 6 months after this second enhancement was +2.00 –2.75 x 175. Again, there was a

Figure 19-15. Horizontal Artemis VHF digital ultrasound B-scan through the visual axis of a cornea 3 months after LASIK for –10.00 that produced a gross overcorrection of +4.00 D. The geometrically correct image is shown above (A) with the raw scan data axially zoomed below (B). The flap is seen to be much thinner centrally (small arrow) than peripherally (large arrow). This unplanned extreme midperipheral deep keratectomy explains the gross overcorrection.

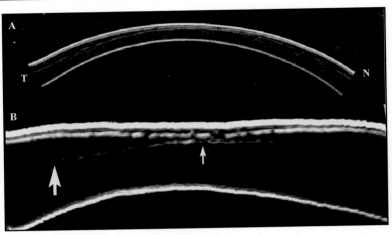

greater-than 100% overcorrection of the cylinder and little change in the spherical equivalent.

The patient was referred to us for evaluation. We were able to obtain electronic files for all Orbscan examinations performed before and after surgery from her original surgeon. After importing these into our Orbscan workstation, we displayed the best-fit sphere back surface maps for preoperative, 3 months postoperative (pre-1st enhancement), and 5 months post-enhancement. All three back surface best-spherical-fit maps were exhibited side-by-side for comparison. We set the fit sphere curvature for all three time points to that of the preoperative back surface best-fit sphere curvature of 6.37 mm (Figure 19-16). The Orbscan back surface maps demonstrate how with each treatment the central radius of curvature of the back surface decreased incrementally. But why would this be occurring, despite the fact that more than 250 µm were predicted (and confirmed by intraoperative measurement) to have been left under the flap?

Artemis VHF digital ultrasound B scanning was performed using the Cornell University arc scan prototype. Figure 19-17 shows the three-dimensional thickness map of the RST demonstrating a thickness centrally of approximately 270 µm, which was more than estimated by calculation based on preoperative parameters but close to what was predicted by the intraoperative pachymetry (305 – 42 = 263 µm). However, the RST 1.5-mm nasal to the center was found to be only 216 µm. (The first enhancement under the flap would have reduced the thickness of the RST at this location by approximately 26 µm, therefore the RST here before the first enhancement was approximately 242 µm.)

The cause of this RST bed asymmetry is evident from inspection of the thickness map of the stromal component of the flap. The stromal component of the flap 1.5 mm

nasally was 139 µm, compared to only 65 µm centrally. The original flap thickness nasally and centrally would have been 189 µm (139 + 50) and 115 µm (65 + 50), respectively. (PRK over the flap would not have removed some tissue from the nasal stromal component of the flap as it was a positive cylinder ablation.)

The asymmetric flap thickness, with an RST below 250 µm in the nasal portion of the cornea, may explain why this patient's cornea was behaving unpredictably on repeated enhancements. Reinstein et al have shown that significant and measurable biomechanical changes occur in the cornea after LASIK with an RST below 290 µm,[26,27] and this asymmetric RST bed may be responsible for unpredicted biomechanical shifts as evidenced by the serial back surface Orbscan exams (Figure 19-16).

Had Artemis VHF digital ultrasound scanning been performed before the first enhancement, it would have been evident that the RST was already below 250 µm nasal to the center after the first treatment. This may have alerted the surgeon to not lift the original flap and remove further tissue from under it, and may have avoided the eventual induction of biomechanically mediated asymmetric astigmatism with monocular diplopia.

In another example, a 33-year-old female underwent simultaneous bilateral LASIK (OS first, OD second) in May 2002 for –6.00 –0.50 x 115 (20/15) OD and –6.00 –0.50 x 20 (20/15) OS. Treatment was carried out with the Hansatome 160-µm head and the MEL70 excimer laser with ablation depths of 99 µm for each eye (6.5-mm fully corrected optical zone). Preoperative Orbscan thicknesses were 54 µm OD and 540 µm OS, yielding predicted RST of 283 µm OD and 281 µm OS. One month UCVA was 20/15-2 in both eyes. Refractions were plano –0.50 x 125 OD and –0.50 D OS. In February 2003, 9 months postoperative UCVA was 20/25 OD and 20/30 OS, refraction was

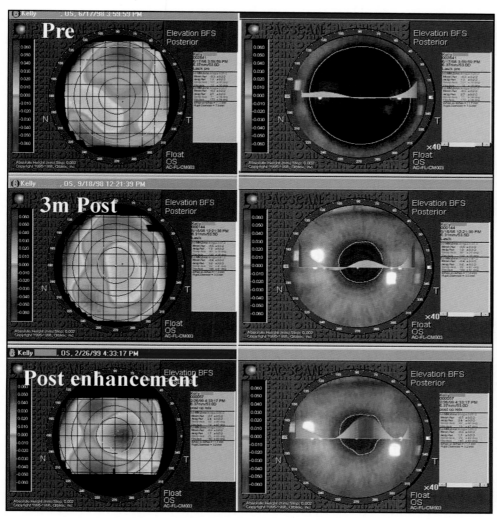

Figure 19-16. Multiple Orbscan back surface best-fit sphere plots before LASIK (top row), 3 months postoperatively (second row), and 6 months after enhancement (bottom row). The best-fit sphere radius for all time stages is user-set to the radius of the central 4-mm zone of the back surface before surgery (6.37 mm) to show back surface shifts in curvature relative to the preoperative state. The first column shows the three-dimensional maps in two-dimensions, while the second column shows horizontal cross-sectional representation of the best-fit to the initial 6.37-mm radius. At 3 months postoperative, the back surface was seen to have decreased a little in radius relative to the preoperative state (relative bulging) and, after enhancement, this back surface bowing is considerably increased.

−0.50 −0.50 x 150 (20/15) OD and −.75 −0.25 x 145 (20/15) OS. As per enhancement protocol in our practice, she underwent Artemis scanning for determination of the RST before enhancement. RST maps for right and left eyes are shown in Figure 19-18. The minimum RST was 278 µm OD and 221 µm OS. Central thickness of the stromal component of the flap was 85 µm OD and 135 µm OS, corresponding to original flap thicknesses of 135 µm OD and 185 µm OS. We reported Artemis VHF digital ultrasound pachymetric mapping of Hansatome flaps created bilaterally using the same blade. The mean (±SD) central thickness for first eyes was 139 (±21.3) µm and second eyes was 122 (±22.4) µm. Second flaps were statistically significantly thinner than first flaps.[31] Therefore, it is not surprising that the right flap was thinner than the left. However, the left (first) flap was approximately 15 µm thicker than expected (185 vs 160). Since the RST was 60 µm thinner than expected, it can be concluded that the Orbscan preoperatively overestimated corneal thickness by approximately 45 µm (original predicted RST – Flap

thickness over 160 – RST achieved = 281 – 5 – 221). Therefore, in this case RST monitoring by direct measurement before what appeared to be a relatively benign enhancement, with adequate tissue reserve, resulted in removing excess tissue from the bed of a cornea already biomechanically compromised with an RST of 221 µm. Had ablation been carried out for the enhancement under the flap, assuming a residual of 283 µm as predicted, ablation in a 7-mm zone of 20 µm would have reduced the RST to approximately 201 µm, with the surgeon assuming that there was still 263 µm of RST. Conceivably this would have led to further biomechanical change and a myopic shift,[26] possibly a second enhancement, and the risk of inducing ectasia,[29] with the surgeon believing that more than 250 µm were being left under the original flap. In fact, many current publications on biomechanical changes and ectasia in the cornea after LASIK are based on the *predicted* value for the RST based on preoperative parameters.[32–34] Our mathematical modeling using Artemis VHF digital-ultrasound–based direct measurement of the RST

Figure 19-17. Three-dimensional pachymetric mapping of the residual stromal layer under the flap and the stromal component of the flap (ie, excluding epithelium) created with a nasal hinge with the Moria LSK "One" using the 130 head. The central thickness of the stromal component of the flap is 65 µm, corresponding to an original flap thickness of approximately 115 µm (65 + 50). However, 2 mm nasal to the center of the flap the stromal component thickness was 139 µm, corresponding to an original flap thickness of 189 µm (139 + 50).

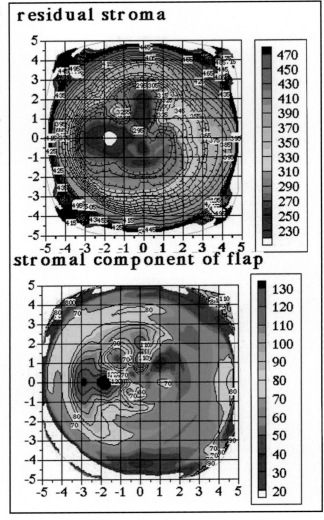

Figure 19-18. Three-dimensional residual stromal thickness maps of the right and left eyes of a patient who had undergone routine LASIK with predicted residual stromal thicknesses of 283 µm OD and 281 µm OS. As seen here, the thinnest points of the residual stromal beds were in fact 278 µm and 221 µm on the right and left eyes, respectively, perhaps accounting for a slightly greater myopic undercorrection on the left due to a biomechanical corneal shift.

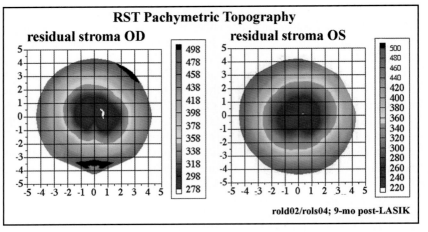

led us to determine that ectasia probably occurs on the average at an RST of 180 μm.[29] We have studied the relative predictability of the RST in LASIK, and found that with modern pachymetry (Orbscan and handheld ultrasound pachymetry), microkeratomes, and laser ablation depths, the RST can be predicted within a standard deviation of 30 μm[35] and hence a range of approximately ±45 μm (95% confidence interval). It is therefore prudent to stay within the Barraquer rule of aiming to leave 250 μm under a lamellar flap,[30] in order to avoid breaching this 180-μm limit.

Given our experience in the subject, our current thinking is that ectasia will occur if either less than 200 μm are left under the flap, or if LASIK is performed in a cornea with undiagnosed keratoconus. Therefore, accurate biometry before LASIK, after LASIK, and before enhancement, as well as cross-interpretation with Orbscan front and back surface shape evaluation, should protect all corneas from ectasia with the exception of those that harbor undiagnosed (or unexpressed) keratoconus.

One of the most unique contributions to ophthalmology by the Artemis 2 will be in the sizing of intraocular lenses (IOLs), particularly phakic intraocular IOLs. The FDA has recently approved the Verisye and Visian phakic IOLs, and so the use of devices such as the Artemis 2 will be paramount in avoiding serious side-effects. Incorrect lens sizing or positioning can lead to long-term complications. One of the main safety hurdles encountered in anterior chamber, angle-supported phakic IOL implantation has been defining the correct amount of haptic force in the angle. If the lens is too large, this can lead to ischemia of the iris, causing iris stromal scarring and pupil ovalization. If too small, the lens may become displaced in the anterior chamber, risking endothelial damage or decrease in the ability to correct astigmatism with toric lenses.

Issues relating to the sizing of posterior chamber lenses exist as well. If the vault of such a lens in the posterior chamber is too large, it can lead to narrowing of the anterior chamber angle. It can also increase the chances of pigment dispersion from the pigment epithelium of the iris with subsequent glaucomatous consequences. If the posterior chamber phakic IOL is too small, excessive contact between it and the crystalline lens may decrease aqueous flow and lens nutrition, as well as directly traumatize the lens surface, leading to cataract.

By providing accurate sulcus-to-sulcus and angle-to-angle measurements, the Artemis 2 has the potential to increase the safety of both anterior and posterior chamber phakic IOLs by improving the accuracy of lens sizing—a crucial issue for long-term safety of these devices (Figure 19-19). Until recently, surgeons have been using the external white-to-white measurement to estimate the internal or sulcus-to-sulcus or angle-to-angle diameters.[36,37] A recent study revealed that either no or insufficient statistical correlation between the external ocular measurements (including white-to-white) and the internal angle-to-angle or sulcus-to-sulcus measurements of the eye, even if other conventional measurements (such as sphere, axial length, anterior chamber depth) were included.[7] This means that the only alternative for ensuring the greatest sizing safety in phakic IOL surgery will be to determine angle-to-angle and sulcus-to-sulcus dimensions by direct measurement. To date, the Artemis 2 is the only technology available that can provide both these measurements directly, in three-dimensions, and under direct visualization for positional confirmation of the location of where measurements are taken. An example is shown in Figure 19-20. Without this feature, it would be relatively easy to measure internal ocular dimensions in the wrong plane.

Improving the safety of phakic IOLs by accurate anatomical surgical planning and postoperative monitoring could position phakic IOLs as a real alternative treatment for correcting lower refractive errors where currently, extraocular corneal refractive surgery is the first-line approach.

Orthopedic surgery was practiced without pre- and postoperative anatomical imaging until the discovery of X-ray imaging in 1895 by Wilhelm Konrad Roentgen. Perhaps layer-by-layer anatomical imaging and biometry of the cornea and anterior segment will have a similar impact on refractive surgery.

REFERENCES

1. Pavlin CJ, Sherar MD, Foster FS. Subsurface ultrasound microscopic imaging of the intact eye. *Ophthalmology.* 1990;97(2):244–250.

2. Reinstein DZ, Silverman RH, Raevsky T, Simoni GJ, Lloyd HO, Najafi DJ, Rondeau MJ, Coleman DJ. A new arc-scanning very high-frequency ultrasound system for 3D pachymetric mapping of corneal epithelium, lamellar flap and residual stromal layer in laser in situ keratomileusis. *J Refract Surg.* 2000;16:414–430.

3. Reinstein DZ, Silverman RH, Coleman DJ. High-frequency ultrasound measurement of the thickness of the corneal epithelium. *Refract Corneal Surg.* 1993;9(5):385–387.

4. Reinstein DZ, Silverman RH, Trokel SL, Coleman DJ. Corneal pachymetric topography. *Ophthalmology.* 1994;101(3):432–438.

5. Reinstein DZ, Silverman RH, Rondeau MJ, Coleman DJ. Epithelial and corneal thickness measurements by high-frequency ultrasound digital signal processing. *Ophthalmology.* 1994;101(1):140–146.

6. Reinstein DZ, Silverman RH, Sutton HF, Coleman DJ. Very high-frequency ultrasound corneal analysis identifies

Figure 19-19. Full anterior segment horizontal Artemis VHF digital ultrasound B-scan encompassing a 15-mm wide sector. The anterior retina can be seen within this scan plane also. The angle-to-angle and sulcus-to-sulcus diameters are easily measured directly. Anterior chamber and posterior chamber volume and dimensions can be studied before insertion of phakic IOLs to predict the separation of such implants from the endothelium of the cornea, or the crystalline lens. Predictive effects on the angle due to posterior chamber phakic IOLs could also be made prospectively to improve patient safety.

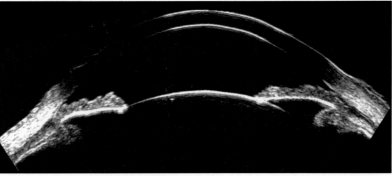

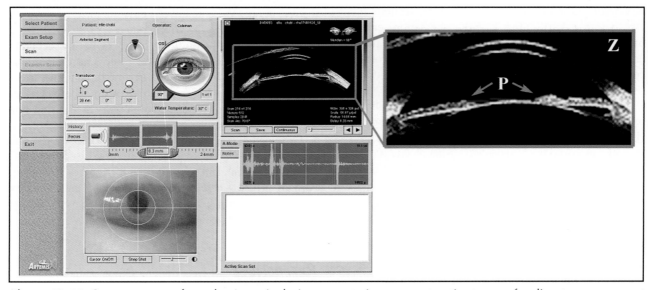

Figure 19-20. Screen capture from the Artemis during an anterior segment patient exam for direct measurement of the sulcus-to-sulcus. Real-time horizontal B-scans are displayed on the upper right quadrant of the screen. The infrared simultaneous video image shows that the position of the horizontal scanning plane is not central or axial. The zoom window (Z) of the B-scan shows a cross-sectional anterior segment representation containing pupil borders (P) that, in the absence of positional information, could have been interpreted as an axial scan, producing a false-low sulcus-to-sulcus diameter. Similarly, the angle-to-angle would have been underestimated falsely. Simultaneous video control is paramount for maximizing the safety of phakic IOL sizing, as improper localization will lead to erroneous biometry and the potential for over-sizing of phakic IOLs.

anatomic correlates of optical complications of lamellar refractive surgery: anatomic diagnosis in lamellar surgery. *Ophthalmology.* 1999;106(3):474–482.

7. Reinstein DZ, Silverman RH, Lloyd OH. Estimation of angle-to-angle or sulcus-to-sulcus from white-to-white and conventional ocular measurements: are there adequate correlations for safe phakic-IOL surgery? In: European Society of Cataract and Refractive Surgery Annual Meeting; September 7–11, 2002; Nice, France.

8. Reinstein DZ, Aslanides IM, Patel S, et al. Epithelial lenticular types of human cornea: classification and analysis of influence on PRK. *Ophthalmology.* 1995;102 (suppl):156.

9. Patel S, Reinstein DZ, Silverman RH, Coleman DJ. The shape of Bowman's layer in the human cornea. *J Refract Surg.* 1998;14(6):636–640.

10. Reinstein DZ, Polack PJ, McCormick S, Rondeau MJ, Coleman DJ. High frequency Ultrasound scanning of corneal scar formation in vivo. *Invest Ophthalmol Vis Sci.* 1992;33(4):1233.

11. Reinstein DZ, Silverman RH, Trokel SL, Allemann N, Coleman DJ. High-frequency ultrasound digital signal processing for biometry of the cornea in planning phototherapeutic keratectomy [letter] [published erratum appears in *Arch Ophthalmol.* 1993;111(7):926]. *Arch Ophthalmol.* 1993;111(4):430–431.

12. Aslanides IM, Reinstein DZ, Silverman RH, Lazzaro DR, Rondeau MJ, Rodriguez HS, Coleman DJ. High-frequency ultrasound spectral parameter imaging of anterior corneal scars. *CLAO J.* 1995;21(4):268–272.

13. Allemann N, Chamon W, Silverman RH, et al. High-frequency ultrasound quantitative analyses of corneal scarring following excimer laser keratectomy. *Arch Ophthalmol.* 1993;111(7):968–973.

14. Lazzaro DR, Aslanides IM, Belmont SC, et al. High frequency ultrasound evaluation of radial keratotomy incisions. *J Cataract Refract Surg.* 1995;21(4):398–401.

15. Silverman RH, Reinstein DZ, Raevsky T, Coleman DJ. Improved system for sonographic imaging and biometry of the cornea. *J Ultrasound Med.* 1997;16(2):117–124.

16. Reinstein DZ, Sutton HFS, Srivannaboon S, Silverman RH, Coleman DJ. Microkeratome efficacy: 3D thickness assessment of corneal lamellar flap accuracy and reproducibility by arc-scanning very high-frequency digital ultrasound. *J Refract Surg.* 2006;In press.

17. Roberts C. The cornea is not a piece of plastic. *J Refract Surg.* 2000;16(4):407–413.

18. Holland SP, Srivannaboon S, Reinstein DZ. Avoiding serious corneal complications of laser assisted in situ keratomileusis and photorefractive keratectomy. *Ophthalmology.* 2000;107(4):640–652.

19. Boscia F, La Tegola MG, Alessio G, Sborgia C. Accuracy of Orbscan optical pachymetry in corneas with haze. *J Cataract Refract Surg.* 2002;28(2):253–258.

20. Prisant O, Calderon N, Chastang P, Gatinel D, Hoang-Xuan T. Reliability of pachymetric measurements using Orbscan after excimer refractive surgery. *Ophthalmology.* 2003;110(3):511–515.

21. Iskander NG, Anderson Penno E, Peters NT, Gimbel HV, Ferensowicz M. Accuracy of Orbscan pachymetry measurements and DHG ultrasound pachymetry in primary laser in situ keratomileusis and LASIK enhancement procedures. *J Cataract Refract Surg.* 2001;27(5):681–685.

22. Patel S, Alio JL, Perez-Santonja JJ. A model to explain the difference between changes in refraction and central ocular surface power after laser in situ keratomileusis. *J Refract Surg.* 2000;16(3):330–335.

23. Gauthier CA, Holden BA, Epstein D, et al. Factors affecting epithelial hyperplasia after photorefractive keratectomy [see comments]. *J Cataract Refract Surg.* 1997; 23(7):1042–1050.

24. Lohmann CP, Reischl U, Marshall J. Regression and epithelial hyperplasia after myopic photorefractive keratectomy in a human cornea. *J Cataract Refract Surg.* 1999;25(5):712–715.

25. Srivannaboon S, Reinstein DZ, Sutton HFS, Silverman RH, Coleman DJ. Effect of epithelial changes on refractive outcome in LASIK. *Invest Ophthalmol Vis Sci.* 1999; 40:S896.

26. Reinstein DZ, Srivannaboon S, Silverman RH, Coleman DJ. Limits of wavefront customized ablation: biomechanical and epithelial factors. *Invest Ophthalmol Vis Sci.* 2002;43:E-Abstract 3942.

27. Patel S, Marshall J, Fitzke FW. Refractive index of the human corneal epithelium and stroma. *J Refract Surg.* 1995;11(2):100–105.

28. Reinstein DZ, Aslanides IM, Silverman RH, Najafi DJ, Brownlow RL, Belmont S, Haight DM, Coleman DJ. Epithelial and corneal 3D ultrasound pachymetric topography post excimer laser surgery. *Invest Ophthalmol Vis Sci.* 1994;35(4):1739.

29. Reinstein DZ, Srivannaboon S, Sutton HFS, Silverman RH, Shaikh A, Coleman DJ. Risk of ectasia in LASIK: revised safety criteria. *Invest Ophthalmol Vis Sci.* 1999; 40(Suppl):S403.

30. Barraquer JI. *Queratomileusis y Queratofakia.* Bogota, Colombia: Instituto Barraquer de America; 1980.

31. Srivannaboon S, Reinstein DZ, Sutton HFS, et al. Hansatome flap consistency analysis by 3D VHF ultrasound pachymetric topography. *Invest Ophthalmol Vis Sci.* 1999;40(4):ARVO abstract.

32. Seitz B, Torres F, Langenbucher A, Behrens A, Suarez E. Posterior corneal curvature changes after myopic laser in situ keratomileusis. *Ophthalmology.* 2001;108(4): 666–672, discussion 73.

33. Pallikaris IG, Kymionis GD, Astyrakakis NI. Corneal ectasia induced by laser in situ keratomileusis. *J Cataract Refract Surg.* 2001;27(11):1796–1802.

34. Seiler T, Koufala K, Richter G. Iatrogenic keratectasia after laser in situ keratomileusis. *J Refract Surg.* 1998; 14(3):312–317.

35. Reinstein DZ, Cremonesi E. Ectasia in routine LASIK: occurrence rate is reduced by one-third when consistently using a thinner flap. *Invest Ophthalmol Vis Sci.* 2001;42(4):S725.

36. Zaldivar R, Oscherow S, Ricur G. The STAAR posterior chamber phakic intraocular lens. *Int Ophthalmol Clin.* 2000;40(3):237–244.

37. Baikoff G. Intraocular phakic implants in the anterior chamber. *Int Ophthalmol Clin.* 2000;40(3):223–235.

Chapter 20

The Keratron and Keratron Scout Corneal Topographers

Renzo Mattioli, PhD and Nancy K. Tripoli, MA

The Keratron family includes the Keratron and the Keratron Scout (Optikon 2000, SpA, Rome, Italy). Both are Placido-based, non-spherically biased, computer-assisted corneal topographers. The Keratron was introduced in 1993 to overcome some limitations in an earlier generation of corneal topographers. The Keratron Scout was introduced in 1999 as a portable, modular version of the Keratron. It can be used hand-held, fitted on a generic slit lamp with a slide adaptor, or positioned intraoperatively with a weight-balanced arm and sterile disposable covers. The Keratron Scout is supplied with full 32-bit software, which can be upgraded from Optikon's web site. Keratrons, including those dating back to 1993 to 1994, can also be operated using the Scout software. An external unit, the Keratron Bridge, provides image grabbing, power supply, and USB interface with any standard PC, either desktop or laptop (Figure 20-1). Both topographers have been recently equipped with corneal wavefront and IR pupillometry, and a number of new accessories.

Before describing these and other Keratron family software features and clinical applications, it is important to understand the unique method of corneal reconstruction that results in Keratron maps that show corneal shape details that are not commonly visible with most other topographers.

THE QUEST FOR ACCURATE CORNEAL TOPOGRAPHY

In the last 2 decades, the color-coded corneal maps produced by corneal topographers, also called computer-assisted videokeratographers (CAVKs), have become an indispensable tool for clinical understanding of corneal shape. The challenge of videokeratoscopy has been to present clinically relevant corneal shape information in pictorials that are well understood so as to discourage over-interpretation. In addition to maps of corneal power, CAVKs have also mapped corneal height and used the height unit to fit contact lenses and predict or evaluate refractive surgical techniques such as photorefractive keratectomy (PRK), laser in-situ keratomileusis (LASIK), laser epithelial keratomileusis (LASEK), and intrastromal rings (ISR).

Since the early 1990s, a new generation of lathes has allowed fabrication of custom contact lenses with far more complex shapes that can conform to the large variety of keratoconic corneas. In the same period, ophthalmic excimer laser technology has been greatly improved by the introduction of flying spot technology and high speed eye-trackers that allow custom modeling and custom retreatments. Both these applications could be linked to CAVKs and guided by corneal topography measurements. However, these applications needed data with higher accuracy and local spatial resolution than could be achieved until then by spherically biased methods.

In the past, Placido-based CAVKs such as the Keratron were criticized as theoretically incapable of producing accurate corneal height information.[1-3] It was argued that the corneal surface description could not be recovered from Placido images without irrevocable limits on accuracy. The Keratron was designed to overcome such criticism. The problems to be solved were (1) accurately measuring the cornea so that the maps and other applications were trustworthy, (2) providing a color-coded map unit that showed corneal shape detail, (3) supporting software processing with precision hardware, (4) rigorously testing the accuracy produced by the hardware/software configuration, and (5) using the configuration to demonstrate as

Figure 20-1. Scout software processes both corneal topography and corneal wavefront maps from either the Keratron Scout or the Keratron.

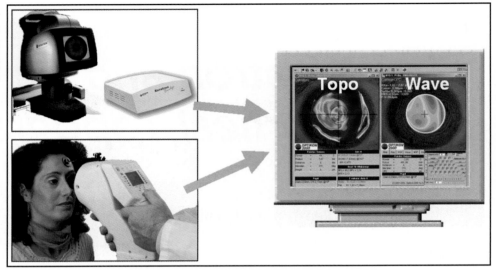

much information as possible to the clinician. This chapter describes the challenges of Placido-based CAVKs and the Keratron's design implementations to meet those challenges.

Clinical Information in a CAVK Color-Coded Map

Prior to the introduction of the Keratron, the leading commercial CAVKs showed maps of "corneal power" as measured along a number of radials. The unit shown was axial power, the mathematical definition of which is the power of a sphere, centered on the CAVK axis, that has the same tangent as the cornea at each measurement position on a corneal profile. Axial power is inversely proportional of the radius of the sphere, using the "thin lens law," D = 337.5/Ra, and that radius is the distance from the surface position to the CAVK's axis measured along a surface normal. Mathematically, it is defined as:

$$Ra = x (1 + (dz/dx)2)^{1/2} / (dz/dx)$$

where z is sagittal height and x is the distance from the axis. Axial power represents the "tilting" of the surface downward from apex to periphery. Its historical relevance lies in its use in the ophthalmometer, and its scientific relevance derives from the fact that the tangent to a surface determines refraction.

Since the corneal surface is smooth, its height changes gradually from position to position. The surface's rate of change, the tangent, reveals more detail about corneal shape than does height. However, the "bending" of the cornea reveals even more details. The geometric unit that describes the bending of the cornea in a given direction

through a given point is the local, also called "tangential" or "meridional" or "instantaneous" curvature, which is the inverse of the radius of a circle whose profile matches the profile of the corneal surface at each measurement position. The radius of the sphere (Ri) is defined as:

$$Ri = (1 + (dz/dx)2)^{3/2} / (d^2x/dx^2)$$

where z is sagittal height and x is the distance from the axis. The sphere used to measure axial power does not have the same instantaneous curvature as the cornea at the same reflective position unless the cornea is spherical. Unlike the sphere, the center of curvature does not necessarily lie on the CAVK axis. Axial power at any point has been shown to be the average of the instantaneous curvature from the center to that point.[4]

Traditional Spherically Biased Methods to Deduct Axial Power from Placido Reflections

Prior to the Keratron, the leading commercial CAVKs derived axial power by (1) measuring the power of the cornea to magnify the image of a mire,[5] or (2) matching the size of a reflected mire to the sizes of mires reflected from a series of spheres.[6,7] The left image in Figure 20-2 shows the problems with these methods. The diagram shows rays from a mire reflecting from a cornea (solid line) and a sphere (dotted line). A point on the sphere (A) and a point on the cornea (B) will reflect the same ray to the lens and form the same image in the reflected mire pattern. However, the sphere and the cornea have different axial radii, heights, and instantaneous curvatures. Traditional axial power measurement records the radius of

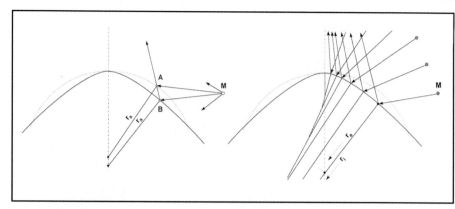

Figure 20-2. (Left) Spherically biased algorithms identify the ray reflected from the cornea as equivalent to a ray from the same mire M reflected on a sphere. (Right) The Keratron arc-step instead reconstructs the whole corneal profile as a continuous sequence of arcs, from vertex to periphery, resulting in higher accuracy of both heights and curvatures.

the sphere as the radius of curvature of the cornea. This results in mild error for axial radii and more extreme error for height and instantaneous curvature.

The false assumption that a sphere and a cornea that reflect the same ray to the lens have the same powers and heights is called "spherical equivalency" or "spherical bias."[6] When the axial power is measured by mire magnification or mire size, corneal height cannot be determined because, for a selected reflection position, an infinite family of combinations of tangents and heights can produce the same axial power. It has been definitively demonstrated that this assumption leads to incorrect height measurement.[6,7] The reliance of early CAVKs on spherically biased measurement techniques resulted in the false assertion that all reflective CAVKs must be inaccurate for measuring height and instantaneous curvature.[1,2]

Corneal Surface Reconstruction Using the Keratron Arc-Step Algorithm

An arc-step algorithm such as that used by the Keratron is a surface reconstruction method that is not spherically biased and is not completely new. It was introduced in 1896 by Allvar Gullstrand[8] and resurrected in different formats 1981 by Doss[9] and others between 1989 and 1992.[10–12] Nevertheless the arc-step was usually assumed to be difficult to implement in a commercial CAVK without smoothing data with polynomial fitting or the like.[13]

The Keratron identifies a continuous sequence of arcs, starting at the vertex, that accurately reconstructs a corneal profile along each of 256 radials, as shown in the right image of Figure 20-2. A cornea reflects rays from each mire through the lens to produce the reflected mire pattern for that cornea. The radii of the arcs in the Keratron's reconstructed profile are adjusted such that they will reflect rays from the appropriate mires to the lens and produce the reflected pattern. The generic arc-step recon-

struction method can describe aspheric corneal profiles because the second and more peripheral arcs need not be centered on the CAVK axis. There is one and only one sequence of arcs that can satisfy a unique sequence of mire reflections.

An unsmoothed arc-step algorithm was implemented on the Keratron to provide accurate height measurements and to produce meaningful maps of instantaneous curvature.[14] When the profile is reconstructed, it yields the instantaneous curvature, height, tangent, and axial power at each intersection of two arcs. This obviates the need for calculating one corneal descriptor from another, since curve-fitting and mathematical derivations necessarily erode measurement accuracy and/or spatial resolution.[15,16]

Keratron Maps of Axial and Curvature Units

Maps that depict unbiased units demonstrate the clinical utility of axial power for traditional reference to optics and instantaneous curvature for shape visualization. The detail that is missing from an axial power map, but is depicted by an instantaneous curvature map, is clinically significant.[17,18] For example, on an axial map of a normal astigmatic cornea such as that in Figure 20-3 (top left), the toricity of regular astigmatism seems to extend to the periphery. When the same cornea is depicted using instantaneous curvature as shown in the same figure, middle left, it now appears that the astigmatism is confined within an approximately circular region of curvature above 37 D, the "corneal cap" (green and yellow). That region is surrounded by a flat peripheral region (blue), which becomes even flatter toward the periphery, reaching a maximum flatness of 15 D (23 mm) or more. The existence of the corneal cap, which appears on most normal corneas, has implications for contact lens fitting and also may prove valuable in early diagnosis of disease. The bottom left diagram in

Figure 20-3. Representations of a normal, astigmatic cornea (left) and a keratoconic cornea (right) include the axial power (top) and curvature maps (middle), and color-coded local curvature along the 9 o'clock corneal profile (bottom).

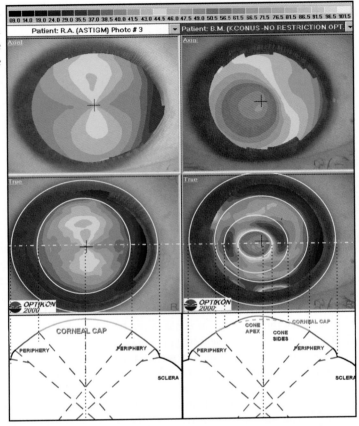

Figure 20-3 represents a corneal profile from nine o'clock to three o'clock. The relatively uniform curvature across the corneal cap in this direction, shown in green and corresponding to the green in the curvature map, changes in the periphery, which is relatively flat, shown in blue corresponding to the blue in the map.

Viewing an axial power map of keratoconus, as shown in Figure 20-3 (top right), can lead to a misinterpretation of shape since a large corneal region seems to be affected by the cone. The instantaneous curvature map (Figure 20-3, middle right) shows that the most highly curved region of the cone is only 2 mm in diameter, and curvature decreases rapidly to a large corneal region that is unaffected by the cone. The bottom right diagram shows that the cone is characterized by a highly curved central region that involves the corneal vertex, surrounded by a somewhat flatter annular region. Much of the corneal cap is unaffected by the cone.

The importance of depicting corneal shape details is well illustrated by maps of a cornea after photorefractive keratectomy (PRK), such as that in Figure 20-4. On this axial map (left), the steepness of the edge appears to involve a large annular region surrounding a generally flat center. On the curvature map (right), the steep bending of the cornea over the ablation's edge can be appreciated.

More importantly, some central island anomalies that are critical to vision following PRK are not visible on the axial map but are seen on the curvature map.

Detecting and understanding corneal warpage caused by contact lenses is also aided by an instantaneous curvature map, as shown in Figure 20-5. On the curvature map (left), the distinctive pattern includes a flat annular region (blue) surrounded by alternating steep (red) and flat (blue) regions. The map on the right side is obtained by subtracting corneal height from the height of a sphere. Although the map contains less detail than either axial or curvature maps, it shows that a highly curved corneal region, indicated by the large cross, differs from the surrounding region by only 5 microns. To reveal this detail requires an operator's option for positioning of the reference sphere and also precise height measurement so that small color steps describe localized corneal shape features.

The Spherical Offset Map

A map of absolute sagittal height, ie, depth with respect to the corneal plane, would always appear as a series of concentric colored doughnuts since the decreases in height from center to periphery are much greater than any circumferential variations in height. Therefore, another surface

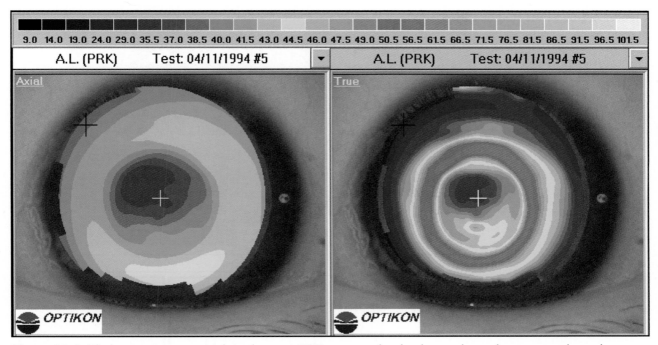

Figure 20-4. The curvature map (right) of a post-PRK cornea clearly shows shape features, such as the steep bending over the edge of the ablation and central islands, which are not clearly visible in the axial power map (left) of the same cornea.

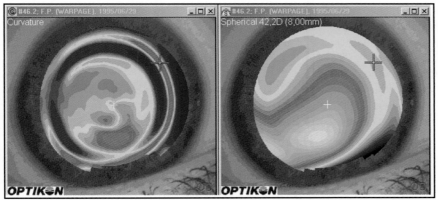

Figure 20-5. Instantaneous curvature map (left) and height or "spherical offset" map (right) of the same cornea with contact lens warpage.

similar to the cornea's must be subtracted and the differences in heights mapped. Simulations of normal corneas have been proposed as the basis for subtraction, but the normative shape of the cornea is disputed, complex, and highly variable, making the use of a single "normal" reference of little value. Therefore, the Keratron subtracts a sphere, a shape that can be easily visualized by users. Difference values near zero are colored yellow and represent positions where the sphere's surface and the cornea's surface coincide. This is illustrated in Figure 20-5. Positions where the cornea rises above the sphere are colored in shades of red, and positions where the cornea dips below the sphere are in shades green-blue. With this convention the map is analogous to a topographic map of the earth.

The positioning of the sphere radically alters the appearance of the map, and users must understand and become accustomed to the alternative views of height. When we first introduced "spherical offset" height maps, users were frequently disappointed by the smooth, general appearance of this kind of map and the lack of detail, even on diseased corneas. To allow them to enhance heights in the region of interest (eg, the apex of a keratoconus, the optical zone of a post-refractive treatment), the Keratron allows the sphere to be fit tangent to the apex (as in Figure 20-6) or to any position selected by the user,

Figure 20-6. The height scale resolution of the spherical offset map can be adjusted to measure detail like this 1.9 micron ectatic scar.

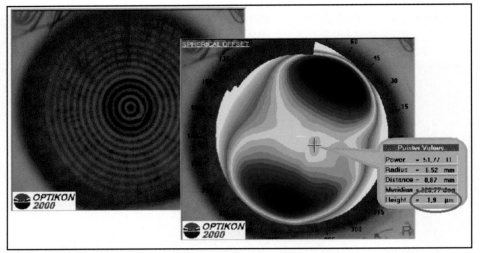

either tangent to a given point or passing through three reference points which is especially useful to align pre-post ablation height differences as in Figure 20-8.

KERATRON FEATURES AND BENEFITS

The accuracy and cost-effectiveness of a measuring instrument depends on the appropriateness of each of its components to the overall objective. To implement the arc-step algorithm on a commercial instrument requires special attention to inherent problems, for example numerical instability and extremely sensitive ring tracing.[2,10] The sub-pixeling and other proprietary numerical methods and design solutions adopted for the Keratron are described in more detail elsewhere.[19] Following is a list of the Keratron's main features and the resulting unique benefits.

Height Accuracy

Earlier CAVKs, which had proven successful in measuring spheres,[7,20–22] were highly inaccurate for measuring aspheres.[5,6] Since 1993 to 1994, the Keratron has been tested by several independent researchers on nonspherical profiles.[23] Tripoli et al[24] measured, on a set of normal prolate, rotationally symmetric surfaces, an error within 0.25 microns within the central 3-mm zone and an error within 1 micron for entire surfaces. Under similar conditions, a TMS-1 (Computed Anatomy, New York, NY) height error was within 85 microns.[5,26] Another frequent criticism of CAVKs is their disregard for the circumferential rise and fall of an astigmatic surface, which theoretically deflects mire reflections. Evidence that this real optical effect produces inconsequential errors in the reconstruction on surfaces with up to 12 diopters of regular astigmatism has been published elsewhere.[25,27]

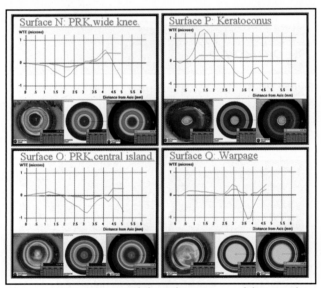

Figure 20-7. Four model surfaces were fabricated to simulate the four clinical conditions shown on the left. Accuracy was always within ± 1.5 microns.

Attempting to measure more complex surfaces that are usually encountered in clinical and surgical practice can lead to even larger height and curvature errors with spherically biased methods.[23,24] The multiple transitions from flat to steep to flat areas present a real challenge for topographic algorithms. Optikon conducted in-house testing on four surfaces that mimicked clinical cases and presented the results at ARVO 1996 (Figure 20-7).[28] In spite of the greater complexity of such shapes, the error remained within less than 1.5 microns. The testing has been repeated on the Keratron Scout with results similar to the Keratron. The examples in Figures 20-3 through 20-7 demonstrate the flexibility of the arc-step for tracking complex profiles without smoothing details.

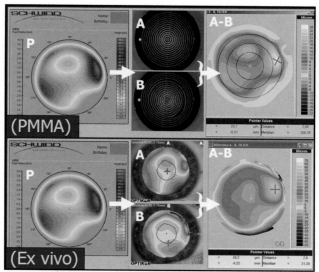

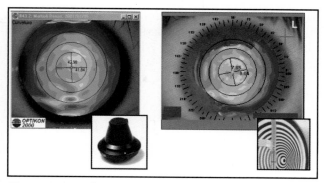

Figure 20-9. The Keratron "Dekking" type cone (left) achieves greater corneal coverage than large "Placido disk" topographers (right), when imaging the same cornea

Figure 20-8. The pre-post height difference (A minus B) after an application of the Schwind ESIRS laser treatment to an aspheric PMMA surface (top row) and to a living eye (bottom row), which shows the accuracy of the Keratron Scout for measuring corneal heights. (Courtesy of Dr. M. Camellin.)

depicts a case by Dr. Camellin, treated with the ESIRIS laser by Schwind Eye-Tech Solutions (Kleinhostheim, Germany) and the "Scout-ORKw" corneal wavefront link.[29]

Corneal Coverage, Focusing, and Positioning

The use of a cone containing lighted mires is not new. As said in a previous section of this book, it was introduced by Dekking in 1930 to place the mire arrangement close to the cornea in order to measure a larger area.[30] The Keratron mire reflections cover about 80% to 90% of a normal cornea in a well-opened eye, illustrated in Figure 20-9. However, the cone can be very sensitive to focal distance. To overcome this theoretical limitation, the Keratrons are equipped with a patented Eye Position Control System (EPCS), pictured in Figure 20-10, composed of an infrared beam that intercepts the corneal vertex. With this system a picture can be taken only when the focusing, ie, "Z" positioning, is within a range as tight as 0.1 mm, which can guarantee a repeatability of ±0.1 diopters or better (see next paragraph and Figure 20-11). Lateral (X, Y) decentering is not critical because of a software method called the Eye Misplacement Control System (EMCS), which recalculates the spatial mire position in the measured direction.[19] Cantera and associates have verified that a misalignment in any direction, up to 1 mm, induces less than 0.1 diopters change in the resulting curvature map.[31]

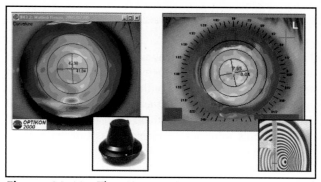

Figure 20-10. The Keratron's Eye Position Control System (EPCS).

In addition to other applications such as custom contact lenses and laser links, the Keratron's height accuracy is very useful for verifying the specified custom laser ablation pattern as implemented, including file transfer, ablation design algorithm, and "fluence." Figure 20-8 shows an example of such a custom ablation pattern (on the left) and the post minus pre-treatment height measurement by a Keratron Scout (on the right). In the top row the ablation was applied on curved plastic surfaces, and the yellow annular zone (difference = 0 microns) corresponds to the untreated zone. The bottom row shows the effect of the same specified ablation on a living eye. This example

Repeatability Check

In spite of EPCS-automated capture enabling, harsh movements and other occurrences (eg, blinking, tear film

Figure 20-11. The Keratron software includes a repeatability check, shown here assessing the stability of acquisition by a surgeon through 7 intraoperative topographic images of the same eye.

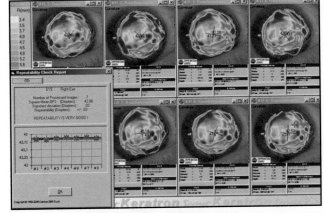

Figure 20-12. The Keratron's mire arrangement and subpixel edging algorithms allow the capture of detail that results in both high resolution and a large range of curvature. In this cornea, curvatures as steep as 2.64 mm (128 D) and as flat as 37.5 mm (9 D) are measured.

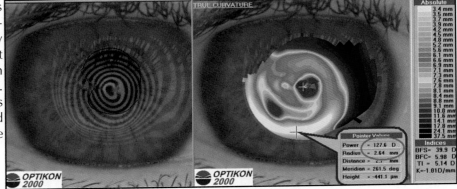

disruption) can still create artifacts that affect overall accuracy, especially in handheld mode. To screen out unacceptable images, a "repeatability check" feedback function was introduced in the Scout software. The repeatability check window, seen in Figure 20-11, can be recalled at any time, or preset to automatic whenever three or more images of the same eye are acquired and processed. Normal eye repeatability is considered "good" with a deviation of the best fit sphere (BFS) of processed maps within 0.24 diopters and "very good" if less than 0.12 diopters. Using this feature for self-training, it is not difficult to obtain repeatability well within 0.1 diopters, thus reducing the acquisition root mean square (RMS) height error to within less than 0.4 micron over a 6 mm zone.

Range of Measurement

Even normal eyes frequently have an instantaneous curvature range between 20 and 50 D. In keratoconus, scars, and post-surgery, corneal curvature often shows a much greater range of power. To achieve their full potential, corneal topographers must also be able to cover such extreme cases without losing too much local information or introducing artifacts. Figure 20-12 shows a case in which the local curvature ranges from less than 10 D (dark blue) in some areas to above 120 D (the measured point =

127.6 D) in others. Mires that are too close together limit an instrument's capability for measuring abrupt changes across the corneal surface. On the other hand, if the mires are too sparse, height reconstruction and detection of local distortion are impaired. With these opposite needs in mind, the Keratron's mire arrangement was optimized both in number and size of steps (28 mires uniformly spaced about 0.166 mm on a 43 D sphere), making use of both black-to-white and white-to-black mire borders. If mires were tracked at the middle of the rings, as in most classic "cone type" videokeratoscopes, an equivalent twice the number of rings would limit instrument curvature measurement range to a maximum of 60 to 70 D.[19] Detecting the borders of alternating black and white mires also ensures accurate tracking of mires even with complex, tangled patterns. In Figure 20-12 only some small edematous areas are unprocessed and were automatically discarded by tracking algorithms as unsuitable. Rarely, special processing functions such as "dots editing" may be needed to recover mires that were automatically tracked incorrectly.

Spatial Resolution

The Keratron's mire arrangement samples an average normal cornea at 166 micron spacing steps. This requires special edging techniques to prevent smoothing and loss of

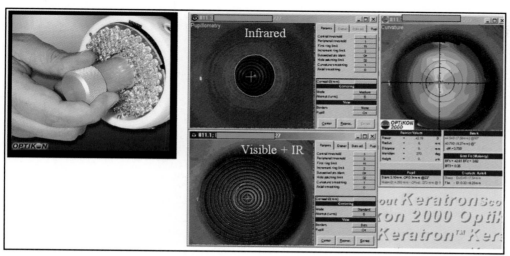

Figure 20-13. The Keratron can track the pupil edge in photopic and mesopic conditions and report it in topographic maps.

important information about localized distortion such as scars. Precise mires tracking is accomplished by the Keratron due to its subpixeling technique. Rather than just searching for black-to-white and white-to-black edge thresholds, the technique uses the entire gray scale information from all the pixels of each profile sector captured by the CCD camera. The resulting equivalent accuracy in detection of a ring position is less than 1/20 of pixel.[19] The small ectasia in Figure 20-6, whose height is less than 2 microns, is detectable because of the crisp mire edge reflections. It could not be detected by nonreflective methods because the confusion in surface-scattered projected lines or slit light edges is typically much larger than this height. The mire's reflections instead naturally amplify even the smallest corneal scar (Figure 20-6, left).

Pupil Tracking

The recent use of links between the corneal wavefront and the excimer laser in which a complex ablation pattern must be precisely aligned with pupil eye-trackers requires accurate measurement of the pupil center and edge, a feature that was less important when corneal topographers were primarily diagnostic instruments. Furthermore a measure of individual natural pupil dilatation at night, or mesopic-scotopic vision conditions, is often required in clinical pre-operative practice. A new illumination system recently has been implemented in new production units to replace both the Scout's "lamp board" (Figure 20-13, left), as well as the Keratron's neon lamp. An assembly of software, firmware, and electronics allows acquisition of the eye image and tracking of the pupil edges in both mesopic and standard photopic light conditions.

The reconstruction of the pupil by the Keratron is performed on an internal reconstruction of a "clean picture"

from the keratoscope image.[19] The mires must have been tracked correctly without induction of artifacts. In some cases a "pupil editor" function can be used for hand correction. The pupil position at the two extreme illumination conditions is measured and represented with respect to corneal vertex. On average in a normal population, the pupil center does not change significantly from photopic to mesopic condition.[32,33] Nevertheless in some cases, the pupil center can be substantially displaced (0.25 mm in the case of Figure 20-13, right). In such a case, although the laser treatments are tracked on the photopic pupil, the ablated zone could be more properly centered on the largest naturally dilated size area.

The "Move Axis"

To measure curvature relative to the virtual pupil, surface measurements must be recalculated relative to a new axis. As with recalculating off-centered images, a lateral translation will result in errors. Instead, the Keratron performs a three-dimensional rotation of the corneal model. The "move axis" feature can also shift the corneal representation to any point desired by the user. This is useful to visualize the symmetry surrounding points of interest such as the keratoconic cone apex shown in Figure 20-14. This example shows also how the flat annular area surrounding the apex (Figure 20-14A) creates a high astigmatism, typically against-the-rule in patients having an inferior keratoconus, because the meridional cut across and perpendicular to the apex are the local flattest and steepest meridians, respectively. Moving the axis to the apex (Figure 20-14B) shows the actual symmetry of the shape of keratoconus

When an image is acquired while a subject gazes at the fixation light, as is shown in Figure 20-15, and the operator

Figure 20-14. Keratron move-axis feature. Different views of the same keratoconus before (A) and after (B) moving the keratoscope axis to the cone center.

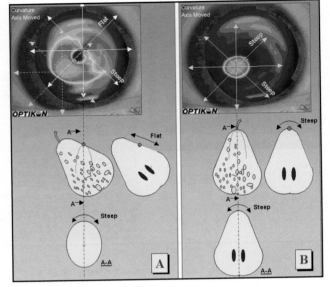

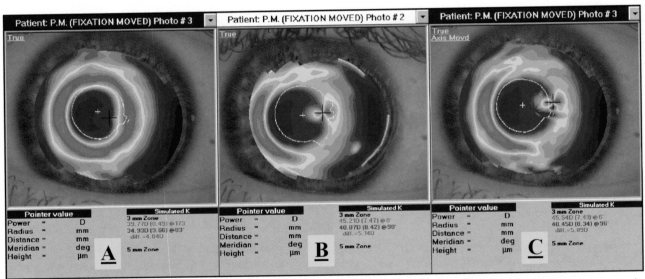

Figure 20-15. In (A), normal function produces a post-ablation "knee" or red ring. Using the Keratron move-axis feature (C) produces the same result as asking the patient to change fixation (B).

moves the axis, the resulting map looks remarkably similar to a map produced by requesting the subject to change his or her gaze. Thus moving the axis produces a virtual rotation of the eye.[34] In Figure 20-15, normal fixation produces a typical post-ablation "knee," a red ring (Figure 20-15A). If the patient is asked to fixate to the side, the vertex moves towards the periphery, and a small "hourglass" indicates the high astigmatism of the "knee zone" (Figure 20-15B). The same image can be created using the Keratron's move-axis feature (Figure 20-15C), showing that the feature mathematically rotates the cornea. The move-axis (Figure 20-15C) preserves the entrance pupil position,

whereas when changing patient fixation (Figure 20-15B), a difficult practice, this important reference is lost. This feature is particularly useful when measuring the actual astigmatism of patients that cannot keep fixation, for example suture distribution after PKP with the intra-operative Keratron Scout.[35]

Process Editing and "Dots Editing"

When CAVK users take a corneal image and are shown only a colored map, they are unaware of the many choices that have been automatically made by the instrument. But all measuring systems can occasionally produce artifacts or skip over regions. The ability to change the parameters that control Keratron processing can be a benefit to the clinician who understands his or her objective. The Keratron offers the user the options to improve ring reconstruction in difficult cases, for example, by changing the sensitivity of borders, or of altering the incremental ring limit, the maximum number of meridians that can be interpolated, the sensitivity for finding the processing center, or the sensitivity for excluding suspected extraneous points. A powerful software feature called "Dots Editing" includes a number of tools to allow the user to re-assign every single B/W (green dots) or W/B threshold (red dots) to its proper ring. A complete removal of artifacts with this tool can be especially important before custom contact lens (CL) height fitting or custom laser link. The user is also permitted to clean a ring pattern by erasing artifactual areas, but is not allowed to add rings or segments of rings.

Intra-Operative Functions

The Keratron Scout can be fitted into an optional weight-balanced trolley, and sterile accessories allow the surgeon to take intra-operative corneal topography, ie, before and after a treatment. While the Scout is sterile sleeved, the surgeon can position and use upside-down buttons to start acquisition for either eye, capture an image, and even browse in the database and save the topography without needing to reach the PC keyboard. The intra-operative Scout has proved very useful in adjusting sutures after PKP and LKP,[35] during PTK treatments, and in measuring pre-op and/or de-epithelialized corneas before and after LASEK topo-link treatments.[36]

WAVEFRONT ANALYSIS WITH THE SCOUT SOFTWARE

Wavefront representations have been implemented in the Keratron Scout software since 2001.[37] These include measuring the corneal wavefront (CW) from Keratron corneal topographies, importing the ocular wavefront (OW) from most commercial aberrometers through data files containing Zernike terms and pupil data, and calculating the internal wavefront (IW) as the linear subtraction of Zernike terms (IW = OW – CW). Other wavefront representations include refraction maps representing Zernike terms and simulating visual function (PSF, MTF) and performance (letter chart, visual acuity, night vision). A more detailed description of these functions,[38,39] as well as wavefront analysis[40] and Zernike polynomials, can be found elsewhere,[41] and in the Scout online help that every

registered Keratron Scout user can download from the Optikon Web site. Below we summarize some basic topics of the new features that allow corneal topographers to "speak the same language" as total wavefront analyzers.

The Corneal Wavefront (CW): A New Way to Represent Corneal Optics

The purpose of wavefront analysis (WA) is to measure wavefront aberrations, and the purpose of corneal topography (CT) is to measure corneal shape. However, more than 70% of the eye's refraction is due to the corneal first surface. Corneal distortion always affects total ocular wavefront aberration more significantly than any other interface. The CW,* the component of the OW due to the cornea, can be calculated from CT height data. The CW can be fit with a Zernike decomposition just as the OW is measured by an aberrometer and fit with Zernikes. Placing the two Zernike representations side-by-side allows inspection of the OW and the contribution of the CW.

Figure 20-16 shows maps of the OW of one of the author's right and left eyes, measured with a Shack-Hartmann (S/H) aberrometer, and of the CW, derived from corneal topography. Only the high order Zernike polynomials from 3rd to 5th radial order are shown. As is often the case, there is similarity between the OW and CW maps. This similarity shows how much high-order aberrations of the cornea affect the total ocular aberrations. However, when total ocular aberrations are very low, there is much less similarity between OW and CW representations of the same eye, and internal aberrations IW become the predominant component in the OW.

From Corneal Geometry to Corneal Wavefront Maps

Since 1994, several authors have made studies of the CW from CAVTs including Howland et al,[42] Hemenger et al,[43] and, in 1997, Schwiegerling and Greivenkamp.[44] A comprehensive collection of CW and IW studies under different patient conditions is among the work of Marcos et al,[45,46] Artal et al,[47–49] and Guirao et al.[50] Figure 20-17 illustrates a model of a simplified procedure based on the optical path difference (OPD), ie, the "least time" Fermat principle, in the "object space."[51,52] If a cornea had an ideal shape and minimal internal aberrations, then rays traced from the fovea would exit parallel from the cornea

---

*The terms corneal or ocular "wavefront" are used here as generic descriptions of either "wavefront error," "wavefront aberration," or "OPD." According to the OSA standard, both units can be used, but the reader must be aware that they are opposite in sign. OPD maps appear similar in color convention to height maps, while WFE maps have opposite colors.

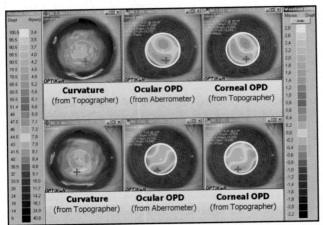

Figure 20-16. Correspondence between high orders of the ocular and corneal wavefronts. The right (top) and left eyes (bottom) of one of the authors are shown as Keratron topography (left), ocular OPD (imported from a S/H aberrometer), and Keratron corneal OPD (right column).

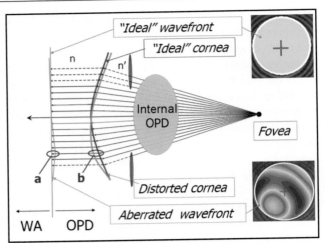

Figure 20-17. A keratoconic cornea accelerates the rays in the superior and retards the rays in the inferior as compared with the ideal cornea. These physical distortions create a mirror aberrated wavefront whose height is scaled about 1:3 to the corneal distortion.

and form a flat wavefront (Figure 20-17, green lines and yellow map on the top right) and the aberrations would be zero. If the cornea is distorted from this ideal shape (example Figure 20-17, orange lines) the rays in one section (the superior) enter the air first where they accelerate. Other rays (the inferior) remain in the cornea for a longer path and are retarded. In the time it takes for a ray to travel about 3 microns in the cornea, it would travel about 4 microns in the air (ie, rays travel $n - 1$ times faster in air than in cornea, where n is the assumed refractive index). For example, in Figure 20-17, a corneal distortion (Figure 20-17B) of 3 microns, will produce an OPD (Figure 20-17A) 1 micron different from the ideal. As a result we can adopt a simple "rule of 3" from corneal elevations:

Every 3 microns of distortion from the ideal shape of the cornea will produce about a +1 micron difference in the OPD map and a −1 micron difference in the wavefront error map.

This simple rule can help estimate the thickness of a soft contact lens to add to the cornea or the amount of corneal tissue to remove from the cornea in order to produce a flat corneal wavefront with no aberration, although some precautions should be followed for different refractive indices. The CW OPD maps (Figure 20-16) closely resemble topographic height maps, but there are conceptual differences between the "spherical offset," which shows a cause, and OPD data, which show the effect. The "ideal cornea" is in fact an ellipsoid centered on the corneal vertex. Its definition depends on refractive indices and pupil position and requires matching the manifest patient refrac-

tion with the corneal curvature at a preset "refractive zone." In fact the Zernike term defocus, Z(2, 0), which depends on the axial length, is the only Zernike term that cannot be measured from the cornea alone and must be input from the manifest spherical equivalent refraction.

Zernike Decomposition of Corneal Wavefront

In the wavefront module of the Scout software, the wavefront surface is calculated from corneal height, and Zernike polynomials up to the 7th order are least-squares best-fit.[53] For an accurate result, all corneal positions within the selected pupil, weighted for their subtended area, are involved in the fitting process. Piston and Tilt components (Zernike radial orders 0 and 1), though calculated, are not usually displayed.

Zernike Selection and Graphical Representations of the Aberrations

The user can select the pupil size, from 3 to 9 mm, and any combination of Zernike terms to be represented by the wavefront map by clicking on specific buttons, arranged as suggested by the OSA standard pyramid.[54] For example, the user can select all orders from 2 to 7, the high orders only, the high orders and astigmatism, only radial orders from 3 to 5, or any combination of individual orders. When the selection is confirmed, the relevant weighted sum of Zernikes is calculated and reported in the map. The ray tracing, the PSF, MTF, or visual simulation, selected in

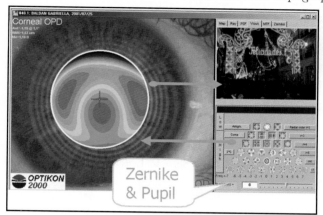

Figure 20-18. Pupil diameter and Zernike data can be selected in a Scout wavefront window affecting the corneal wavefront map, which further generates a simulation of the patient's vision

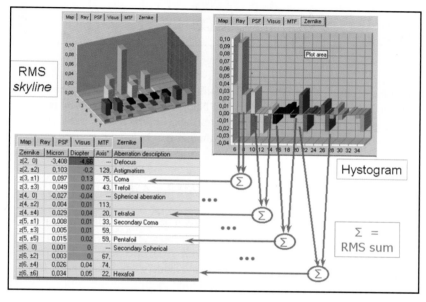

Figure 20-19. A number of alternative Zernike term formats have been proposed and are shown by the Keratron software.

the display panel at the top right in Figure 20-18, are updated to show the effect of using only the selected Zernike terms. Such a decomposition of the wavefront into selected Zernike "ingredients" can support the clinician's understanding of how individual or combined aberrations affect vision. In the "Zernike" display panel (Figure 20-19), a spectrum of the selected Zernike polynomials can be pictorially illustrated by selecting from the five different formats ("Histogram," "Color boxes," "RMS skyline," "Zernike list," or "Aberration summary").

A clinically relevant representation is the "Aberration summary." Here the aberrations at the opposite sides of the OSA pyramid (sine + cosine, or positive and negative F index) are presented not as individual Zernike terms, but as their RMS sum. This sum is expressed in microns as well as in "equivalent defocus" diopters and axis. For example in the case in Figure 20-19, the amount of primary coma is 0.13 D at 75 degrees, or 0.097 microns RMS (or the combination of sine and cosine terms) at the select-

ed pupil size. The equivalent defocus proposed by Thibos[55] expresses the wavefront variance in familiar dioptric terms. Reporting the Zernike terms in defocus equivalent diopters has the further advantage that diopters are fairly independent of pupil size, as shown in a study by Indiana University.[56] A green-yellow-red pattern in Figure 20-19 suggests a likely normality of individual aberrations.

From the Wavefront to PSF, MTF, and Visual Simulations

The calculation of the point spread function (PSF), the modulation transfer function (MTF), the visual simulation of two different letter charts (from 20/500 to 20/100, and from 20/100 to 20/20), and pictures of night vision are not done by simple ray-tracing, but by complex mathematics using Fourier optics on the pupil size area, and the Fast Fourier Transform (FFT), as summarized in Figure 20-20.

Figure 20-20. From wavefront OPD maps the point spread function (PSF), the modular transfer function (MTF), and visual simulations are calculated using Fast Fourier Transforms.

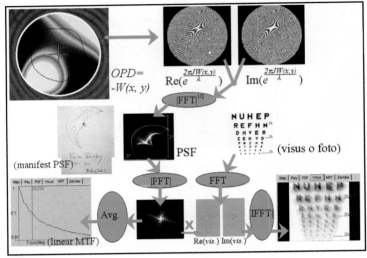

Only this process produces faithful simulations,[57] by including the effect of both the wave propagation and the diffraction created by the pupil edge. Simplified patterns or retinal spot-diagrams should not be confused with the real PSF.

The Clinical Utility of CW Measurement

CW measurement is not intended to replace WA. This new representation has special clinical utility because it evaluates corneal optics using the same "language" as wavefront analyzers, and can be decomposed by Zernike fitting into representations analogous to WA including simulated visual acuity, PSF, MTF, and other quantities that assess quality of vision. In this respect the CW is a more sensible representation of corneal optics than either axial or refractive maps. Unlike WA, CT data allow investigators to assess the CW under varying conditions such as pupil size and position.

CW analysis can help clinicians to understand patient comfort or discomfort despite apparently bad or good corneal conditions, may aid the design of surgical interventions, and/or may predict the efficiency of strategies that concentrate on removing only extremely disturbing aberrations. Visual simulations of the CW are not to be regarded as a curiosity but as new, very powerful tools for clinicians. In addition to internal aberrations, light scattering, media opacity, and retinal problems may cause these simulations to differ from reality. However in an example (Figure 20-21), we can appreciate how well the corneal PSF matches the patient's drawing of a small spot of light. Both the CW and the drawing were made under the same lighting, and therefore pupil, conditions. This example

shows that the CW simulations, which directly derive from the corneal PSF, can be especially realistic in the presence of high corneal aberrations, in which case a direct measurement by an aberrometer can be very difficult.

LINKS WITH EXCIMER LASERS

Keratron height data can be output to files for any third-party software application. Specific links have been developed in agreement with Schwind Eye-Tech Solutions (Kleinostheim, Germany) and Nidek (Gamagori, Japan). These include a "topo-link" with Schwind "ORK-t" software (now obsolete) and a versatile link with Nidek "FinalFit." Optikon pioneered with Schwind the adaptation of CW features to link a Keratron CAVK with an excimer laser system. The Scout software's CW was linked to the ORKw (optimized refractive keratectomy–wavefront), a software program that had been previously developed by Schwind for ocular wavefront links with ESIRIS. The first case of a photo-ablative treatment using a corneal-wavefront link was made by Dr. M. Camellin in February 2002.[29] Other medical researchers extended this experience in the next few years, including Bonci,[58] Dr. Carmen Barraquer (Bogotá, Colombia), Arbelaez,[59] Rummelt,[60,61] Siganos,[62] and others. (For a more complete and updated documentation please contact the Schwind APM department and see the web site: www.eye-tech-solutions.com.)

In principle, the advantages of a CW link with respect to topography, OW, or both, are as follows:

1. Optimization of the ablation pattern volume
2. Simpler comparison of results with the target

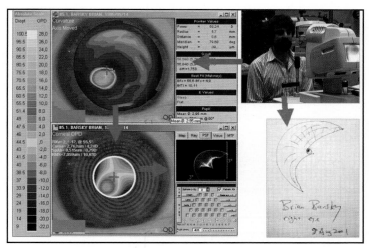

Figure 20-21. Example of a simulated point spread function (PSF) from a corneal wavefront map (OPD), compared with a drawing of the equivalent manifest PSF by the subject in scotopic conditions. (Courtesy Prof. B. Barsky)[67]

3. Overcoming some limits of Munnerlyn formulas[63,64]

4. The possibility of aberration management

5. The possibility of interaction with aberrometers

A more detailed description of these arguments can be found in quoted papers, and in a book recently edited by Camellin on LASEK and ASA.[65]

FITTING CONTACT LENSES WITH THE KERATRON SOFTWARE

Thanks to their accuracy in tracking both small local and peripheral corneal distortion, height-difference fluorescein pattern algorithms allow the Keratron and Scout to guide their users through easy design and simulation of contact lens fitting in several ways. The user interface has been made ergonomic for easy familiarization, even for old-fashioned practitioners. Classic methods that allow users to select or fit lenses according to central K-readings and corneal diameter are still available. However the major leap introduced by the Scout is its Contact Lens Editor (CLE), which comprises a number of height-fitting methods and protocols.

The CLE is an integral part of the Scout software. To activate this module, select any map from the screen, or a processed image directly from the database, and click on the Contact Lens Editor button in the Scout toolbar. Although maps usually cover 80% to 90% of the cornea, a preliminary extrapolation, placing three points around the limbal edge, is required to both fill the gaps and to measure corneal diameter at the same time.

Some specially automated "lens-family protocols" are provided to guide the user through a large number of virtual trial-sets. Such "family protocols" were first made for Horus (Verona, Italy) contact lenses[66] to include a selection of the geometry based on some corneal parameters and manufacturer's algorithms. Similar "family protocols" are also in progress with manufacturers including TS (Milano, Italy) and Soleko (Pontecorvo, Italy).

The Scout Contact Lens Editor

The Keratron and Keratron Scout CLE windows and menu offer several choices. You can choose to:

- **Select a virtual trial set**, to be chosen among a wide number of CL manufacturers (registered users, see Scout DC-ROM or Optikon Web site) to simulate the fitting of a lens

- **Fit a custom multi-curve contact lens** according to classical criteria "Contour" and "OC+2"

- **Fit a custom lens using a "height fitting" method**: multi-curve (up to 5 zones), multi-conic (Figure 20-22), toric (up to 4 zones) or Ortho-K lens (5 zones, inverse geometry, Figure 20-23)

A number of tools allow the user to evaluate and optimize fitting and design:

1. A **Clearance Panel** (eg, bottom right in Figures 20-22B and 20-22C) plots the cross sectional vertical distance between the lens and the cornea, in microns. Clicking on the map is sufficient to select the meridian and see how the relevant clearance section changes.

2. **Moving the lens** to any point on the cornea to simulate real lens movement on the eye allows the user to find the point of maximum symmetry and is always recommended as the first step. To move the

Figure 20-22. Contact lens fitting to a keratoconic cornea using the Scout Contact Lens Editor.

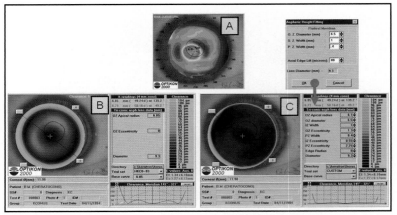

Figure 20-23. Ortho-K contact lens fitting on a young patient.

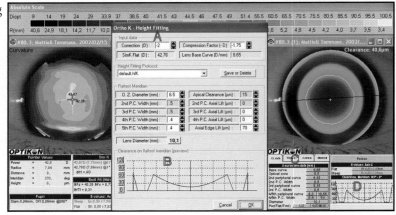

lens just double-click-drag-and-drop the lens on the fluorescein map.

3. **Tilting the lens** along the flattest and steepest meridians, using 4 buttons on the map, allows the user to simulate the effects of blinking and gravity.

4. **Indenting the lens**, ie, pushing in or pulling the lens out, simulates the effect of indentation and compares this with the pattern of a tight lens.

5. Programming the **Lens Selection Protocol**, ie, the way the lens is first chosen within any trial-set. The protocol can be either classical curvature (ie, according to K-readings and toricity) or height criteria. Default setting is a "height-fitting" protocol, which leaves an "apical clearance" of 10 microns.

6. Evaluating the residual cylinder of a front spherical lens, or designing the ideal front toric with a **Lens Power Input & Calculator** panel.

Figure 20-22 shows contact lens fitting to a keratoconic cornea (Figure 20-22A) using the Scout Contact Lens Editor and two different methods: (1) a lens selected from a "virtual trial set" (Figure 20-22B) and (2) a custom designed tri-conic lens created automatically with the Height Fitting (Aspheric) feature (Figure 20-22C). The

Clearance Panel shows how well the contact lens conforms to the flat corneal meridian when the lens is properly placed on the cone's apex.

Figure 20-23 shows an example of Ortho-K contact lens fitting. The user can create or select from among the available "height fitting protocols" and modify his or her data. The protocol in this example projects a 10.1 mm lens to get 15 microns clearance at the apex and a parallel fit in the midperiphery, with a compression factor of −1.75 D. The operator must then input only the desired correction in the panel (Figure 20-23A), click OK, and the software will automatically calculate the parameters reported in panel (Figure 20-23C) of a 5-curve CL. Note the similarity between the desired (Figure 20-23B) and achieved clearance plots (Figure 20-23D), despite natural corneal asymmetries. It is noticeable in this method, unique to the Scout, that all geometric components of the lens are not empirically extrapolated from "sim-k" or "Ro and e" values, but are calculated on actual corneal heights, measured by Keratron's arc-step on the flat meridian. This optimizes the design, even with complex shaped and asymmetric corneas.

Lens designs can be saved and attached to the relevant corneal topography, up to 8 different designs per image.

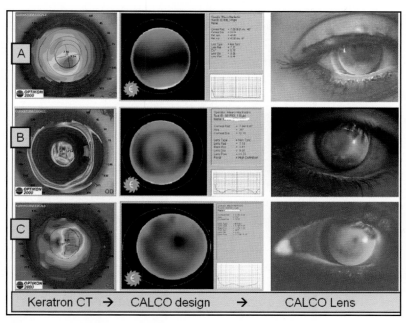

Figure 20-24. Examples of CALCO lens designs.

The CLE fluorescein simulations are not just equivalent to real fluorescein testing at the slit lamp. A good quality design can in fact be better evaluated with the CLE than with real trial-set testing, because the topographers "virtual reality" fitting is static and does not stress the cornea. A physical test can hide how much the cornea is fitting itself to the lens as the lens shapes the cornea, before incurring in patient discomfort and warpages like those shown in Figure 20-5.

As a general result, many optometrists using a Keratron corneal topographer have improved their RGP first lens success fitting rate from 30% to 40% to 80% to 90% and higher. Another advantage is of course that these optometrists may support medical centers, thus screening a wider population for keratoconus and other corneal pathologies.

CALCO Lenses and Other Third-Party Links

Beside Berkeley UC's OPTICAL project,[67] Eikon's CALCO (Firenze, Italy) has been the first among commercial third-party software providers to manufacture fully custom contact lenses based on Keratron's data beginning in 1996. In Latin, "calco" means "cast." The basic idea that stands behind the CALCO Lens Designs is that of a strict integration between corneal topography and contact lens fitting. The earliest contact lens manufacturing lathes were designed to cut sphere-based geometries. The cutting tool was mounted on a rotation axis so that machining performance was optimized for spherical surfaces. New generation lathes (eg, the Rank-Pneumo Optoform, by Taylor Hobson UK, now Precitech, Keene, NH, USA) overcame these limitations by designing complex aspherical profiles made of a large number of small steps, with a resolution down to 10 nanometers. Such geometries can significantly improve comfort and global performance of a rigid (gas permeable) lens. A natural evolution was to manufacture contact lenses based on accurate elevation corneal geometry data from the Scout, using the computer to manage a lens geometry optimized to fit each cornea. This was not intended to subsume the fitter's job, but rather to give him or her the capability of designing an aspheric lens according to fitting parameters instead of complex geometric ones. In fact, the first step of a lens design is to define the desired tear layer shape (Figure 20-24). The Tear Layer page comprises data describing how a lens fits a semi-meridian of the cornea. The lens design is controlled by the clearance between cornea and lens, and not by lens base curve, etc. Operators can choose diameters and lifts in order to design optimized lens completing all data: power, thickness, optic zone, correction of lens spherical aberrations, and multi-focal optic options. It is worth noting that this approach allows full control of the design because the parameter of clearance between cornea and lens is much closer to fitting philosophy than the parameter of eccentricity. Moreover, working with clearance frees the fitter from the overhead of managing complex geometrical parameters. The use of the CALCO lens design has dramatically improved first fit success rate and patient comfort in a number of complex situations.

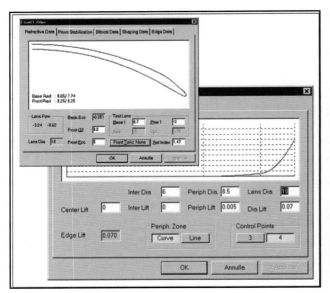

Figure 20-25. CALCO windows.

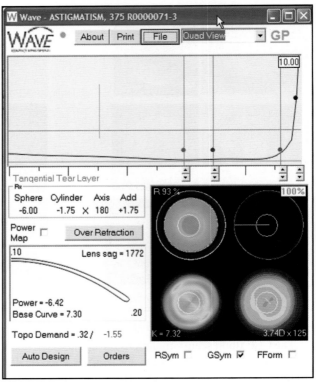

Figure 20-26. A screen shot of the WAVE program (www.wavecontactlenses.com).

Figure 20-25 illustrates some examples:

- Panel A: Early stage keratoconus—The design is chosen as a conform fit, moderately flat. The image of the lens at the slit lamp confirms comfortable wear.

- Panel B: Post hyperopic PRK treatment—Design is made to leave a small central clearance—The slit lamp image shows lens stability and good physiological response.

- Panel C: A rare superior keratoconus–axial symmetry design—The patient and the slit lamp lens image confirm good positioning, high visual acuity, and comfort.

Following Eikons' CALCO,[68–70] other fully custom methods designed to link the Scout with third-party software have been independently developed by companies all over the world. Among others are Edward's Wave[71,72] (Figure 20-26), which is very popular especially in the USA, as well as Europeans ProCornea's EyeLite and Ing. Liffredo's Focal Points.[73] These programs import the complete corneal geometry, diameter, and other data from the Keratron Scout software and design lens files that specialized labs, eg, Eikon (Firenze, Italy), VerkerOptik (now Optiek Verkerk, Amersfoort, The Netherlands), ProCornea (Eerbeek, The Netherlands), Essilor (Wiener Neudorf, Austria), No7 (East Sussex, UK), Eyequip (Jacksonville, FL, USA), etc, can import to manufacture fully custom lenses. Thus lenses having more versatile shapes than classical multicurve or multi-conic geometries can be uniquely and individually designed for each eye.

CONCLUSIONS

Thousands of users and researchers from around the world have been using the Keratron and Keratron Scout since 1993 in their clinical practice and studies. Since then, the Optikon Keratron team has never stopped improving the software and hardware of this family of corneal topographers. We hope that all current and future Keratron users will continue to appreciate our commitment to maintain our state-of-the-art topographic system for over a decade.

REFERENCES

1. Wilson SE, Wang JY, Klyce SD. Quantification and mathematical analysis of photokeratoscopic images. In: Shanzlin DJ, Robin JB, eds. *Corneal Topography: Measuring and Modifying the Cornea*. New York: Springer-Verlag; 1991:1–9.

2. Klyce SD, Wang JY. Considerations in corneal surface reconstruction from keratoscope images. In: Masters BR, ed. *Noninvasive Diagnostic Techniques in Ophthalmology*. New York: Springer-Verlag, New York; 1990:76.

3. Merlin U. I cheratoscopi: caratteristiche e attendibilita. In: Buratto L, Cantera E, Dal Fiume E, Genisi C, Merlin U, eds. *Topografia Corneale.* Milan, Italy: CAMO; 1995:43–56.

4. Klein SA, Mandell RB. Axial and instantaneous power conversion in corneal topography. *Invest Ophthalmol Vis Sci.* 1995;36:2155–2159.

5. Cohen KL, Tripoli NK, Holmgren DE, Coggins JM. Assessment of the power and height of radial aspheres reported by a computer-assisted keratoscope. *Am J Ophthalmol.* 1995;119:723–732.

6. Roberts C. Characterization of the inherent error in a spherically biased corneal topography system in mapping a radially aspheric surface. *J Refract Corneal Surg.* 1994;10:103–116.

7. Koch DD, Foulks GN, Moran CT, Wakil JS. The corneal EyeSys system: accuracy analysis and reproducibility of first-generation prototype. *J Refract Corneal Surg.* 1989; 6:423–429.

8. Gullstrand A. Photographic-ophthalmometric and clinical investigations of corneal refraction. *Am J Optom Arch Am Acad Optom.* 1966;43:143–214.

9. Doss JD, Hutson RL, Rowsey JJ, Brown R. Method for calculation of corneal profile and power distribution. *Arch Ophthalmol.* 1981;99:1261–1265.

10. Wang J, Rice DA, Klyce SD. A new reconstruction algorithm for improvement of corneal topographical analysis. *J Corn Refract Surg.* 1989;5:379–387.

11. van Saarloos PP, Constable, IJ. Improved method for calculation of corneal topography for any photokeratoscopic geometry. *Optom and Vis Sci.* 1991;68:957–965.

12. Klein SA. A corneal topography algorithm that produces continuous curvature. *Optom Vis Sci.* 1992;69:829–834.

13. Campbell C. Reconstruction of the corneal shape with the MasterVue corneal topography system. *Optom Vis Sci.* 1997;74:901.

14. Mattioli R, Carones F, Cantera E. New algorithms to improve the reconstruction of corneal geometry on the Keratron videokeratographer. *Invest Ophthalmol Vis Sci.* 1995;36(suppl):1400.

15. El Hage SG. The computerized corneal topographer EH-270. In: Shanzlin DJ, Robin JB, eds. *Corneal Topography: Measuring and Modifying the Cornea.* New York: Springer-Verlag; 1991:11–24.

16. El-Hage SG. Suggested new methods for photoker-atoscopy: a comparison of their validities. *I Am J Optom Arch Am Acad Optom.* 1971;48:897–912.

17. Brancato R, Carones F. *Topografia Corneale Computerizzata.* Milan, Italy: Fogliazza; 1994:2.12–17.3.

18. Chan WK, Carones F, Maloney RK. Corneal topographic maps: a clinical comparison. In: *International Society of Refractive Keratoplasty—Abstract Book.* Pre-Academy Meeting of the ISRK, San Fancisco, October 28–November 3, 1994.

19. Mattioli R., Tripoli N. Corneal geometry reconstruction with the Keratron videokeratographer. *Optom Vis Sci.* 1997;74:881–894.

20. Hannush SB, Crawford SL, Waring GO III, Gemmill MC, Lynn MJ, Nizam A. Accuracy and precision of keratometry, photokeratoscopy and corneal modeling on calibrated steel balls. *Arch Ophthalmol.* 1989;107:1235–1239.

21. Maguire LJ, Wilson SE, Camp JJ, Verity S. Evaluating the reproducibility of topography systems on spherical surfaces. *Arch Ophthalmol.* 1993;111:259–262.

22. Wilson SE, Verity SM, Conger DL. Accuracy and precision of the Corneal Analysis System and the Topographic Modeling System. *Cornea.* 1992;11:28–35.

23. Carones F, Gobbi PG, Brancato R, Venturi E. Comparison between two computer-assisted keratoscopes in measuring aspheric surfaces. *Invest Ophtalmol Vis Sci.* 1994;35 (suppl):3748.

24. Tripoli NK, Cohen KL, Holmgren DE, Coggins JM. Assessment of radial aspheres by the Keratron keratoscope using an arc-step algorithm. *Am J Ophthalmol.* 1995;120:658–664.

25. Tripoli NK, Cohen KL, Obla P, Coggins JM, Holmgren DE. Height measurement of astigmatic test surfaces by a keratoscope that uses plane geometry reconstruction. *Am J Ophthalmol.* 1996;121:668–676.

26. Cohen KL, Tripoli NK, Holmgren DE, Coggins JM. Assessment of the height of radial aspheres reported by a computer-assisted keratoscope. *Invest Ophthalmol Vis Sci.* 1993;34(suppl):1217.

27. Wang JY, Rice DA, Klyce SD. Analysis of the effects of astigmatism and misalignment on corneal surface reconstruction from photokeratoscopic data. *Refrac Corn Surg.* 1991;7(2):129–140.

28. Mattioli R, Carones F. How accurately can corneal profiles heights be measured by Placido-based videokeratography? *Invest Ophthalmol Vis Sci.* 1996;37(suppl):4273.

29. Camellin M, Federici R, Federici S. Clinical applications of the aberrometric functions of the Keratron Scout. In: Caimi F, Brancato R, eds. *The Aberrometers.* Canelli, Italy: Fabiano; 2003:259–268.

30. Dekking HM. Zur Photographie der Hornhautoberfl-Eche. *Graefes Arch Ophthalmol.* 1930;124:708–730.

31. Cantera E, Carones F, Brancato R, Cantera I, Neuschuler R. Evaluation of a new autofocus device for computer-assisted corneal topography. *Invest Ophtalmol Vis Sci.* 1994;35(suppl):2063.

32. Walsh G. The effect of mydriasis on the pupillary centration of the human eye. *Ophthalmic Physiol Opt.* 1988; 8:178–182.

33. Wyatt HJ. The form of the human pupil. *Vision Res.* 1995; 35:2021–2036.

34. Mattioli R, Carones F. An algorithm to recalculate topographic maps from any axis for computer assisted videokeratography. In: *ISRS—Abstract book*. International Society of Refractive Surgery Meeting, Atlanta, October 29–November 3, 1995.

35. Mattioli R, Federici R. Intra-operatory corneal topography—tools and applications. Acts from the congress Refractive on Line, Milan: ICH; Sept. 2001. Available at: www.refractiveonline.it/2001/eng/01_federici/default.htm and CD-ROM.

36. Vinciguerra P. *Smoothing Highly Aberrated Eyes Into a Clinically Measurable and Treatable Range*. Paper presented at 5th ICWS-ORCwavefront congress, Whistler, BC, Canada; Feb. 2004. Avaliable at: www.opt.uh.edu/research/voi/WavefrontCongress/2004/presentations/26Vinciguerra.swf.

37. Mattioli R, Representation of corneal wavefront from corneal topography. Acts from the congress Refractive on Line, Milan: ICH; Sept. 2001. Available at: www.refractiveonline.it/2001/eng/02_mattioli/default.htm and CD-ROM of the congress.

38. Mattioli R. Corneal topography and wavefront analysis. In: Caimi F, Brancato R, eds. *The Aberrometers*. Canelli, Italy: Fabiano; 2003:113–132.

39. Mattioli R, Frondizi S, Rubeo A, Saldutti M. The Keratron Scout and wavefront analysis. In: Caimi F, Brancato R, eds. *The Aberrometers*. Canelli, Italy: Fabiano; 2003:243–257.

40. Marcos S. Aberrations and optical quality of the eye: what the clinician needs to know. In: Caimi F, Brancato R, eds. *The Aberrometers*. Canelli, Italy: Fabiano; 2003:15–26.

41. Tripoli NK. The Zernike polynomials. In: Caimi F, Brancato R, eds. *The Aberrometers*. Canelli, Italy: Fabiano; 2003:51–64.

42. Howland H, Buettner J, Applegate R. Computation of the shapes of normal corneas and their monochromatic aberrations from videokeratometric measurements: vision science and its applications. *Technical Digest Series*. 1994;2:54–57.

43. Hemenger RP, Tomlinson A, Oliver K. Corneal optics from videokeratographs. *Ophthalmic Physiol Opt*. 1995; 15:63–68.

44. Schwiegerling J, Greivenkamp JE. Using corneal height maps and polynomial decomposition to determine corneal aberrations. *Optom Vis Sci*. 1997;74:906–916.

45. Marcos S. Aberrations and visual performance following standard laser vision correction. *J Refract Surgery* 2001; 17:596–601.

46. Marcos S, Barbero B, Llorente L, Merayo-Lloves J. Optical response to LASIK for myopia from total and corneal aberrations. *Invest Ophthalmol Vis Sci*. 2001; 42:3349–3356.

47. Artal P, Guirao A, Berrio E. Compensation of corneal aberrations by the internal optics in the human eye. *Journal of Vision*. 2001;1:1–8.

48. Artal P, Berrio E, Guirao A, Piers P. Contribution of the cornea and internal surfaces to the change of ocular aberrations with age. J *Opt Soc Am: A*. 2002;19:137–143.

49. Artal P, Guirao A. Contributions of the cornea and the lens to the aberrations of the human eye. *Optics Letters*. 1998; 23:1713–1715.

50. Guirao A, Gonzalez C, Redondo M, Geraghty E, Norrby S, Artal P. Average optical performance of the human eye as a function of age in a normal population. *Inv Ophth Vis Sci*.1999;40:203–213.

51. Hemenger RP, Tomlinson A, Oliver K. Corneal optics from videokeratographs. *Ophthalmic Physiol Opt*. 1995; 15:63–68.

52. Guirao A, Artal P. Corneal wave aberration from videokeratography: accuracy and limitations of the procedure. *J Opt Soc Am A*. 2000;17:955–965.

53. Malacara D. *Optical Shop Testing*. 2nd ed. New York: John Wiley & Sons; 1992:472–488.

54. Thibos LN, Applegate RA, Schwiegerling JT, Webb RH, VST Members. Standards for reporting the optical aberrations of eyes: vision science and its applications. *OSA Trends in Optics & Photonics*. 2000;35:110–130.

55. Thibos LN. Wavefront data reporting and terminology. *J Refract Surgery*. 2001;17(suppl):578–583.

56. Thibos LN. Indiana aberration study. *J Opt Soc Am A*. In press.

57. Smith S. Digital *Signal Processing*. 2nd ed.1999. San Diego: California Technical Publishing; 1999: Chapters 18–24.

58. Bonci P. Decentramenti in chirurgia rifrattiva. In: Buratto L, Picardo V, eds. *Focal Points*. Novara, Italy: Fabiano; 2003:11–25.

59. Arbelaez MC. Early work shows safety and efficacy. *Ophthalmology Management*. 2003; March:56–58.

60. Rummelt V. *Neuer Perspektiven zur Darstellung der Kornea*. Available at: http://www.eye-tech-solutions.de/docs/CornealWavefront.PDF

61. Rummelt V. Selective corneal wavefront diagnosis and excimer laser treatment for vision improvement. *Highlights of Ophthalmology*. 2003;31(5):27–30.

62. Siganos D. Quality of vision improved with ORK-W system. *Euro Times*. May 2003;16. Available at: www.escrs.org/eurotimes/May2003/quality.asp.

63. Munnerlyn CR, Koons J. Photorefractive keratectomy: a technique for laser refractive surgery. *J Cat Refract Surgery*. 1988;14:46–52.

64. Gatinel D, Hoang-Xuan T, Azar DT. Determination of corneal asphericity after myopia surgery with the excimer laser: a mathematical model. *Invest Ophthalmol & Vis Sci*. 2001;42:1736.

65. Mattioli R, Camellin M. La aberrometria corneale ed il link "topo aberrometrico." In: Camellin M, ed. *LASEK ed ASA*. Canelli, Italy: Fabiano; 2004:231–253.

66. Risoldi U, Venturini S, De Nicolò N. LAC RGP Horus e topografo corneale, una soluzione integrata, moderna ed efficace. *Professional Optometry—Dogma SV, Italy.* 1996;8:32, 41.

67. Garcia D, Barsky B, Bolles B. The Optical Project at UC Berkeley (SIGGRAPH '96 electronic theatre video). Available at: http://www.cs.berkeley.edu/optical/SIG-GRAPH96_ET.html.

68. Manganotti A, Pedrotti E, Sbabo A. Lenti a contatto RGP Custom Made con link topografico a risparmio apicale nel cheratocono: nostra esperienza e confronto con lenti tradizionali. *Euvision.* 2004; 3:6–13.

69. Manganotti A. "L'evoluzione applicativa delle lenti a contatto RGP: dalle lenti a contatto su misura tradizionali, alle LAC Custom Made realizzate mediante link informatico con topografo corneale. *Euvision.* 2003;1:8–14.

70. Manfredini M. La topografia corneale nella pratica contattologia. Contact Lens Manual—A comprehensive study and reference guide (Contact Lens Society of America). Capitolo 17, Parte 1(suppl):397-408. Ottico. 2001;293 (suppl):19–34.

71. Maller K. Using CAD/CAM lenses for orthokeratology. *Review of Contact Lenses.* 2004;April:16–20.

72. Linton G. Software increased one OD's RGP fit. *Contact Lens Spectrum.* 2000;November:60.

73. Focal Points® in a prescription laboratory. Boston update (news and info from Polymer Technology Co.). 2001;10(Summer):1–3.

Chapter 21

The Tomey TMS Corneal Topographer

Stephen D. Klyce, PhD

The analysis of corneal topography is now the standard of care in anterior segment practices. The first corneal topographer commercially available was the Computed Anatomy, Inc. (New York, NY) Corneal Modeling System in 1987.[1,2] It incorporated many of the LSU Eye Center research laboratory findings in its implementation;[3] of greatest impact was the incorporation of the color-coded display of corneal surface curvature.[4] This device had limited commercial success owing to its cost but was remarkable in that it measured both anterior corneal curvature and corneal thickness profiles, capabilities subsequently available in the Bausch and Lomb (Rochester, NY) model Orbscan II. Computed Anatomy was acquired by the Tomey Corporation (Nagoya, Japan) in the early 1990s following the introduction of the Computed Anatomy Topography Modeling System, the TMS-1. This model became the earliest "work horse" corneal topographer, supplanted eventually by subsequent Tomey models. At the time of this writing, the Tomey TMS-4 is commercially available with software version 3.5C. This chapter will review the features of the TMS-4 as well as the capabilities of the software. It should be noted that not every capability of the TMS-4 software will be covered here; priority is given to those of most frequent clinical use.

GENERAL CHARACTERISTICS

Several methodologies have been used to measure corneal curvature, including interferometry, profilometry, and Placido disk reflective methods. While interferometry has the greatest potential sensitivity of measurement, interference produces fringes according to the deviation of a measured surface from a reference surface. If the distortions in the measured surface become much greater than a few wavelengths of the measuring light wavelength, the fringes produced will merge and become indistinguishable. In essence, interferometry is too sensitive a measurement technique to apply to the imperfect optics of the eye. Profilometry is the technique used by slit-based topographers and fluorescein-stained tear film techniques (raster stereography). The early version Orbscan I used anterior corneal surface data obtained with a scanning slit to estimate corneal topography, while the Oculus (Lynnfield, Wash) Pentacam uses a rotating slit to obtain this data. However, direct measurement of the corneal profile does not provide sufficient resolution for the accurate depiction of corneal topography. Placido reflective technology appears to have the requisite sensitivity of measurement and is employed by all of the commercially successful corneal topographers, including the upgraded Orbscan II.

There are two basic approaches used with the Placido disks. Some use a large faceplate with a large working distance to project images of mires onto the corneal surface. This approach has the advantage of less critical focus and the disadvantage of corneal shadows created by the brow and the nose of the patient, which can obscure portions of the peripheral mire images. Other corneal topographers use a small cone-shaped Placido disk target with a short working distance. The advantage of this arrangement is a greater potential coverage of the corneal surface; the disadvantage is more sensitivity to error in focus. Both types have seen commercial success. All of the Tomey models have used the small, cone-type Placido disk.

Topographic Displays

Corneal topographers project a Placido pattern onto the corneal surface, capture this with a CCD camera, determine

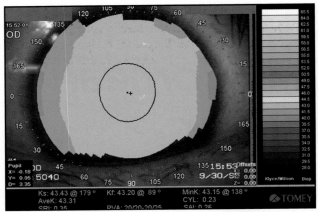

Figure 21-1. The Tomey TMS-4 single standard power map using the Klyce/Wilson scale. This is a cornea from a normal eye. This map conveys all the characteristics of a normal cornea: uniform central powers tapering toward the limbus, relatively smooth contours, and K readings near 43 D. An outline of the pupil is shown with its location and diameter noted in the lower left-hand corner. The central cross indicates the position of the vertex normal at the alignment axis of the TMS-4. The central small square represents the position of the pupil center. Corneal statistics are displayed in the lower panel. SimK1 is labeled Ks and SimK2 is labeled Kf in this version of the software. These and the other indices are described in the text.

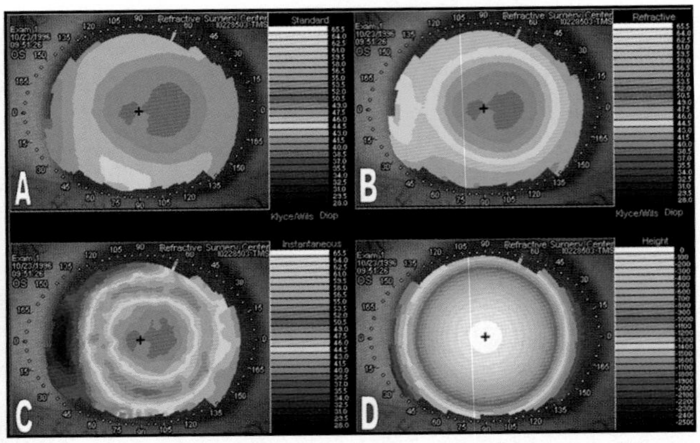

Figure 21-2. The TMS-4 multimap display is used here to illustrate the appearance of a single exam (cornea after PRK) with the 3 different power maps and the height map. (A) The standard power display. (B) The refractive power map. Note the central powers are the same as A, but allowing for spherical aberration steepens the peripheral powers. (C) The instantaneous map shows the "red ring" in the transition zone, which modern algorithms have overcome for the most part. Note the additional noise compared to A. (D) Without amplification, the true height map is unable to show useful detail of the shape changes responsible for the power maps.

the precise location of each of the mires, and convert these positions into curvature at each measurement point. The curvature data is expressed in a number of ways; millimeters are often used for contact lens applications, while diopters are most often used for clinical diagnostics. The curvature data available from corneal topographers is generally conditioned with the keratometric index (1.3375) such that the values presented include the dioptric power of the tear film/air interface (about 48 D) and the dioptric power of the endothelial/aqueous humor interface (about −5 D). This makes dioptric power values equivalent to total corneal power and conveniently correspondent to keratometry.

The scales available on the TMS-4 include the absolute scale, the Klyce/Wilson scale, the Maguire/Waring scale, a user-adjustable scale, and a normalized scale. Normal clinical use of the TMS-4 involves use of one of the 1.5 D contour interval scales (absolute or Klyce/Wilson), which show the relevant topographic features without overemphasizing details.[5] The scales are implemented with a color palette that consists of contrasting colors that make the contour boundaries obvious so that corneal topographic irregularities are not masked. This strategy of a combination of a fixed range, a fixed interval, and a well-select-

ed color palette are essential for proper interpretation of corneal topography. Further emphasis on the importance of proper topographic scale choice is presented in Chapter 6 of this book.

Curvature data is commonly calculated with three different approaches. The *standard map* with the TMS-4 displays corneal surface dioptric power with a spherical approximation method commonly referred to as axial power (Figures 21-1 and 21-2A). This is the baseline map ordinarily used in routine clinical screening. The strength of this method for calculating and displaying corneal topography is that it removes the corneal positive spherical aberration component from the power calculation. The remaining curvature displayed retains more of the shape characteristics seen in the normal cornea: steeper (higher power) in the central region and flatter (lower power) in the periphery.

A second display of corneal curvature available on the TMS-4 is the *refractive power map* (Figure 21-2B). This method for calculating corneal power uses Snell's Law, which is necessary for accurate ray tracing in order to evaluate the corneal contribution to the aberrations measured with wavefront sensors. Note that the negative spherical aberration of the natural lens (as well as the modern

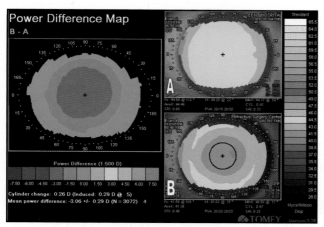

Figure 21-3. The TMS-4 power difference map is useful for examining the actual effect of a refractive surgical procedure on the corneal topography. (A) The preoperative cornea. (B) The postoperative result. (C) The difference between preoperative and postoperative examinations.

aspheric intraocular lenses [IOLs]) compensates to some extent for the positive spherical aberration of the cornea.

A third display of corneal curvature available on the TMS-4 is the *instantaneous map* (Figure 21-2C). This label is shortened from "instantaneous radius of curvature," which offers the most detailed look at local changes in the corneal curvature. Because of the method of calculation, the instantaneous map contains significant noise artifacts that may mislead the user to assume that a cornea has an abnormally high amount of higher-order aberrations (HOAs). However, the instantaneous map increases the detail of curvature changes, particularly in the corneal periphery, and may be the only means by which to evaluate the peripheral optics of the cornea after myopic refractive surgery. Generally, amplifying the corneal power distribution beyond that shown with the standard axial power map shows details that are not of consequence to vision or to diagnostics. However, the instantaneous map clearly shows the transition zone characteristics after refractive surgery, and these may be responsible for night vision complaints after refractive surgery (Figure 21-2C).

The final map type available on the TMS-4 is the *height map* (Figure 21-2D). The raw height map is of itself not useful diagnostically except in extremely aberrated corneas. The main component of the height data is a sphere, and this masks the small curvature changes that are clearly shown with the power maps. However, the TMS-4 offers two additional displays that allow inspection of distortions in true cornea shape. The *enhanced height map* is created by subtracting an average sphere that fits the raw height data. The enhanced height map produces an aberration structure, which bears a similarity to wavefront dis-

plays because both are in units of microns. A second routine, the *height difference map*, displays the difference in height data between two corneal examinations. This allows the change in shape induced by refractive surgery to be displayed, which can be useful when comparing planned versus achieved shape changes.

A difference map is also available to show changes in corneal power with time or condition. As with the height change map, the *power difference map* permits the evaluation of changes in corneal power induced by refractive surgery or another condition (Figure 21-3).

Each of the maps available on the TMS-4 embodies a number of user-selectable features. The cursor can be moved around on a map to view the radius and power at any measured point. The same routine can be used to estimate the distance and difference in power between any two points. This same ruler function can be used to obtain a calibrated "white to white" measurement. The TMS-4 measures the margins of the pupil in the video image it captures, and the pupil outline can be superimposed on any of the maps, as noted in Figure 21-1. Astigmatism is calculated in a number of ways: orthogonal, instantaneous, and zonal. Orthogonal astigmatism is similar to standard keratometry; instantaneous astigmatism gives an indication of corneal irregularity; zonal astigmatism is useful for planning astigmatic surgery and for contact lens applications. Other features that are user-selectable include the presence or absence of the eye image, a routine for verifying the accuracy of the mire tracking, a slide making utility, exam backup, import and export, and several grid overlays for measurement.

By itself, the color-coded contour map is useful for classifying corneal topography, but it does not lend itself directly to quantitative evaluation of specific values of clinical interest. A number of corneal topographic indices are available on the TMS-4; some, such as the simulated keratometry data, were designed for direct clinical use. Other indices were designed primarily for use in automatic discrimination software, described below. Each of the indices was evaluated for a group of normal corneal topographies to determine the mean and standard deviation for the normal population. To assist the user in distinguishing among normal, potentially abnormal (suspect), and clearly abnormal corneal topography, each index is color-coded. A green-colored index indicates a value that is within ±2 standard deviations of the normal average. A yellow-colored index indicates a caution: that an index is 2 to 3 standard deviations from the normal average. A red-colored index indicates a value that is more than 3 standard deviations away from the normal average. Some of the statistical indices can be displayed on the standard maps, as in Figure 21-1. More extensive statistics are found on the statistics display (Figure 21-4).

The first indices enumerated for the TMS-4 and now standard on all corneal topographers are those associated with simulated keratometry (SimK).[6,7] SimK1 gives the dioptric power and associated angle of the principle meridian; SimK2 gives the dioptric power and associated angle of the meridian orthogonal to the principle meridian; and MinK gives the dioptric power and associated angle of the meridian with the lowest overall dioptric power. The simulated keratometric cylinder of the corneal surface (Cyl) is obtained from the SimK readings. The surface asymmetry index (SAI) measures the difference in corneal powers at every ring (180 degrees apart) over the entire corneal surface.[6,7] The SAI is often higher than normal in keratoconus, penetrating keratoplasty, decentered myopic refractive surgical procedures, trauma, and contact lens warpage. Adequate spectacle correction is often not achieved when SAI is high.

The surface regularity index (SRI) is a correlate to potential visual acuity and is a measure of local fluctuations in central corneal power.[6,7] When SRI is elevated, the corneal surface ahead of the entrance pupil will be irregular, leading to a reduction in best spectacle-corrected visual acuity. High SRI values are found with dry eyes, contact lens wear, trauma, and penetrating keratoplasty. The potential visual acuity (PVA) is derived from a clinical correlation[7] of SRI versus the best spectacle-corrected visual acuity. The PVA is given as the range of best spectacle-corrected Snellen visual acuity that might be expected from a functionally normal eye with the topographical characteristics of the analyzed cornea. Diagnostic evaluation should consider the fact that tear film breakup can greatly influence PVA (and SRI). Prolonged gazing at a fixation target by a patient without blinking can produce tear film breakup, transiently reduced vision, and abnormal values of PVA and SRI. With proper blinking, abnormal values of PVA are associated with true irregular corneal astigmatism, as is often observed with keratoconjunctivitis sicca, contact lens warpage, lamellar keratoplasty, and herpes keratitis. SRI and PVA are extremely valuable diagnostically to differentiate visual deficit: if an eye exhibits good corneal potential but suffers visual loss when best-corrected, the deficit will be associated with compromised internal optics, retinal disease, or neural deficit.

The average corneal power (ACP) is an area-corrected average of the corneal power ahead of the entrance pupil.[8,9] This value is generally a more accurate measurement to use for IOL calculations than keratometry values, particularly in postsurgical corneas. The corneal eccentricity index (CEI) is a measure of corneal eccentricity, a global shape factor. A positive (normal) value is obtained for a prolate surface, a nil value for a sphere, and a negative value is used to indicate an oblate surface. Higher than

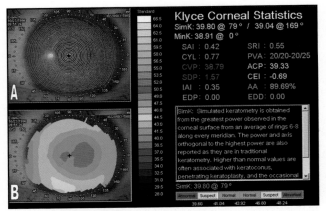

Figure 21-4. TMS-4 statistics display. (A) A raw image of the eye with the mires overlaid with the green rings found by the computer; this is useful for verifying the accuracy of the processing. (B) The standard map display of corneal topography. The right half of the figure displays the statistics calculated for the examination. Indices that are green in color indicate values within ±2 standard deviations of the value found in normals. Those yellow in color indicate suspect values that lie between 2 and 3 standard deviations from the normal. Those red in color represent abnormal values more than 3 standard deviations from the normal. The cutoff values are indicted for every statistic in the scale at the bottom of the panel. These change appropriately for each statistic by moving the mouse cursor over one of the statistics. The definition for each statistic is obtained in the same manner.

normal values are found with keratoconus, and negative values are often found with symptomatic contact lens wear and myopic refractive surgical corrections. The standard deviation of corneal power (SDP) is calculated from the distribution of all corneal powers in an examination.[10] The coefficient of variation of corneal power (CVP) is calculated from SDP divided by the grand average of corneal powers. This fundamental statistic is high when there is a broad range of powers in the corneal surface and has been found to be a good measure of corneal multifocality. High values of CVP are found in moderate to severe keratoconic corneas as well as after corneal transplants, in the early postoperative period. Manifest refraction of an eye with high CVP will be difficult to achieve, but attention to refraction is important in such a patient to attain spectacle tolerance. The CVP value given has been scaled up by a factor of 1000.

The irregular astigmatism index (IAI) is an area-compensated average summation of inter-ring power variations along every meridian for the entire corneal surface analyzed.[11] The IAI increases as local irregular astigmatism

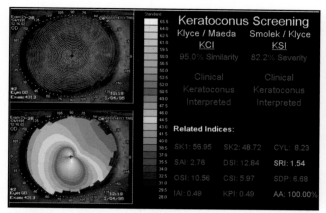

Figure 21-5. The TMS-4 keratoconus screening tool analyzing a cornea with moderate keratoconus. The statistical indices presented are fully described in the text.

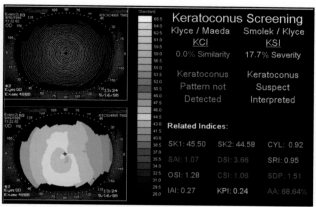

Figure 21-6. The TMS-4 keratoconus screening tool analyzing a cornea that is suspect keratoconus. Note that the Klyce/Maeda method reports the absence of clinical keratoconus, while the Smolek/Klyce method reports the presence of suspect keratoconus. This is not a contradication: the Klyce/Maeda method only recognizes clinical keratoconus; suspect keratoconus was not part of its training.

in the corneal surface increases. IAI is high in corneal transplants shortly after surgery; persistence often heralds suboptimal best spectacle corrected vision.

The analyzed area (AA) gives the fraction of the corneal area covered by the mires that could be processed by the TMS-4 software. AA is lower than normal for corneas with gross, irregular astigmatism, which causes the mires to break up and not be resolved. A lower than normal AA is found with early postopertive corneal transplants, advanced keratoconus, and trauma. AA can also be artificially low during a squint or when the eyes are not opened wide.

The elevation/depression diameter (EDD) is the equivalent diameter of the area found to contain powers within the pupil 1 D or more from the mode. It is calculated from twice the square root of this area divided by Pi. The units are millimeters. The elevation/depression power (EDP) calculates the average power of apparent islands (or peninsulas) and valleys for those areas of the cornea that are within the demarcated pupil. If the pupil is not available for a given exam, EDP is calculated from an area 4 mm in diameter, centered on the corneal topographer axis. Together with EDD, EDP can be used to estimate the size of so-called central islands after excimer laser sculpting. Any power within the pupil that is 1 D or more beyond the mode (most frequently occurring power) is multiplied by the cornea local area it represents (area compensation); this total is then divided by the total area of the summed powers. The units are Diopters. Normal corneas with high cylinder, corneal grafts, and clinical keratoconus will also exhibit degrees of abnormal EDP and EDD.

Modern corneal topography algorithms and devices offer reliable and repeatable measurements of surface curvature. In addition to the basic features described above, the TMS-4 offers several advanced features that take advantage of the consistent examinations that can be obtained.

Screening Software

The presence of the keratoconus or suspect keratoconus pattern in corneal topography is a contraindication for standard refractive surgery because it puts the cornea at risk for developing keratectasia. This is a particular concern for laser in situ keratomileusis (LASIK), where keratectasia can occur 6 to 18 months after surgery in corneas exhibiting suspect keratoconus topography,[12] as well as for photorefractive keratectomy (PRK), where keratectasia can occur 4 to 5 years after surgery in such corneas (R. Zaldivar, personal communication). Corneal topography is the most sensitive method for detecting suspect keratoconus, and because of this, often there are no other signs, although careful retinoscopy may reveal a slight scissoring of the light reflex in these cases. Suspect keratoconus topographic patterns often present as a subtle asymmetry in corneal power. Since all corneas exhibit some degree of asymmetry, in order to differentiate between these normal variations and changes consistent with suspect keratoconus, a quantitative analysis is indicated. The TMS-4 has two keratoconus screening programs (Figure 21-5). The Klyce/Maeda method[11] uses discriminant analysis and a decision tree to report the similarity in percent of a corneal topography to clinical keratoconus. The Smolek/Klyce[13] method extends this approach using neural networks to assign a similarity value to corneas with clinical kerato-conus and gives a severity index of the pathology. In addition, the latter method was also trained on suspect kerato-conus topographies (Figure 21-6). A number of complementary corneal topographic indices were developed to aid in the discrimination of keratoconus from other corneal pathologies in order to increase the specificity of the tests.[11] The opposite sector index (OSI) represents the maximum difference between average corneal powers between any 2 opposite sectors. The differential sector index (DSI) represents the maximum difference between average corneal powers between any two sectors. The center/surround index (CSI) is the difference in average corneal power between the central 3-mm diameter of an analyzed area and an annulus surrounding this central area from an inner radius of 1.5 mm to an outer radius of 3 mm. This index is used to capture central keratoconus. These and other indices already described are used in the calculation of the keratoconus index (KCI) and the keratoconus severity index (KSI).

Here is one caveat in the use of these screening utilities: although the training sets of topography examinations contained a number of different types of corneal topographic anomalies in addition to normal corneas and those with keratoconus, they were trained to detect only keratoconus. Hence, when presented with a clear example of topographic pellucid marginal degeneration, the screening utilities will each report the absence of keratoconus, with keratoconus indices colored green. Therefore, it is important that these utilities not be used as general screening programs for refractive surgery, since abnormal corneal conditions other than keratoconus are also contraindications for conventional refractive surgical techniques.

Hjortdal and co-workers[14] were the first to show the utility of Fourier decomposition in corneal topography analysis. They demonstrated that the average power, cylinder, and irregular astigmatism could be extracted from each mire. The TMS-4 implements a Fourier decomposition display (Figure 21-7) along the lines suggested by these authors. With this implementation, the power values along each of the mires are fit sequentially with a one-dimensional Fourier series analysis, which provides a radial microzonal analysis. This routine decomposes corneal power data into zonal spherical equivalent, zonal cylinder, zonal asymmetry, and zonal higher-order irregularity. In addition, each of these variables is given for 3 and 6 mm zones. These data can be useful for the analysis of the quality of refractive outcomes for different approaches. This approach has been used to evaluate corneal topographic effects of cataract surgery,[15] irregular astigmatism and contrast sensitivity after photorefractive keratecto-my,[16] keratoconus progression,[17] to establish normative data for normal corneas versus those with pathology or

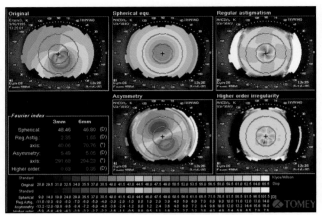

Figure 21-7. The TMS-4 Fourier decomposition display. Here a keratoconic cornea is decomposed into spherical, cylindrical, asymmetrical, and higher-order irregularity components. Because the analysis is done on a ring-by-ring basis, the cylinder component is not radially linear.

surgery,[18] to examine the effects of overnight wear of contact lenses worn for orthokeratology,[19] and to evaluate visual acuity after penetrating keratoplasty.[20]

The TMS-4 has contact lens fitting software that has evolved from the TMS-1 program, one of the first such utilities available on a corneal topographer. Using elevation and position data allows a three-dimensional representation of the cornea to be analyzed for a contact lens fit using several rules similar to those used by contact lens fitters. Eccentricity and keratometry readings are available from the corneal statistics, and these are used to select an initial contact lens fitted to the corneal surface from those lens characteristics that are stored on the TMS-4. The contact lens is then mathematically lowered onto the corneal surface by properly controlling the lens tip and tilt. This allows the clearance between the contact lens and the corneal surface to be calculated, and the amount of clearance is indicated using a simulated fluorescein exam (Figure 21-8). If necessary or desired, the operator can then make adjustments to the lens design, such as base curve and diameter, while observing the effect on the fit. This program has been used successfully to obtain good fits with rigid gas-permeable contact lenses for both normal and irregular corneas.[21,22]

SUMMARY AND CONCLUSIONS

The TMS-4 is the latest Tomey corneal topographer; its predecessors included the very first clinical device capable of producing a data-rich map of corneal shape, the

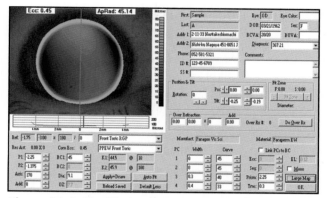

Figure 21-8. The TMS-4 has an extensive contact lens program with a large built-in library of commercial contact lenses as well as customizable one-off routines. The map simulates the clinical fluorescein test and is useful for inspecting the lens clearance. It updates if base curve or other parameters are adjusted.

Computed Anatomy corneal modeling system (CMS). Nearly all of the advances in corneal topography were made with the CMS topographer and its descendants, including the following: scales and color palettes that promote rapid and accurate interpretation, display types that allow the clinician to examine topography in greater detail and to appreciate changes over time, topographic statistical indices that provide quantitative assessment of corneal shape factors and corneal optical quality, and screening programs that differentiate suspect keratoconus and clinical keratoconus from normal individual variations in corneal shape. Corneal topography analysis has made huge strides from the early 1980s, when keratometry and keratoscopy were state of the art. Without this essential tool, which has become the standard of care in anterior segment practice, there is no doubt that refractive surgery would have remained underdeveloped and would not have achieved the enormous success it has today. It was the corneal topographer that taught us that small functional optical zones, central islands and peninsulas, and decentrations are clear detractors of visual quality. It was the corneal topographer that detected suspect and early keratoconus to classify these patients as ineligible for standard refractive surgical procedures. These are just a few of the many advancements that define the critical role the TMS corneal topographer has played in the development of corneal shape analysis, a science that has provided both the clinician and the refractive surgery patient with better information, safer surgery, and ultimately, clearer vision for the past 20 years. It will continue to do so in the years to come.

ACKNOWLEDGMENTS

This work was supported in part by US Public Health Service grants EY03311 from the National Eye Institute (National Institutes of Health, Bethesda, Md). The author is indebted to Marguerite B. McDonald, MD (Southern Vision Institute, New Orleans, La) for providing the patient examinations used to illustrate this chapter.

Dr. Klyce has no financial interest in any product discussed in this chapter.

REFERENCES

1. Gormley DJ, Gersten M, Koplin RS, Lubkin V. Corneal modeling. *Cornea.* 1988;7:30–35.

2. Mammone RJ, Gersten M, Gormley DJ, Koplin RS, Lubkin VL. 3-D corneal modeling system. *IEEE Trans Biomed Eng.* 1990;37:66–72.

3. Klyce SD. Computer-assisted corneal topography: high resolution graphical presentation and analysis of keratoscopy. *Invest Ophthalmol Vis Sci.* 1984;25:1426–1435.

4. Maguire LJ, Singer DE, Klyce SD. Graphic presentation of computer–analyzed keratoscope photographs. *Arch Ophthalmol.* 1987;105:223–230.

5. Wilson SE, Klyce SD, Husseini ZM. Standardized color-coded maps for corneal topography. *Ophthalmology.* 1993;100:1723–1727.

6. Dingeldein SA, Klyce SD, Wilson SE. Quantitative descriptors of corneal shape derived from computer-assisted analysis of photokeratographs. *Refractive & Corneal Surgery.* 1989;5:372–378.

7. Wilson SE, Klyce SD. Quantitative descriptors of corneal topography: a clinical study. *Arch Ophthalmol.* 1991;109:349–353.

8. Alimisi S, Miltsakakis D, Klyce S. Corneal topography for intraocular lens power calculations. *J Refract Surg.* 1996;12:S309–S311.

9. Maeda N, Klyce SD, Smolek MK, McDonald MB. Disparity of keratometry readings and corneal power within the pupil after refractive surgery for myopia. *Cornea.* 1997;16:517–524.

10. Mafra CH, Dave A, Wilson SE, Klyce SD. Extracapsular cataract surgery: corneal topographic alterations. *Invest Ophthalmol Vis Sci.* 1993;34:1248.

11. Maeda N, Klyce SD, Smolek MK, Thompson HW. Automated keratoconus screening with corneal topography analysis. *Invest Ophthalmol Vis Sci.* 1994;35:2749–2757.

12. Randleman JB, Russell B, Ward MA, Thompson KP, Stulting RD. Risk factors and prognosis for corneal ectasia after LASIK. *Ophthalmology.* 2003;110:267–275.

13. Smolek MK, Klyce SD. Current keratoconus detection methods compared with a neural network approach. *Invest Ophthalmol Vis Sci.* 1997;38:2290–2299.

14. Hjortdal JO, Erdmann L, Bek T. Fourier analysis of videokeratographic data. A tool for separation of spherical, regular astigmatic and irregular astigmatic corneal power components. *Ophthalmic Physiol Opt.* 1995;15:171–185.

15. Olsen T, Dam-Johansen M, Bek T, Hjortdal JO. Evaluating surgically induced astigmatism by Fourier analysis of corneal topography data. *J Cataract Refract Surg.* 1996;22:318–323.

16. Tomidokoro A, Soya K, Miyata K, Armin B, Tanaka S, Amano S, Oshika T. Corneal irregular astigmatism and contrast sensitivity after photorefractive keratectomy. *Ophthalmology.* 2001;108:2209–2212.

17. Oshika T, Tanabe T, Tomidokoro A, Amano S. Progression of keratoconus assessed by Fourier analysis of videokeratography data. *Ophthalmology.* 2002;109:339–342.

18. Tanabe T, Tomidokoro A, Samejima T, Miyata K, Sato M, Kaji Y, Oshika T. Corneal regular and irregular astigmatism assessed by Fourier analysis of videokeratography data in normal and pathologic eyes. *Ophthalmology.* 2004;111:752–757.

19. Hiraoka T, Furuya A, Matsumoto Y, Okamoto F, Sakata N, Hiratsuka K, Kakita T, Oshika T. Quantitative evaluation of regular and irregular corneal astigmatism in patients having overnight orthokeratology. *J Cataract Refract Surg.* 2004;30:1425–1429.

20. Miyai T, Miyata K, Nejima R, Samejima T, Hiraoka T, Kiuchi T, Kaji Y, Oshika T. Visual acuity measurements using Fourier series harmonic analysis of videokeratography data in eyes after penetrating keratoplasty. *Ophthalmology.* 2005;112:420–424.

21. Szczotka LB, Reinhart W. Computerized videokeratoscopy contact lens software for RGP fitting in a bilateral postkeratoplasty patient: a clinical case report. *CLAO J.* 1995;21:52–56.

22. Bufidis T, Konstas AG, Mamtziou E. The role of computerized corneal topography in rigid gas permeable contact lens fitting. *CLAO J.* 1998;24:206–209.

Chapter 22

Topcon KR-9000PW

Naoyuki Maeda, MD

With advancements in refractive surgery, cataract surgery, and contact lenses, there is a huge demand to evaluate quality of vision objectively. Corneal topographic analysis is very useful in showing the optical quality of corneas following refractive surgery or the optical quality of those with corneal diseases such as keratoconus.[1–3] Interpretation of color-coded maps reveals corneal irregular astigmatism qualitatively.[4] Topographic indices such as SRI,[5] or the results of Fourier analysis[6] and Zernike analysis[3] can show the effects of corneal irregular astigmatism on vision quantitatively.

Recently, the compensational association between cornea and internal optics became obvious not only for regular astigmatism but also for irregular astigmatism or HOAs.[7] For this reason, an instrument that can measure both corneal and ocular HOAs may be useful for the comprehensive evaluation of the optical system of the eye.

MAIN FEATURES

The Topcon KR-9000PW Wavefront Analyzer (Tokyo, Japan) (Figure 22-1) provides four functions: autokeratometry, autorefractometry, videokeratography, and wavefront sensing. These four kinds of measurements can be performed sequentially in a session. Table 22-1 indicates the specifications of the machine. Many original articles and reviews about this instrument have already been published.[8–25]

KERATOMETRY AND REFRACTOMETRY

Keratometry and refractometry can be performed in a similar fashion to the conventional autorefractometers or autokeratometers. The principles are identical, and the results can be printed out in the conventional fashion without a personal computer (PC) (Figure 22-2). In addition to conventional autorefractometry, this machine can provide better objective refractions with the aid of wavefront technology. Although the conventional refractometer obtains sphere and cylinder values based on the values at the paracentral zone only, the wavefront sensor can calculate the sphere and cylinder using data within the entire pupillary zone. Though the difference between these two methods may be small in normal eyes, the difference will increase dramatically in cases following refractive surgery with a decentered optical zone, a smaller optical zone, or in postkeratoplasty cases.

CORNEAL TOPOGRAPHY

As a corneal topographer, this machine utilizes Placido ring technology. Infrared illumination projects a Placido ring to minimize miosis of the pupil during wavefront sensing and to improve patient fixation by reducing luminance.

Output of corneal topography with this machine consists of a mire image, corneal power map, and corneal HOA map (Figure 22-3). Although the instantaneous power map is also available, the axial power map with the Smolek/Klyce scale[26] is the default. This is because the absolute scale with a 1.5 D step can make clear any clinically significant abnormality in corneal shape and can screen clinically insignificant differences in topography.[27] With such a standard scale, it is easy for the conventional videokeratoscope users to perform visual inspection of these topographic maps.

In addition to the conventional display of corneal power distribution, KR-9000PW enables us to check corneal

Figure 22-1. The external appearance of KR-9000PW.

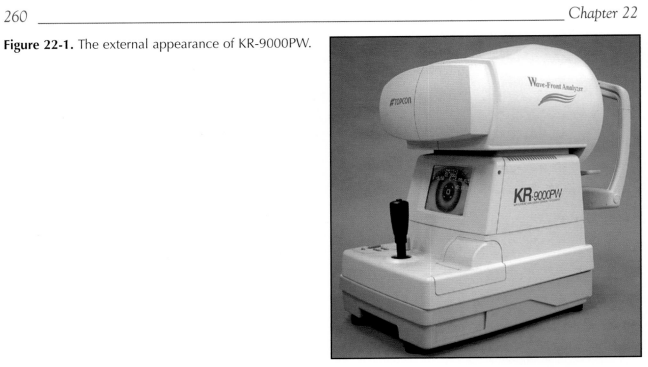

TABLE 22-1

SPECIFICATIONS OF KR-9000PW

Refractive power measurement Measuring range	Hyperopia: 0 to +22 D, 0.25 D step display (switchable to 0.12 D step display)
	Myopia: 0 to –25 D, 0.25 D step display (switchable to 0.12 D step display)
	Astigmatism: 0 to 8 D (+ or –), 0.25 D step display (switchable to 0.12 D step display)
	Axial angle: 0 to 180 degrees, 1 degree step display (switchable to 5 degree step display)
Corneal curvature measurement Measuring range	Radius of corneal curvature: 5.00 to 10.00 mm, 0.01 mm step display
	Corneal refractory power: 67.50 to 33.75 D, 0.25 D step display (switchable to 0.12 D step display)(corneal refractive index = 1.3375)
	Corneal astigmatic power: 0 to 10 D (+ or –), 0.25 D step display (switchable to 0.12 D step display)
	Corneal astigmatic axial angle: 0 to 180 degrees (1 degree step display)
Ocular higher-order aberration measurement	Hartmann-Shack wavefront aberrometer
	Higher-order aberration: Zernike polynomial up to 6th order or up to 4th order
	Aberration Display: Total aberration, higher order aberration
	Measuring range: 0 ± 15 D
	Measuring area: 7.0 mm
Corneal topography/Corneal high-order aberrations measurement	Number of Placido rings: 11
	Number of measurement sampling points: 3,960
	Radius of corneal curvature: 5.00 to 10.00 mm
	Corneal refractive power: 67.50 to 33.75 D (keratometric index = 1.3375)
	Measuring area (diameter): 0.8 mm to 9.2 mm (radius of corneal curvature = 8 mm)
	Axial power map
	Higher-order aberration : Zernike polynomial up to 6th order or up to 4th order.
Minimum pupil diameter measurable (REF)	2.0 mm
Target fixation	Auto fog system
PD measurement	85 mm measuring range max, 1 mm display unit
Dimensions	310 (W) x 475 (D) x 500 (H) mm
Weight	23 kg

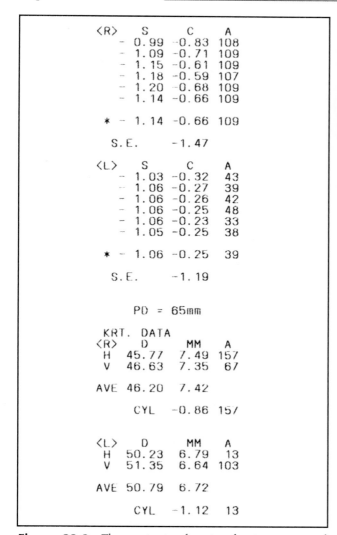

```
<R>    S     C     A
    - 0.99 -0.83 108
    - 1.09 -0.71 109
    - 1.15 -0.61 109
    - 1.18 -0.59 107
    - 1.20 -0.68 109
    - 1.14 -0.66 109

*   - 1.14 -0.66 109

    S.E.    -1.47

<L>    S     C     A
    - 1.03 -0.32  43
    - 1.06 -0.27  39
    - 1.06 -0.26  42
    - 1.06 -0.25  48
    - 1.06 -0.23  33
    - 1.05 -0.25  38

*   - 1.06 -0.25  39

    S.E.    -1.19


    PD = 65mm

KRT. DATA
<R>    D    MM    A
  H  45.77 7.49 157
  V  46.63 7.35  67

AVE 46.20 7.42

       CYL  -0.86 157


<L>    D    MM    A
  H  50.23 6.79  13
  V  51.35 6.64 103

AVE 50.79 6.72

       CYL  -1.12  13
```

Figure 22-2. The output of autorefractometry and autokeratometry.

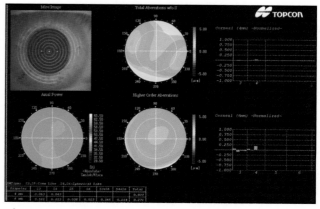

Figure 22-3. The display for corneal topography: mire image, corneal power map, and corneal HOA map.

HOAs qualitatively and quantitatively. Figure 22-3 shows a color-coded map of the corneal HOA. The absolute scale is also used for the display to show clinically significant HOAs or irregular corneal astigmatism with rapid pattern recognition. Unlike with the conventional axial power map, we can easily separate the irregular astigmatism component from sphere and cylinder with this corneal HOA map. By comparing the corneal HOA map and the ocular HOA map, the origin of irregular astigmatism (ie, due to anterior corneal surface or due to internal optics of the eye) can be identified. The details of HOAs will be explained in the following section.

ABERROMETER

The purpose of wavefront sensing is to evaluate the optical quality of the eye by analyzing the shape of its wavefront.[8,9] The optical quality of a wavefront is usually expressed as wavefront aberration, which is defined as the deviation between the wavefront that comes from an ideal optic system and the wavefront that originates from an actual optical system. The unit used for wavefront analysis is microns and is usually expressed as the root mean square (RMS) value.

The principle of the Hartmann-Shack sensor is demonstrated in Figure 22-4. A very narrow beam of super luminescent diode is projected onto the retina, and the light that exits from the eye is focused on a CCD camera by a lenslet of the Hartmann plate, creating a spot pattern. Displacements of lenslet images (Hartmann image) from their reference positions are used to calculate the shape of the wavefront. Wavefront aberrations are calculated by expanding the wavefront into sets of Zernike polynomials. Zernike polynomials are the combination of independent trigonometric functions. The terms of the Zernike polynomials (Figure 22-5) are useful in showing the wavefront aberrations because of their orthogonality. For example, the second order includes three terms that represent defocus and regular astigmatism. The third order has four terms that represent coma and trefoil. Spectacles can correct only second-order aberrations; they cannot correct third or higher orders, which represent irregular astigmatism.

The wavefront can be displayed as color-coded maps. The advancing part of a wavefront is represented by warmer colors, and the trailing part of the wavefront is represented by cooler colors.

Figure 22-4. The principle of the Hartmann-Shack sensor.

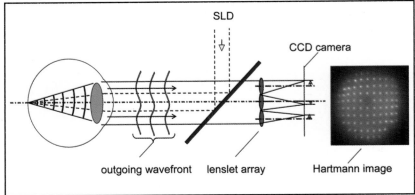

Figure 22-5. Zernike pyramid up to the sixth order.

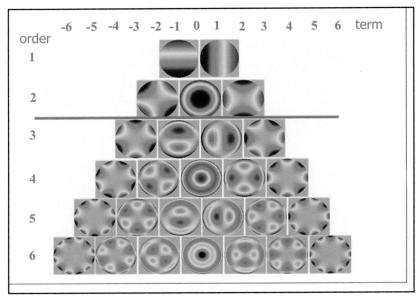

The ocular total aberration map shows all refractive errors of the eye, including defocus (sphere), regular astigmatism (cylinder), and irregular astigmatism (Figure 22-6 lower center). The relationship between defocus errors (myopia and hyperopia) and the topographic pattern in the ocular total aberration map is shown in Figure 22-7. One can also easily estimate uncorrected visual acuity (UCVA) of the eye using the total aberration map of the eye.

The ocular HOA map (Figure 22-6 lower right) includes only HOAs. Therefore, the severity of irregular astigmatism is shown in the map. The BSCVA can be easily speculated by a visual inspection of the ocular HOA map.

In addition to ocular total or HOA maps, the RMS values of each Zernike term are represented quantitatively in a bar graph (Figure 22-8). Point spread function (PSF), modulation transfer function (MTF), and simulated retinal images of Landolt rings are also represented (Figure 22-9).

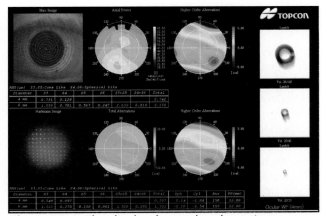

Figure 22-6. The display for ocular aberration.

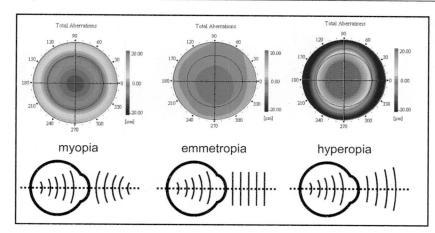

Figure 22-7. Defocus and ocular total aberration map.

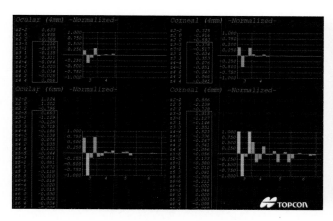

Figure 22-8. Bar graph of Zernike terms.

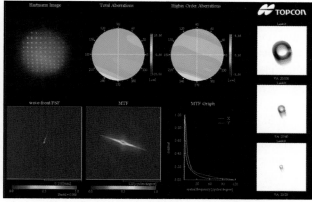

Figure 22-9. Point spread function, modulation transfer function, and simulated retinal images of Landolt rings.

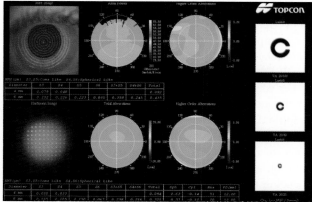

Figure 22-10. Emmetropic eye.

REPRESENTATIVE CASES

Emmetropia

The result of a typical emmetropic eye is shown in Figure 22-10. The mire image (upper left) consists of a smooth concentric circle, and the axial power map (upper center) indicates no regular or irregular astigmatism. The corneal HOA map (upper right) shows a flat wavefront that reveals no irregular astigmatism at the anterior corneal surface. The Hartmann image (lower left) is consistent with a regular grid pattern. Uniform patterns are seen in the ocular total aberration map (lower center), indicating emmetropia. The ocular HOA map (lower right) reveals no clinically significant irregular astigmatism.

Myopic Astigmatism

Figure 22-11 shows a case of myopic astigmatism. A vertical bowtie pattern indicates regular astigmatism with

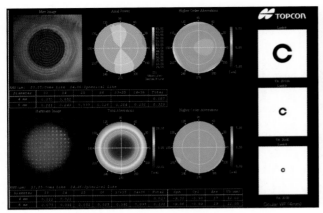

Figure 22-11. Myopia astigmatism.

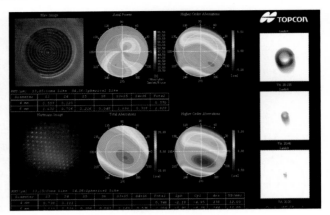

Figure 22-12. Keratoconus.

prolate asphericity in the corneal axial power map. The ocular total aberration shows an oval wavefront in the center, indicating myopic regular astigmatism. Flat wavefronts in the corneal and ocular HOA maps showed no obvious HOAs at the cornea or internal optics.

Keratoconus

The distorted mires and localized abnormal steepening in Figure 22-12 show that this is the typical keratoconic eye. The ocular total aberration map is similar to that in Figure 22-9, showing this keratoconic eye also has myopic astigmatism. The corneal HOA map reveals the combination of an advanced wavefront in the upper part and a delayed wavefront in the lower part. This asymmetric pattern indicates that the eye has vertical coma.[16] A similar pattern in the ocular HOA map shows that the source of irregular astigmatism is the cornea. The simulated retinal images are blurred and look like comets due to coma aberration.

Conventional LASIK for Myopia

An example of a conventional myopic LASIK case is shown in Figure 22-13. The flat area is shown in the center of the axial power map, and the flat wavefront is shown in the ocular total aberration map due to myopic correction. In the corneal and ocular HOA maps, the advanced wavefront in the center indicates that a mild increase of spherical aberration is shown in both maps.

ZERNIKE VECTOR MAP

Because HOA maps consist of a combination of several Zernike terms, it is sometimes difficult to perform a visual inspection of wavefront maps. The existence of

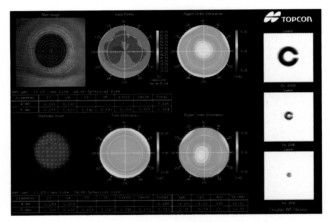

Figure 22-13. Conventional LASIK for myopia.

pairs in Zernike terms, such as in trefoil and coma, also makes it difficult to analyze the characteristics of ocular HOAs quantitatively. Describing the Zernike terms as vector components with a magnitude and orientation approach, similar to the cylinder power and axis, may help to solve these problems.

For each pair of standard Zernike terms, a single magnitude and axis value were calculated using Campbell's simplified Zernike functions,[28] as shown in Figure 22-14.

In the Zernike vector map, the magnitudes and orientations of coma, trefoil, secondary astigmatism, and tetrafoil, in addition to spherical aberration, were shown. Glancing at the map, the character of the HOA in each clinical case can be easily distinguished. In a myopic patient (Figure 22-15), the map for the total HOA (top) shows mild but complex patterns. On the other hand, Zernike vector maps (bottom) clearly show that the pattern is due to the combination of a small amount of trefoil and a small amount of spherical aberration. Figure 22-16 reveals the Zernike vector analysis in a patient with keratoconus. The output of the Zernike vector maps indicates

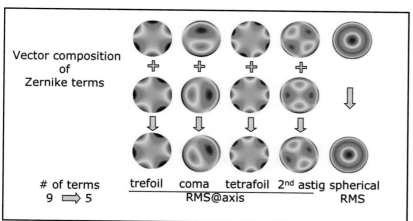

Figure 22-14. The vector analysis of Zernike terms.

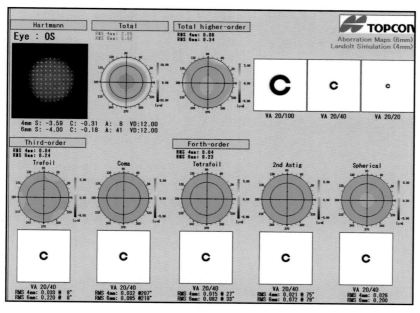

Figure 22-15. Zernike vector map in a patient with myopia.

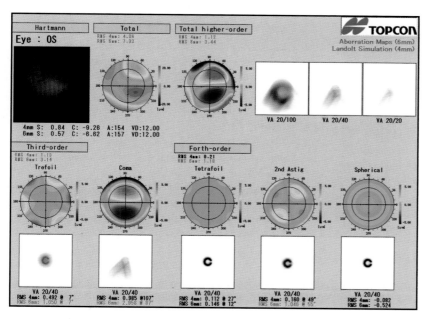

Figure 22-16. Zernike vector map in a patient with keratoconus.

Figure 22-17. The changes in spherical aberration and the Zernike vector map.

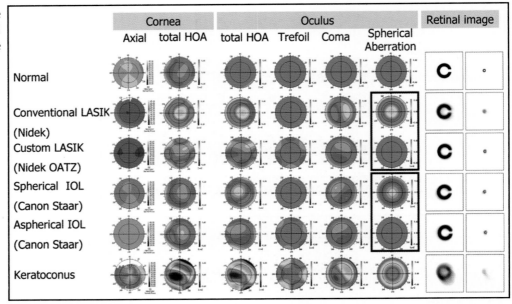

the magnitudes and angles for each term. It is obvious that the coma aberration is dominant, followed by trefoil and secondary astigmatism, in this eye. Figure 22-17 shows the difference between conventional LASIK and custom LASIK or between spherical IOLs and aspheric IOLs with respect to HOAs.

In summary, detailed information about corneal and ocular HOAs can be obtained in the clinic using a combination of a Placido disk-based corneal topographer and a Hartmann-Shack wavefront sensor.

REFERENCES

1. Klyce SD, Maeda N, Byrd TJ. Corneal topography. In: *The Cornea.* 2nd ed. Boston, Mass: Butterworth-Heinemann; 1998:1055–1075.

2. Applegate RA, Hilmantel G, Howland HC, et al. Corneal first surface optical aberrations and visual performance. *J Refract Surg.* 2000;16:507–514.

3. Maeda N. Evaluation of optical quality of corneas using corneal topographers. *Cornea.* 2002;21:S75–S78.

4. Maguire LJ, Singer DE, Klyce SD. Graphic presentation of computer-analyzed keratoscope photographs. *Arch Ophthalmol.* 1987;105:223–230.

5. Wilson SE, Klyce SD. Quantitative descriptors of corneal topography. A clinical study. *Arch Ophthalmol.* 1991; 109:349–353.

6. Oshika T, Tomidokoro A, Maruo K, Tokunaga T, Miyata N. Quantitative evaluation of irregular astigmatism by Fourier series harmonic analysis of videokeratography data. *Invest Ophthalmol Vis Sci.* 1998;39:705–709.

7. Artal P, Guirao A, Berrio E, Williams DR. Compensation of corneal aberrations by the internal optics in the human eye. *J Vis.* 2001;1:1–8.

8. Maeda N. Wavefront technology in ophthalmology. *Current Opinion in Ophthalmology.* 2001;12:294–299.

9. Maeda N. Wavefront technology and LASIK application. In: Dimitri AT, Koch DD, eds. *LASIK: Fundamentals, Surgical Techniques, and Complications.* New York, NY: Marcel Dekker, Inc; 2002:139–151.

10. Kuroda T, Fujikado T, et al. Wavefront analysis in eyes with nuclear or cortical cataract. *Am J Ophthalmol.* 2002; 134:1–9.

11. Koh S, Maeda N, Kuroda T, et al. Effect of tear film break-up on higher-order aberrations measured with wavefront sensor. *Am J Ophthalmol.* 2002;134:115–117.

12. Kuroda T, Fujikado T, et al. Wavefront analysis of higher-order aberrations in patients with cataract. *J Cataract Refract Surg.* 2002;28:438–44.

13. Kuroda T, Fujikado T, et al. Effect of aging on ocular light scatter and higher order aberrations. *J Refract Surg.* 2002; 18:S598–S602.

14. Ninomiya S, Fujikado T, et al. Changes of ocular aberration with accommodation. *Am J Ophthalmol.* 2002;134: 924–926.

15. Ninomiya S, Maeda N, et al. Evaluation of lenticular irregular astigmatism using wavefront analysis in patients with lenticonus. *Arch Ophthalmol.* 2002;120:1388–1393.

16. Maeda N, Fujikado T, et al. Wavefront aberrations measured with Hartmann-Shack sensor in patients with keratoconus. *Ophthalmology.* 2002;109:1996–2003.

17. Ninomiya S, Fujikado T, et al. Wavefront analysis in eyes with accommodative spasm. *Am J Ophthalmol.* 2003; 136:1161–1163.

18. Kelly JE, Mihashi T, Howland HC. Compensation of corneal horizontal/vertical astigmatism, lateral coma, and spherical aberration by internal optics of the eye. *J Vis.* 2004;4:262–271.

19. Fujikado T, Kuroda T, et al. Wavefront analysis of an eye with monocular triplopia and nuclear cataract. *Am J Ophthalmol.* 2004;137:361–363.

20. Fujikado T, Kuroda T, et al. Light scattering and optical aberrations as objective parameters to predict visual deterioration in eyes with cataracts. *J Cataract Refract Surg.* 2004;30:1198–1208.

21. Amano S, Amano Y, et al. Age-related changes in corneal and ocular higher-order wavefront aberrations. *Am J Ophthalmol.* 2004;137:988–992.

22. Tanabe T, Miyata K, et al. Influence of wavefront aberration and corneal subepithelial haze on low-contrast visual acuity after photorefractive keratectomy. *Am J Ophthalmol.* 2004;138:620–624.

23. Yamane N, Miyata K, et al. Ocular higher-order aberrations and contrast sensitivity after conventional laser in situ keratomileusis. *Invest Ophthalmol Vis Sci.* 2004; 45:3986–3990.

24. Fujikado T, Kuroda T, et al. Age-related changes in ocular and corneal aberrations. *Am J Ophthalmol.* 2004;138:143–146.

25. Bellucci R, Morselli S, Piers P. Comparison of wavefront aberrations and optical quality of eyes implanted with five different intraocular lenses. *J Refract Surg.* 2004;20:297–306.

26. Smolek MK, Klyce SD, Hovis JK. The Universal Standard Scale: proposed improvements to the American National Standards Institute (ANSI) scale for corneal topography. *Ophthalmology.* 2002;109:361–369.

27. Wilson SE, Klyce SD, Husseini ZM. Standardized color-coded maps for corneal topography. *Ophthalmology.* 1993;100:1723–1727.

28. Campbell CE. A new method for describing the aberrations of the eye using Zernike polynomials. *Optom Vis Sci.* 2003;80:79–83.

Chapter 23

Three-Dimensional Stereo Corneal Topographic System: The AstraMax

Ming Wang, MD, PhD; Shawna Hill, OD; and Tracy Swartz, OD, MS

Multi-dimensional imaging reveals significantly more information not detected by single-dimensional imaging. Traditional x-ray imaging is limited, while multi-dimensional imaging, such as CAT (computed axial tomography) scans and magnetic resonance imaging, yields far more diagnostic insight. Multi-dimensional imaging as such has ushered in a new era of medicine with unprecedented cross-sectional imaging of the human body and brain with unprecedented resolution. Similar to traditional x-ray films, corneal topography in general is computer data processed from several sets of single-dimensional images. Customized treatment and higher visual expectations after surgery have increased demands on the corneal imaging system capabilities. These demands include reliability, repeatability, validity, and increased sensitivity over a wide range of curvatures.

The rate of successful data capture needs to be reliable, even for complex irregular corneas after keratorefractive surgery. Traditional corneal topographic systems are designed to image regular, prolate corneal surfaces. After keratorefractive surgery, the corneal surface can be extremely irregular. Many of the intrinsic mathematical assumptions inherent to traditional corneal topographic systems result in errors or complete failure.[1]

Instrument repeatability needs to be strong. Variability increases when imaging complex corneal surfaces, since directionality of reflected light beams, as well as the quality of the reflection, varies on irregular surfaces.

Validity may be in question when ocular surface diseases, such as dry eye, cause aberrant artifactual readings. Corneal opacities, such as PRK haze, may cause false topography readings in slit-scanning systems, as the opacities change scattering patterns of detecting light beams.[2,3]

Keratorefractive surgery has greatly expanded the range of architectural parameters of the cornea. Physiological keratometric readings of a normal cornea range between 39 and 46 D. Following keratorefractive surgery, that range expands to the low-30s and mid-50s. Since most of the traditional corneal topography systems are designed to operate in a linear range that corresponds to the physiological cornea keratometric range, they tend to break down in eyes with extreme flat or steep diopter curvature.

The above-mentioned limitations of commonly used corneal topographic systems result in limited sensitivity and specificity when imaging irregular corneal surfaces. Typical systems lack the sophistication required by modern keratorefractive surgery to accurately measure preoperative corneal surfaces and formulate laser treatment plans for primary treatment. More importantly, typical systems are less likely to reliably identify topography etiologies responsible for reduced visual quality in patients after keratorefractive surgery and may not be sensitive enough to design laser treatment plans for complex corneal surfaces.

Multi-dimensional imaging of the cornea delivers an increased level of sensitivity and specificity of imaging data in complex corneal surfaces with larger dynamic ranges of corneal architectural parameters. A protypical system of multi-dimensional corneal imaging is the AstraMax (Winter Park, FL) three-dimensional stereo corneal image system.

The AstraMax three-dimensional stereo corneal topographic system (Figure 23-1) employs three cameras rather than one central camera, as is used in all traditional unidimensional systems. A highly detailed grid (Figure 23-2) is projected onto the cornea. Three cameras detect the reflections of this grid, creating a three-dimensional image of the cornea (Figure 23-3). Compared with traditional unidimensional corneal topographic systems, the multicamera system has the following advantages:

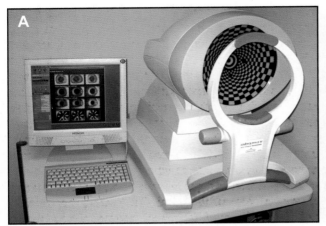

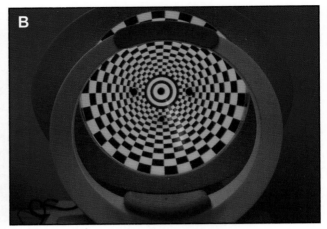

Figure 23-1. (A) The AstraMax system. (B) The illuminated grid showing the location of the cameras.

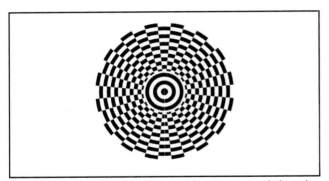

Figure 23-2. The Placido grid target used by the AstraMax system.

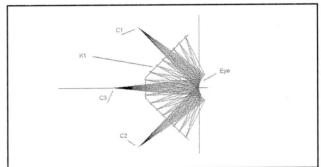

Figure 23-3. The camera placement used by the AstraMax system.

- Three cameras simultaneously capture three independent data sets, generating 35,000 data points in a single shot and far surpassing the data output of a traditional one-dimensional corneal topographer.

- Overlay of the reflected grid pattern using the multiple cameras creates a true three-dimensional image, which is more useful in elevation mapping.

- Unlike the slit-scanning corneal topographic system, which requires up to two seconds for data acquisition and thus can be prone to issues with dry eye and eye movement, the AstraMax employs rapid data acquisition using all three cameras in as little as 0.2 seconds.

- The AstraMax projects a cross-slit pattern, which is simultaneously captured by all three cameras, generating data and allowing for evaluation of the posterior surface and pachymetry.

Clinical Cases

The following are clinical cases in which AstraMax helped identify causes of visual problems in keratorefractive surgery patients. These include identification of topographic irregular astigmatism.

Case I

A patient S/P myopic LASIK, who later underwent a hyperopic LASIK enhancement OS, presented with monocular diplopia uncorrectable with glasses or gas permeable lenses. Topographical analysis revealed a sharp demarcation along the temporal edge on both curvature and elevation maps using the AstraMax (Figure 23-4). This edge pulled the gas permeable lens nasally, making contact lens wear problematic. The shape pattern was less

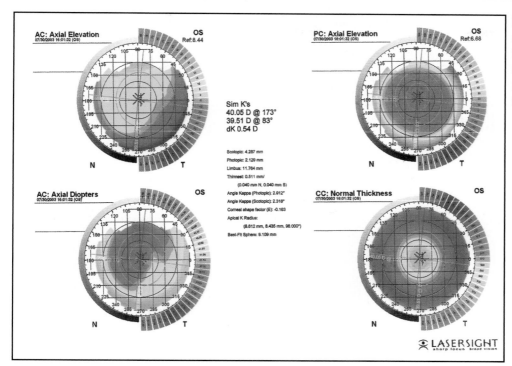

Figure 23-4. A sharp demarcation along the temporal edge on both curvature and elevation maps was found using the AstraMax.

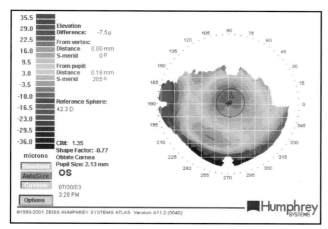

Figure 23-5. Conventional Placido disk topographic maps failed to identify the topographic irregularity noted in Figure 23-4.

obvious using a traditional Placido disk topographer, while other systems failed to identify the topographic abnormality (Figures 23-5 and 23-6). Coma accounted for the multiple images reported by the patient, as measured by the WaveScan (Figure 23-7). We recommended advanced fitting with larger gas permeable lenses and await technology to allow custom ablation.

Case II

A patient S/P myopic LASIK for monovision presented complaining of blurry vision and ghost images in each eye. He suffered from DLK greater in the right eye following his surgery, which was treated medically. Topographical analysis by the AstraMax successfully revealed a decentered ablation zone with a central island (Figure 23-8). However, the curvature map of a traditional slit-scanning topographer (Figure 23-9) showed only a small amount of astigmatism. Figure 23-10 shows a traditional Placido disk elevation map illustrating the patient's irregular surface. We treated the irregular surface using punctal plugs in the lower lid, and for the residual refractive error, we enhanced the eye, resulting in a substantial increase in visual acuity.

Case III

A patient presented complaining of blurred vision. BCSVA was 20/20 (–0.75 DS). Topographical analysis by AstraMax showed significant steepening in the inferior cornea on both curvature and elevation maps (Figure 23-11). Analysis by traditional slit-scanning and Placido disk topographers showed no significant corneal steepening on the axial maps (Figures 23-12 and 23-13). Three months later, all topographers showed inferior steepening. AstraMax best identified the early diagnosis of pellucid marginal degeneration.

Case IV

A patient S/P myopic LASIK who later underwent a hyperopic LASIK enhancement presented complaining of

Figure 23-6. Slit scanning topographic maps failed to identify the topographic irregularity noted in Figure 23-4.

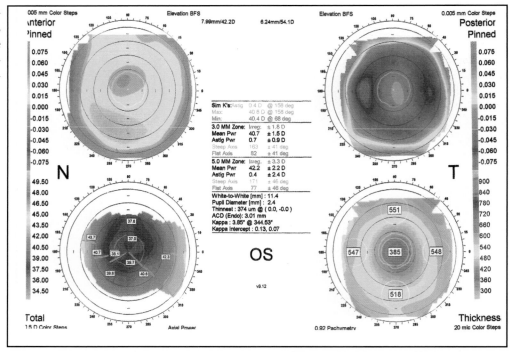

Figure 23-7. Coma accounted for the multiple images reported by the same patient.

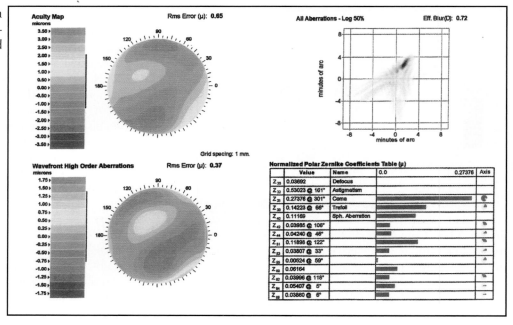

blurry vision and ghost images. Topographical analysis revealed irregular steepening on both curvature and elevation maps using the AstraMax (Figure 23-14). Using a traditional Placido disk system, steepening was noted on the axial map (Figure 23-15) but not the elevation map (Figure 23-16). We diagnosed the patient with irregular astigmatism, and he underwent a third enhancement to correct the residual refractive error without complication.

Case V

A patient S/P hyperopic PRK who later underwent a hyperopic PRK enhancement presented complaining of blurry vision with a monocular double image. Topographical analysis demonstrated astigmatism on both the AstraMax (Figure 23-17) and a slit-scanning topographer (Figure 23-18). However, compared with ultrasound

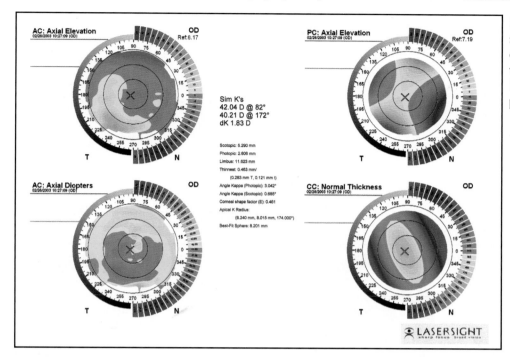

Figure 23-8. AstraMax successfully revealed a decentered ablation zone with a central island following repeated LASIK procedures.

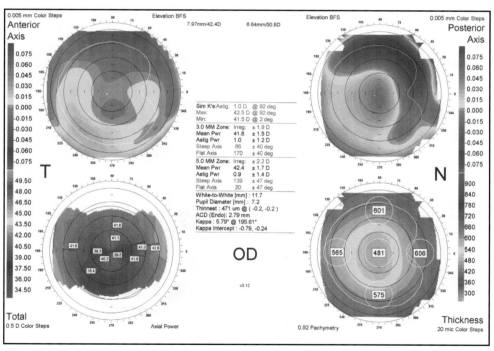

Figure 23-9. Scanning slit topography's curvature map found only mild astigmatism.

pachymetry of 466 μm, the AstraMax closely estimated the corneal thickness (460 to 500 μm) unlike the scanning slit system, which grossly underestimated the corneal thickness (369 μm). The patient will require an enhancement for the large amount of residual cylinder.

Case VI

A patient S/P hyperopic LASIK presented complaining of fluctuating vision and difficulty focusing. Topographical analysis by traditional Placido disk (Figure 23-19) and a

Figure 23-10. Placido disk elevation map illustrating the patient's irregular surface.

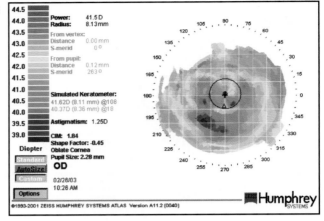

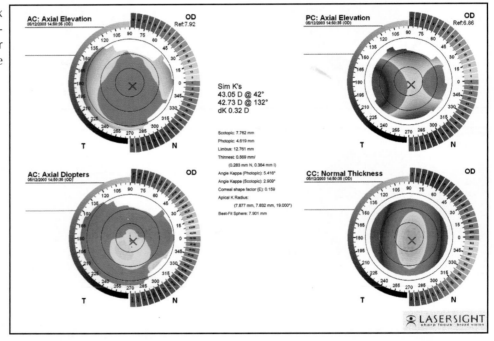

Figure 23-11. AstraMax showed significant steepening in the inferior cornea on both curvature and elevation maps.

slit-scanning system (Figure 23-20) showed central steepening on an elevation map, characteristic of a hyperopic treatment. The elevation map of the AstraMax (Figure 23-21) demonstrated the corneal multifocality, the main contributing cause to the patient's accommodative instability.

Case VII

Topographical analysis by the AstraMax revealed steepening along the horizontal meridian on the curvature map (Figure 23-22). The slit-scanning curvature map appears uniformly steep according to color (Figure 23-23). We diagnosed the patient with atypical pellucid marginal degeneration.

CONCLUSION

The advantages to the multi-dimensional corneal imaging used in three-dimensional stereo corneal topography are similar to that of CAT scans (a multi-dimensional x-ray) over traditional x-ray machines. In detecting topographic etiologies, this multi-dimensional technology has shown enhanced sensitivity to visual problems following keratorefractive surgery as well as detecting changes due to early corneal disease. Continued research and investigation resulting in refinement of this new multi-dimensional corneal topographic technology will improve our corneal imaging capability as well as our efforts to improve visual quality in patients undergoing keratorefractive surgery.

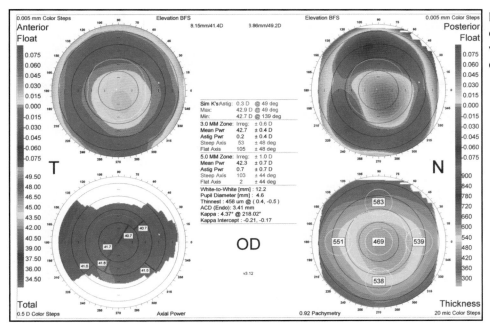

Figure 23-12. No significant corneal steepening was noted on the axial map of a slit-scanning system.

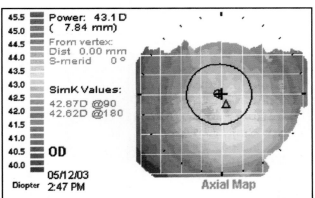

Figure 23-13. No significant corneal steepening on the axial maps of a traditional Placido disk system.

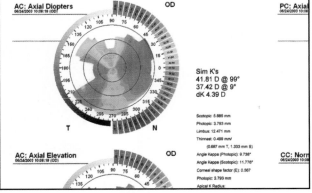

Figure 23-14. Irregular steepening on both curvature and elevation maps from the AstraMax.

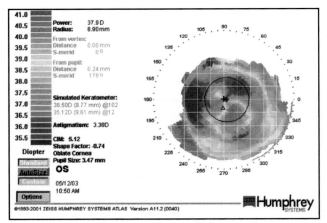

Figure 23-15. Using a traditional Placido disk system, steepening was noted on the axial map.

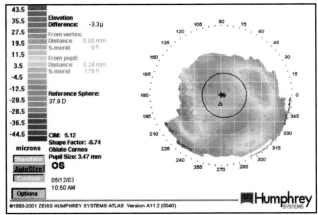

Figure 23-16. The irregularity seen in Figure 23-15 was not noted on this corresponding elevation map using traditional Placido disk technology.

Figure 23-17. Pachymetry was in the same range as the ultrasound pachymetry of 466 µm.

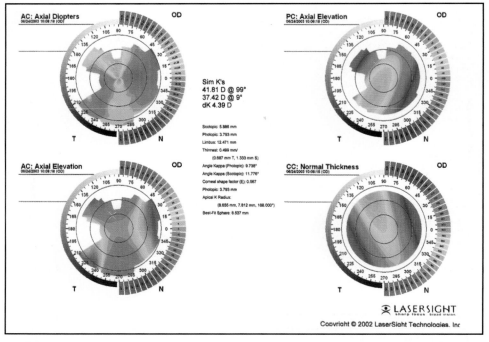

Figure 23-18. Slit-scanning pachymetry measurements were significantly lower than ultrasound.

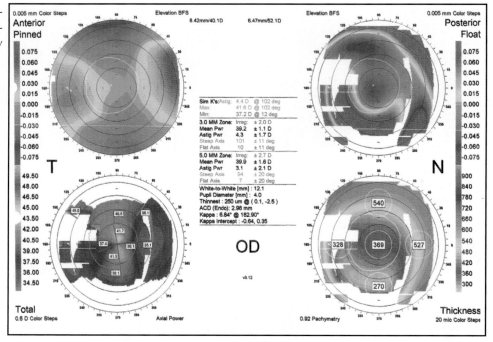

REFERENCES

1. Roberts C. Characterization of the inherent error in a spherically-based corneal topography system in mapping a radially aspheric surface. *J Refract Corneal Surg.* 1994;10:103–111.

2. Boyd BF. Topography system. In: Boyd B, Agarwal A, Alio J, Krueger R, Wilson S, eds. *Wavefront Analysis, Aberrometers, and Corneal Topography.* El Dorado, Paname: Highlights of Ophthalmology International; 2003:112.

3. Boscia F, La Tegola MG, Alessio G, Sborgia C. Accuracy of Orbscan optical pachymetry in corneas with haze. *J Cataract Refract Surg.* 2002;28:253–258.

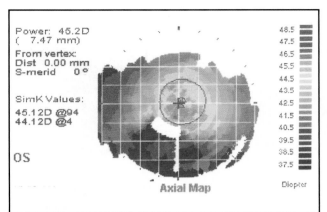

Figure 23-19. Central steepening characteristic of a hyperopic LASIK treatment using Placido disk topography.

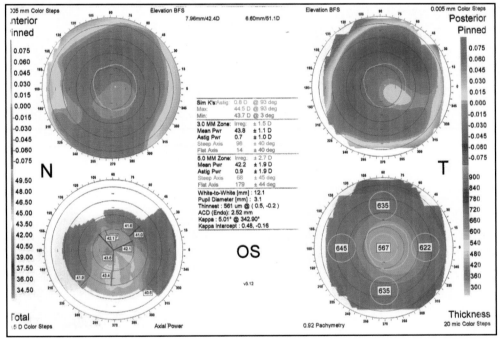

Figure 23-20. Central steepening characteristic of a hyperopic LASIK treatment using slit-scanning topography.

Figure 23-21. Multifocality, identified by the AstraMax system, was the etiology for the patients focusing difficulties.

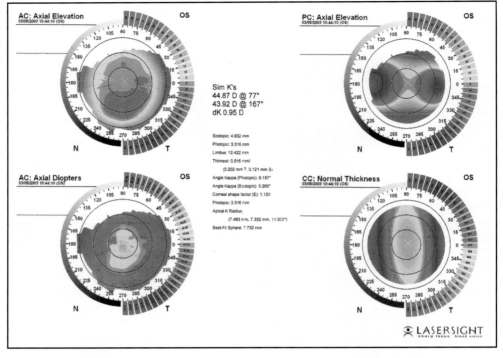

Figure 23-22. AstraMax revealed steepening along the horizontal meridian on the curvature map.

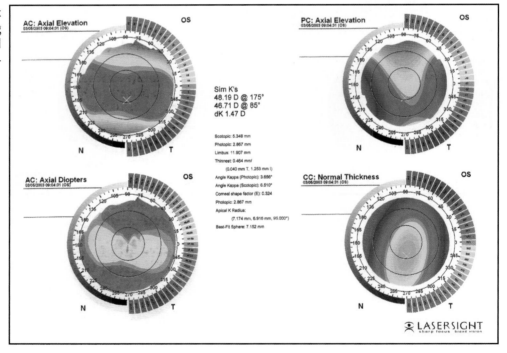

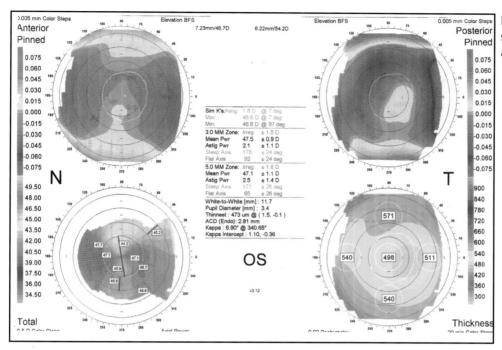

Figure 23-23. The slit-scanning curvature map appears uniformly steep.

Pentacam

Matthias Maus, MD; Stephan Kröber; Tracy Swartz, OD, MS; Michael W. Belin, MD;
Marc Michaelson, MD; John Sutphin, MD; and Ming Wang, MD, PhD

The Pentacam eye scanner (Figure 24-1) (Oculus USA, Lynnwood, Wash) utilizes Scheimpflug imaging, a principle named after and patented by the Austrian Theodor Scheimpflug in Vienna in 1904. To appreciate the advantages of a Scheimpflug camera for ophthalmologic purposes, it is appropriate to first review the basic principles and limitations of an ordinary camera.

A camera uses three planes: the film plane, the lens plane, and the plane of sharp focus. All three planes are imaginary surfaces. A camera's film is fixed on the film plane. The lens plane passes through the optical center of the lens and is perpendicular to the lens axis. The lens will depict any object that is positioned on the plane of sharp focus crisply onto the film plane (Figure 24-2). For an ordinary camera, these three planes are all parallel to each other, and therefore, all three planes are perpendicular to the lens axis. As long as a given application only calls for limited depth of focus, this setup works well. The depth of focus is the range over which the film plane can be moved while maintaining an image of acceptable sharpness.

Ophthalmologic applications require an extended depth of focus to effectively image the entire anterior segment. In Scheimpflug imaging, the three planes are not parallel but slanted so they intersect in a line, or simplified, in a point of intersection. Put more elaborately, the Scheimpflug principle states that if the lens is tilted in a way that the resulting lens plane intersects the film plane, then the plane of sharp focus, due to its dependence upon the lens plane, must also pass through that same line of intersection. This line is sometimes referred to as the "Scheimpflug line." The benefit this setup brings is extended depth of focus. However, the extended depth of focus has a trade-off: distortion of the image (Figure 24-3).

The Pentacam computes the acquired picture to compensate for this distortion.

The Pentacam is a rotating Scheimpflug camera that provides 25 to 50 Scheimpflug images during one scan in less than 2 seconds, yielding 500 true elevation points per image. The system integrates two cameras. One is located in the center for the purposes of detection of the size and orientation of the pupil and to control fixation. The second is mounted on the rotating wheel to capture images of the anterior segment. The Scheimpflug image is a complete picture from the anterior surface of the cornea to the posterior surface of the lens (Figure 24-4). It generates up to 25,000 true elevation points for each surface, including the area of the center of the cornea. Fixation is controlled by a second camera, which captures and corrects eye movements.

To capture images of the anterior segment, the rotating wheel takes slit images in three dimensions. The slit images are photographed on an angle from 0 to 180 degrees to avoid shadows from the nose. Every picture is a complete image through the cornea in the specific angle, so a real 360-degree image of the anterior segment of the eye is acquired. Because the images are taken rotating around the corneal center, more measurement points are obtained from the center of the cornea. The period of time required to complete the measurement of the anterior segment is 2 seconds for 50 single slit images. From every single slit image, 500 points are evaluated. Therefore, for 50 Scheimpflug images, 25,000 true elevation points are measured. An exact three-dimensional model of the anterior segment is created from the evaluation data and displayed in a default "overview" presentation (Figure 24-5). An exact three-dimensional model of the anterior segment is created from the evaluation data. Figure 24-6 shows a

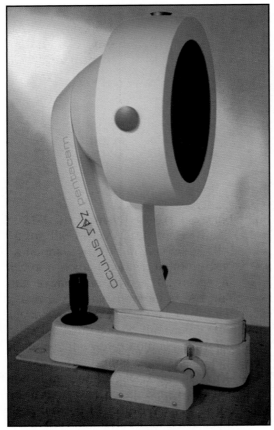

Figure 24-1. The Pentacam comprehensive eye scanner. (Courtesy of Michael Belin, MD.)

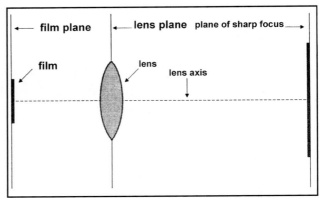

Figure 24-2. Diagram of an ordinary camera. (Courtesy of Matthias Maus, MD.)

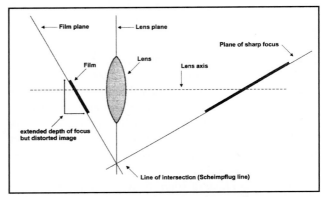

Figure 24-3. Diagram of a Scheimpflug camera. (Courtesy of Matthias Maus, MD.)

pseudophakic posterior chamber IOL viewed tomographically.

This technology allows a comprehensive scan of the anterior segment and holds several advantages over current topographic technology. Placido disk technology utilizes assumptions inherent to power calculation and paracentral measurement of the cornea. Placido disk topographers and keratometers, which are limited to the anterior surface, are not able to measure true corneal power. Instruments typically assume that the posterior surface radius is 82% of the anterior surface when calculating the net power of the cornea. This natural ratio is no longer valid following keratorefractive surgery such as LASIK, and significant error results. Because the Pentacam measures the elevation data directly, true power maps are attainable.

Placido disk systems also create error by using paracentral measurements. In the eye S/P keratorefractive surgery, the variability of the central compared to the peripheral cornea may be substantial. Scheimpflug imaging allows for a more complete analysis of the anterior segment,

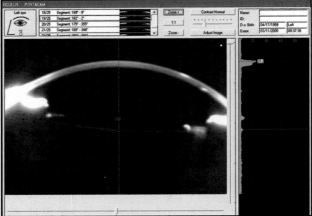

Figure 24-4. Scheimpflug image of the anterior segment of an eye with a posterior chamber IOL. (Courtesy of Marc Michelson, MD.)

including lens transmission and determination of the anterior chamber architecture.

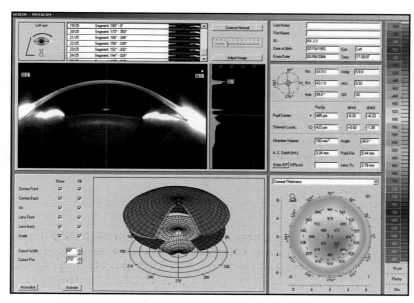

Figure 24-5. Images of a patient with keratoconus are created from the height data and displayed in the overview. (Courtesy of John Sutphin, MD).

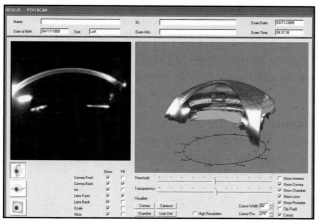

Figure 24-6. An exact three-dimensional model of the anterior segment is created from the evaluation data. (Courtesy of Marc Michelson, MD.)

DATA CAPTURE AND IMAGING

Dilation of the pupil is not required for topography, pachymetry, and anterior corneal analysis. For evaluation of IOLs and densitometry, dilating the pupil is indicated in most cases. The Pentacam automatically starts capturing images, but if necessary, a manual scanning release can be initiated. When the scan is imminent, the patient is asked to widely open his eyes in order to allow for an unobscured view of the eye. While scanning, a second camera tracks eye position to compensate for saccadic eye movements.

The Pentacam captures 50 grayscale images that depict the entire anterior segment from the cornea to the posterior lens surface. There is the option to limit the amount of pictures taken to either 12 or 25, although this decreases resolution. The default 50 images is preferable to create the most accurate three-dimensional rendering of the cornea.

Once the Scheimpflug images are captured, a "virtual eye" of the anterior eye segment is computed. The virtual eye is displayed onscreen, where it can be manipulated. The underlying mathematical model is the basis for all subsequent calculations, such as anterior chamber analysis, topography, and pachymetry.

As with most kinds of keratometers, areas that were obscured in some way during the measurement are marked appropriately. The data points in that area are then interpolated. In such a case, it is best to repeat the measurement. The Pentacam utilizes a "quality factor," a judgment of whether or not a particular measurement is useable. A quality factor higher than 95 indicates a good measurement.

If an examination calls for only one Scheimpflug image to be taken, the exact camera position can be defined. For densitometric assessment of the lens, 5, 10, or 15 Scheimpflug images can be taken from a single camera position. The mean value of the captured images is computed into a single image that is then displayed. This technique is known as "enhanced dynamic Scheimpflug imaging." A blue illumination light can be switched on to aid with the evaluation of the lens without having to dilate the patient's pupil.

Once the images are displayed, the Pentacam offers basic image-enhancing functions similar to Adobe Photoshop (San Jose, Calif). Image changes can be saved for later review. These features come in handy when dealing with more challenging cases. They are especially

Figure 24-7. An overview display of a patient with an ICL. (Courtesy of Matthias Maus, MD.)

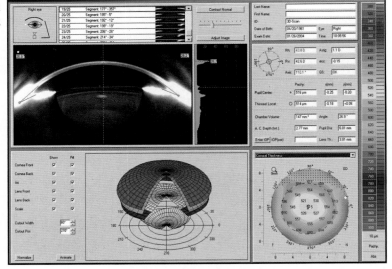

Figure 24-8. Typical topographical quad map for a patient with keratoconus. (Courtesy of Michael Belin, MD.)

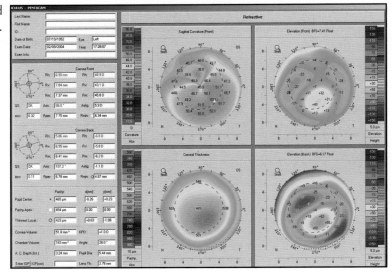

helpful when using the Pentacam's densitometry function. Densitometry will be described in more detail below. It is important to note that these changes only affect the images that are onscreen at the time of image editing.

An overview display of a patient S/P ICL implantation contains a set of different representations (Figure 24-7); the most frequently needed data is displayed alongside the virtual eye and the actual Scheimpflug images. The more sophisticated counterparts of the smaller comprehensive representations may be selected for enlargement and manipulation.

COMPREHENSIVE ANTERIOR SEGMENT EVALUATION

The Pentacam provides a complete analysis of the anterior and posterior surface topography of the cornea derived from true elevation measurements, allowing for computations of anterior and posterior sagittal (axial) and tangential (local or instantaneous) curvature, anterior and posterior elevation maps with comparisons to a best fit sphere, ellipsoid or toric-ellipsoid, and full corneal pachymetry. The Scheimpflug principle allows for data capture in patients with significant keratoconus and severe irregular astigmatism, which may prevent successful Placido imaging. Typical topographical quad map of a patient with keratoconus is shown in Figure 24-8.

An additional tool for the refractive surgeon is the elevation-based keratoconus detection program. As opposed to other programs that rely solely on the anterior corneal surface or curvature, this program compares rate of change and location of the pachymetry values by utilizing data from both the anterior and posterior corneal surfaces. Figure 24-9 illustrates results from the topography-based keratoconus detection program. This figure shows the

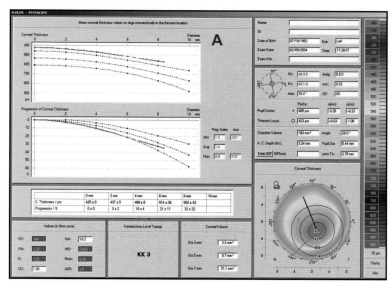

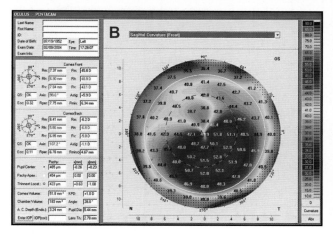

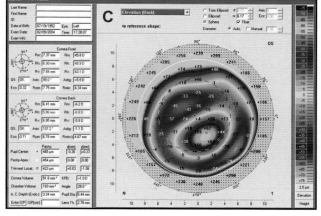

Figure 24-9. Topography-based keratoconus detection program: (A) the keratoconus indices display; (B) a sagittal map; and (C) a posterior elevation map of the same eye. (Courtesy of Marc Michelson, MD.)

(A) keratoconus indices display, (B) a sagittal map, and (C) a posterior elevation map of the same eye.

The TrueNetPower map (Figure 24-10) reflects the true power of the cornea in its entirety. Figure 24-10 shows the image of an eye S/P LASIK where epithelial ingrowth induced 7 D of central astigmatism.

The Pentacam enables evaluation of the anterior chamber angle, height, volume, and depth and calculates a colored anterior chamber depth map (Figure 24-11). The anterior chamber values are calculated from the three-dimensional model.

The Pentacam calculates the pachymetry of the cornea from limbus to limbus with an accuracy of +/–5 µm and displays corneal thickness in a colored map. An example is shown in Figure 24-12, an eye with ectasia following LASIK.

The evaluation of the crystalline lens, including the subscapular layer, is also possible with this technology, which offers an objective quantification of lens densitom-

etry to follow the development of cataracts (Figure 24-13). The densitometry becomes visible through the illumination using blue light.

The Pentacam also provides a corneal wavefront analysis for both surfaces using Zernike indices to detect high-order aberrations attributable to the corneal surfaces. Zernike functions and higher-order aberrations are demonstrated in a patient undercorrected with LASIK in Figure 24-14.

APPLICATIONS FOR ANTERIOR SEGMENT EVALUATION

The Pentacam possesses a variety of features, allowing the physician to use it for multiple purposes. These include prekeratorefractive surgery considerations, keratoconus screening, phakic intraocular lens (PIOL) planning,

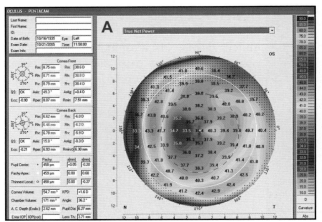

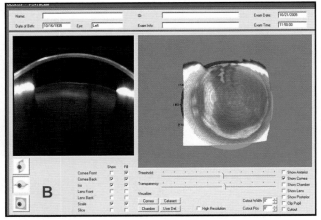

Figure 24-10. True net power map in an eye S/P LASIK where (A) epithelial ingrowth induced 7 D of central astigmatism. (B) The ingrowth can be seen on the raw image. (Courtesy of Marc Michelson, MD.)

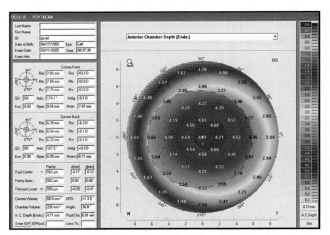

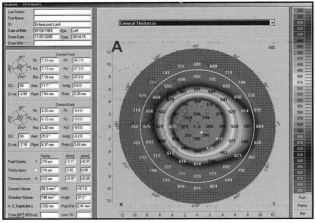

Figure 24-11. Anterior chamber depth map. (Courtesy of Marc Michelson, MD.)

Figure 24-12A. The pachymetry map details the pachymetry of the cornea from limbus to limbus in an eye with ectasia following LASIK.

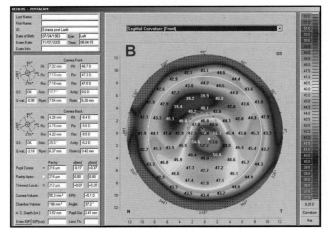

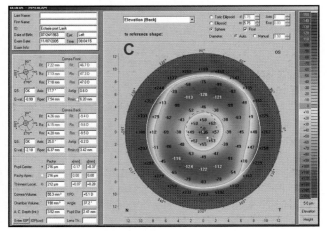

Figure 24-12B–C. (B) The anterior curvature map and (C) the posterior float also show the ectasia. (Courtesy of Marc Michelson, MD.)

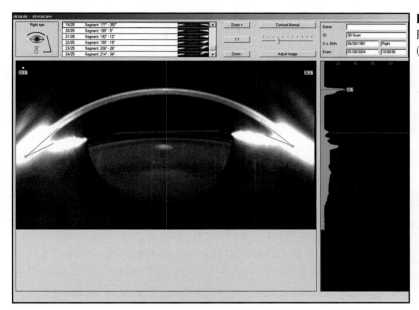

Figure 24-13. Lens evaluation using the Pentacam. Note the lens opacities. (Courtesy of John Sutphin, MD.)

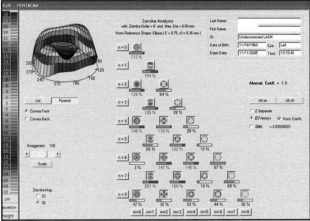

Figure 24-14. Wavefront analysis in a patient undercorrected by LASIK. (Courtesy of Marc Michelson, MD.)

calculation of post-refractive surgery IOL power, and densitometry of the lens. The Pentacam also aids in the correct diagnosis of glaucoma. These features make it a valuable asset for thoroughly assessing the anterior segment in an efficient manner. As an added bonus, its impressive images and graphical rendering of the anterior segment make it a potent marketing tool.

Prekeratorefractive Surgery Considerations

In keratorefractive corneal surgery, screening patients for conditions that may negatively affect long-term corneal stability is important for successful treatments. Patients seeking evaluation for a keratorefractive procedure need to be assessed for sufficient corneal thickness and the presence of corneal disorders, most notably keratoconus.

For most cases, the procedure of choice is LASIK. For myopic treatment, tissue is removed centrally in order to flatten the cornea, reducing its refractive power. In hyperopic treatment, the laser ablates in a peripheral circular fashion to steepen the cornea. Central tissue removal is minimal for a hyperopic treatment.

It is commonly accepted that after tissue ablation, a residual central stromal thickness under the flap of at least 250 μm should remain in order to avoid iatrogenic ectasia, a condition in which the cornea bulges forward, causing myopia. In severe cases, keratoplasty may become necessary. Pentacam's pachymetry module is a good choice for pre-LASIK assessment. It has the capability of mapping the corneal thickness over the complete ablation zone.

In total, the Pentacam collects corneal pachymetry data from an array of 25,000 points. The location of the pupil center, corneal apex, and the thinnest point of the cornea are displayed, as these are useful to refractive surgeons to ensure candidacy. The Pentacam's measurements are accurate to ±5 μm. Studies have shown that the Pentacam's measurements compare reasonably well with measurements taken with A-scan ultrasonography.[1,2]

Based on pachymetry, the patient can be informed as to which refractive procedure is best or if they should refrain from any kind of keratorefractive surgery. For those with higher refractive errors, an enhancement procedure might become necessary. Ensuring that sufficient stroma remains for a possible enhancement procedure is also important prior to procedure.

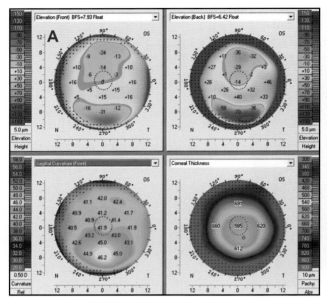

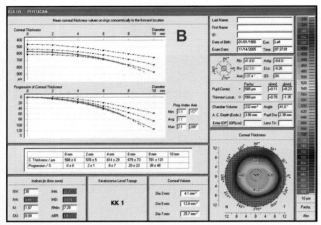

Figure 24-15. (A) The Quad map and (B) the indices display show increased inferior steepening in this case of forme fruste keratoconus. (Courtesy of Jason Stahl, MD.)

Should the patient elect to undergo a refractive procedure, proper surgical planning requires in-depth knowledge of pachymetry. Higher ablation depths necessitate thin flaps, and may require the use of a femtosecond laser-assisted LASIK. Differences in ablation depth among ablation profiles, such as wavefront-guided, wavefront-optimized, topography-guided, or asphericity-adjusting profiles, can be significant. The size of the optical zone also significantly influences ablation depth.

Keratoconus Screening

Keratoconus is a condition in which the cornea becomes progressively thinner, causing corneal distortion and vision loss. While diagnosing a more advanced form of keratoconus may be simple, early stages are challenging. Patients' complaints in manifest keratoconus may range from photophobia, halos, glare, and image distortion to diplopia or polyopia. However, patients in early stages are typically asymptomatic.

The Pentacam aids in finding subtle signs of early keratoconus, such as the invagination of the cornea's posterior surface and forward movement of Bowman's membrane. Furthermore, the Pentacam facilitates diagnosis of forme fruste keratoconus. While a forme fruste keratoconus can be corrected using spectacles and contact lenses, regular monitoring is required.

Traditional Placido-based keratometry systems safely recognize most cases of keratoconus. Unfortunately, they have a high false-positive rate. The problem with Placido-based systems is that they interpolate a lot of data (ie, they make many assumptions and simplify in some regards).[3]

Placido-based devices assume that the corneal apex, line of sight, and the reference axis of the keratometer from which the measurements are taken are identical. Thus, a normal cornea with a decentered apex may be diagnosed with keratoconus.

The Pentacam has a different approach. Its high resolution yields a true elevation map, independent of the reference axis. Placido-based systems suffer from a central "blind-spot," while the Pentacam excels in the central area due to a high density of data points obtained from the Scheimpflug camera rotating around the center of the cornea. The central deviation of the cornea's anterior elevation of more than +15 μm is indicative of keratoconus. Anterior elevation differences of less than +12 μm are considered normal. Values between +12 to +15 μm are suspicious and should prompt further investigation. It is very important to locate the thinnest point of the cornea because it will correspond to the most elevated area. Theoretically, the evaluation of posterior elevation is also possible. Values tend to be higher by about 5 μm. However, experience with the assessment of posterior elevation is limited.

We will use several cases to demonstrate the diagnostic power of the Pentacam:

A 40-year-old male with a manifest refraction of –3.25 –1.00 x 85 yielding 20/15 visual acuity OS was diagnosed with forme fruste keratoconus. Maps and indices are displayed in Figure 24-15. Both net power and anterior sagittal maps show the increase inferior Ks. The keratometric indices detail the irregularity. LASIK was avoided, and the patient underwent successful PRK.

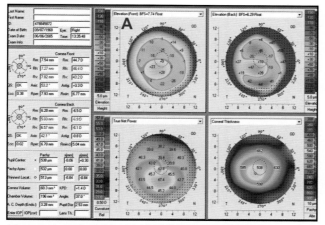
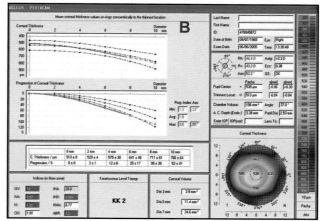

Figure 24-16. An example of a patient with keratoconus: (A) Quad map display and (B) keratoconus indices display. (Courtesy of Marc Michelson, MD.)

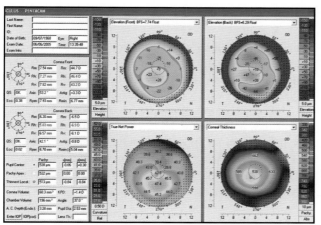

Figure 24-17. Early keratoconus in a 37-year-old female. (Courtesy of Jason Stahl, MD.)

A patient with keratoconus is shown in Figure 24-16. Posterior float and sagittal curvatures are characteristic for keratoconus.

A 37-year-old female with a manifest refraction of OD +0.50 –4.75 x 59 yielding 20/25 visual acuity diagnosed with early keratoconus based on maps is shown in Figure 24-17.

Treating keratoconus has thus far been limited to catering for the best possible vision correction until a transplant is required. Usually, this requires fitting of rigid gas permeable (RGP) contact lenses to correct irregular astigmatism. However, in more advanced cases, contact lens wear can become impossible due to the irregular corneal surface. Contact lenses will simply not adhere to the eye. Sometimes, InTacs (Addition Technology Inc, Fremont, Calif) are used to stabilize keratoconus. Their proper position can be evaluated nicely using the Pentacam's imaging capabilities. In extreme cases of keratoconus, a corneal

transplant may become necessary. Recently, a procedure called "corneal crosslinking" has been proposed by Prof. Dr. Theo Seiler. In corneal crosslinking, ultraviolet (UV) light in conjunction with riboflavin is used to crosslink stromal collagen fibers in order to stabilize the cornea mechanically. It can be expected that the Pentacam will be used as a means to assess the results of the procedure.

In addition to detecting early keratoconus, contact lens warpage resulting from excessive contact lens wear and irregular astigmatism secondary to keratorefractive surgery can be diagnosed using the Pentacam. A posterior elevation map of a patient 7 years postoperative LASIK and LRI with astigmatism is shown in Figure 24-18A. The patient has severe superior and inferior posterior floats corresponding to the steep meridional axis. A sagital frontal pentacam image detailing over 5 D of central astigmatism keratometrically is shown in Figure 24-18B.

Phakic Lens Implantation Surgical Planning

Managing cases of high ametropia frequently includes the placement of IOLs. Exact knowledge of the available intraocular space is paramount for appropriate candidate selection and counseling. A refractive or phakic lens implant is recommended whenever keratorefractive procedures are impossible due to insufficient corneal thickness or corneal architecture. In refractive lens exchange (RLE), replacing the natural unclouded lens with an implant makes accommodation impossible. A phakic lens implant retains the ability to accommodate since the natural lens remains. The Pentacam allows assessment of the anterior chamber depth required for phakic lens planning.

The iris-claw phakic IOL (ie, Verisyse [Advanced Medical Optics, Santa Ana, Calif]) is a widely chosen option. Before such a lens is implanted, Nd:YAG iridotomy

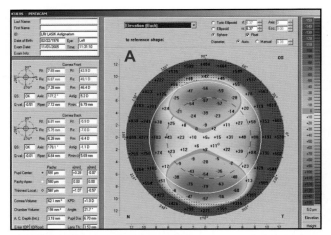
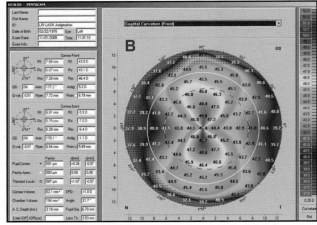

Figure 24-18. (A) Posterior elevation map of a patient 7 years postoperative LASIK and LRI with residual astigmatism. (B) A sagittal frontal Pentacam image detailing over 5 D of central astigmatism keratometrically. (Courtesy of Jason Stahl, MD.)

is routinely performed to prevent glaucoma. The Pentacam facilitates monitoring the results of this procedure. The Pentacam measures the distance from the anterior surface of the crystalline lens to the corneal endothelium. Once an implant is in place, the Pentacam helps in monitoring its settlement and refractive power change.

Calculation of Postrefractive Surgery Intraocular Lens Power

Keratorefractive surgery alters the curvature of the anterior surface of the cornea. With the growing popularity of cornea-altering refractive surgery, devising a reliable method to calculate true corneal power becomes increasingly important. Exact knowledge of corneal power is important to correctly calculate IOLs. Traditional Placido-based topographers and keratometers only measure the anterior surface of the cornea. To calculate the corneal power, it is assumed that the radius of the posterior surface is approximately 82% of the anterior radius. However, this relationship changes with refractive surgery, and error results.

Some Placido-based devices are unable to accurately measure the central 1 to 1.5 mm of the cornea, or offer only low resolution. If a cornea has been altered, paracentral measurements are no longer valid for interpolating central data introducing a second source of error. The combined errors account for a deviation from the true value of approximately 25%.

Unlike Placido systems, the Pentacam supplies true, high-resolution data from the corneal center. This is especially important for measuring corneas S/P myopic excimer treatment, which have been flattened centrally. For calculating the true net power of a surgically altered

cornea, both the anterior and posterior surfaces need to be measured individually. Based on these measurements, the Pentacam calculates the cornea's true net power. The Pentacam comes with a dedicated software module called the "Holladay Report," developed in conjunction with Jack T. Holladay, MD. Figure 24-19 shows a Holladay Report for a patient pre- and postoperatively. It displays five colored maps: the anterior refractive power, tangential curvature and elevation, posterior elevation, and corneal thickness.

Densitometry

The Pentacam's densitometry function quantifies lens density on a scale from 0 to 100, 100 being completely opaque. The grayscale image of a Scheimpflug image is the basis for this densitometric quantification. The density of the lens can be measured at any point enabling assessment of the different layers of the lens. A dotted white vertical line represents the plane of the displayed values. Clicking into the representation of the values highlights the respective point of measurement in the Scheimpflug image. By default, the plane of measurement intersects the corneal apex. Aspects like lens thickness can also be assessed from the acquired Scheimpflug image.

Evaluation of the lens using the Pentacam allows for examination of the lens in patients presenting for LASIK who may be better suited for RLE. Figure 24-20 shows a 52-year-old male who presented with nuclear sclerosis. IOL was recommended for both eyes rather than keratorefractive surgery. The left eye was performed first. It would be a mistake to perform LASIK on this type of patient because the patient will blame the cataracts on the LASIK procedure. With the densitometry/photo, it is easy to show

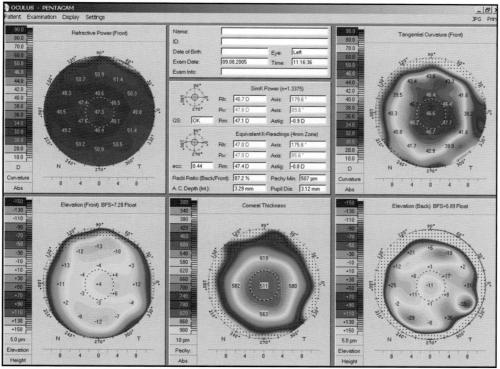

Figure 24-19A. The Holladay report presents five color maps: anterior refractive power, tangential curvature, anterior elevation, posterior elevation, and corneal thickness. This map was taken of a high myope pre-LASIK. (Courtesy of Matthias Maus, MD.)

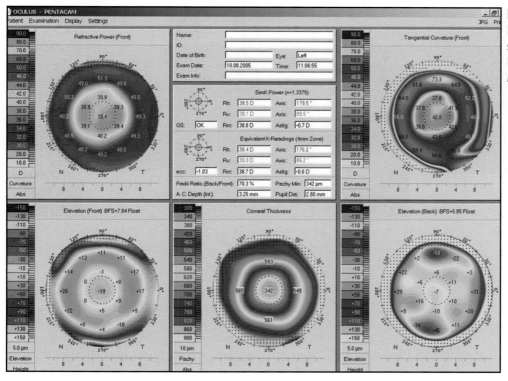

Figure 24-19B. The Holladay report for the same eye 1 day post-op LASIK. (Courtesy of Matthias Maus, MD.)

Figure 24-19C. The Holladay report for the same eye 1.5 months postop LASIK. (Courtesy of Matthias Maus, MD.)

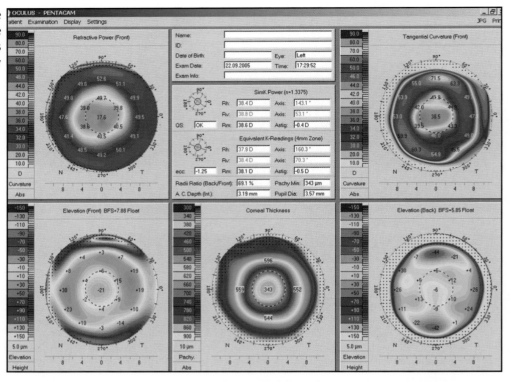

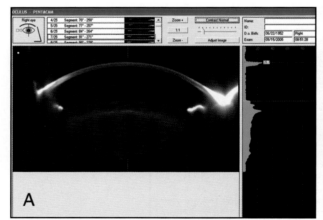

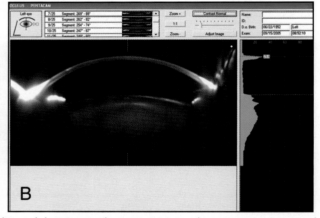

Figure 24-20. Densitometry facilitates patients understanding of their aging lens: (A) OD and (B) OS. (Courtesy of Jason Stahl, MD.)

patients their aging lens, which helps them understand why they should avoid LASIK.

Glaucoma Diagnosis

The Pentacam is an outstanding tool for monitoring the effects of IOP-lowering drugs on the anterior chamber angle over time. An image of the anterior chamber angle can be seen in Figure 24-21. The patient can be shown the positive effects of the drug to promote patient compliance and enhance therapeutic long-term success.

Corneal thickness influences tonometry measurements, such that intraocular pressure (IOP) measurement may not reflect the true IOP. Performing tonometry on a thin cornea results in a lower value due to ease of applanation, causing a false sense of safety for both the physician and his or her patient. A thicker cornea results in a higher measurement, possibly triggering premature glaucoma therapy. The Pentacam offers the possibility to enter an IOP value to determine a corrected IOP.

The Pentacam as a Marketing Tool

Those interested in surgical correction of their ammetropia are often well-informed and demanding customers looking not only for a skilled and experienced sur-

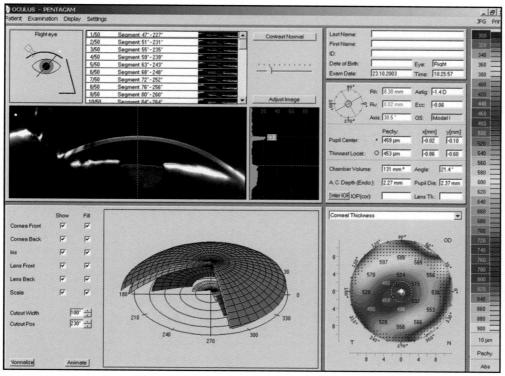

Figure 24-21. Narrow anterior chamber as viewed with Scheimpflug imaging.

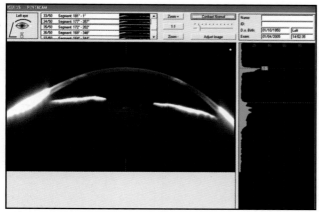

Figure 24-22. Scheimpflug image of showing CK spots. (Courtesy of Matthias Maus, MD.)

geon, but also for the latest technology. Surgeon competence and the will to do the very best for each patient needs to be conveyed to patients.

The Pentacam promotes the competence of a practice. Colorful maps and animated three-dimensional models are great visual aids. A patient presenting for LASIK whose Pentacam results reveal keratoconus may better understand why elective procedures are to be avoided with visual demonstration of their abnormality. Surgical procedures may be better explained as well. For example, the effect of conductive keratoplasty is demonstrated in Figure 24-22. This image was obtained from a 55-year-old female S/P

CK 2 years ago for presbyopia. Her MR has remained –1.50 D OS and her UCVA-near is J2.

Dispensing printouts is also a wonderful idea since patients can refer to their measurements at home and better remember what the physician has explained to them. They might show friends and family, promoting your practice.

Besides serving as a marketing tool, the Pentacam can also strengthen the doctor–patient relationship. Pachymetry without topical proparacaine is beneficial to patients. Follow-up visits may be less stressful. Since the operation of the Pentacam can be delegated to the practice's personnel, physicians have more time for other tasks.

REFERENCES

1. Barkana Y, Gerber Y, Elbaz U, et al. Central corneal thickness measurement with the Pentacam Scheimpflug system, optical low-coherence reflectometry pachymeter, and ultrasound pachymetry. *J Cataract Refract Surg.* 2005; 31(9):1729–1735.

2. O'Donnell C, Maldonado-Codina C. Agreement and repeatability of central thickness measurement in normal corneas using ultrasound pachymetry and the OCULUS Pentacam. *Cornea.* 2005;24(8):920–924.

3. Tang W, Collins MJ, Carney L, Davis B. Compare: The accuracy and precision performance of four videokeratoscopes in measuring test surfaces. *Optometry & Vision Science.* 2000;77(9):483–491.

Chapter 25

Precisio

Tracy Swartz, OD, MS; Charles Wm. Stewart, OD; Giuseppe Bellezza, MD;
Vincenzo Marchi, MD; Giuseppe D'Ippolito, DrIng; and Ming Wang, MD, PhD

Precisio topography is an elevation-based system utilizing the Scheimpflug principle. It is improved from previous Scheimpflug products in that Precisio uses off-axis projection through the center of the cornea to eliminate data loss caused by reflections off the center of the cornea. Precisio provides high-definition elevation data using over 39,000 data points per surface. Structures measured include anterior and posterior cornea, pachymetry, and anterior chamber. Importantly, Precisio used as the basis for surgery provides exceptional repeatability.

A precise slice of white light is projected at an angle of 20 degrees while being rotated about the visual axis (Figure 25-1). The patient's visual axis is auto-aligned with the axis of rotation of the system using software-controlled four-axis motion. This further minimizes data variability that may be operator induced.

The cross sectional images shown in Figure 25-2 are recorded at high speed by two synchronized video systems: the main camera and the focus camera.

The main camera provides the high-resolution images that yield data to analyze the shape of the anterior and posterior cornea, iris, and chamber angle. Fifty images are acquired in 1 second, each covering the anterior segment limbus to limbus. Data points are collected with repeatability typically better than 3 μm.

The focus camera provides integrative and positional data to complete the triangulation necessary for high definition tomography (Figure 25-3). Integration of the data from the main camera is further augmented from the integrated eye-tracking technology used during the acquisition process.

Limbal vessel architecture is included within the data set for use in positive eye identification and rotational position registration of elevation data when used with the surgical laser delivery system. An example can be seen in Figure 25-4.

Unlike topography systems, which estimate elevation from curvature or refractive data, the Precisio high-definition data was specifically engineered to meet the demands of corneal surgery. Default displays include the anterior elevation (Figure 25-5), posterior elevation (Figure 25-6), and pachymetry maps (Figure 25-7). Three-dimensional maps are also displayed (Figure 25-8) and are easily manipulated to demonstrate irregularities in corneal shape.

Currently, Precisio can be used to guide excimer procedures using corneal interactive programmed topographic ablation (CIPTA) and corneal lamellar ablation for transplantation (CLAT). The customized treatment strategy is chosen based on the patient's corneal stability. In virgin eyes, or in cases of irregular astigmatism due to scarring, previous refractive surgery, or trauma where the corneal shape is unchanging, CIPTA can be used to regularize the cornea and address the refractive error, if the surgeon so chooses. In cases of corneal instability due to ectasia, corneal disease, or previous refractive surgery requiring corneal transplant, CLAT is used.

CORNEAL INTERACTIVE PROGRAMMED TOPOGRAPHIC ABLATION

CIPTA is the synthesis of true corneal shape data, detailed refraction, and dynamic pupillometry, creating custom refractive surgery. When using CIPTA, the volume of the planned ablation is described by the intersection of the anterior surface of the cornea and the ideal aconic corneal surface. The ablation takes into account the patient's true anterior corneal surface, not a derived surface based on mathematical calculation. The transition zone guarantees a constant slope in all radial directions

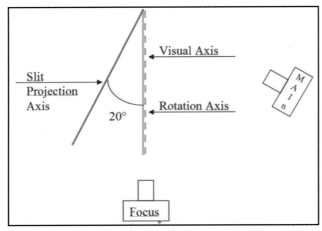

Figure 25-1. Precisio system diagram.

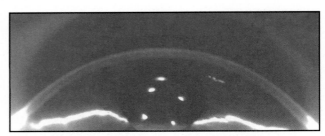

Figure 25-2. High-definition cross-sectional images.

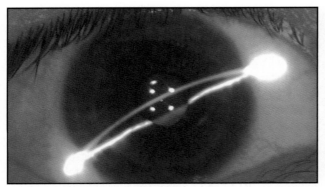

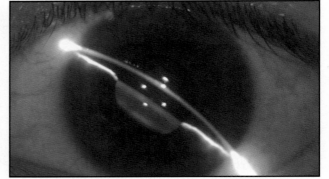

Figure 25-3. Positioning data for triangulation is obtained from these images taken by the focus camera.

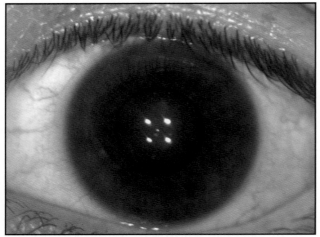

Figure 25-4. Limbal vessel detail used for operative rotational positioning and eye identification.

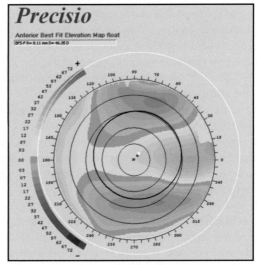

Figure 25-5. An anterior elevation map.

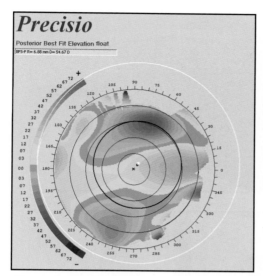

Figure 25-6. A posterior elevation map.

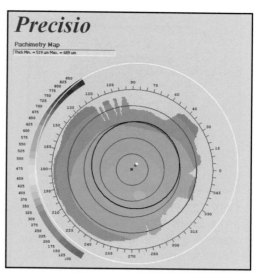

Figure 25-7. A pachymetry map.

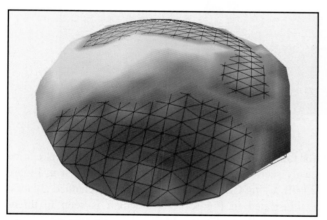

Figure 25-8. Three-dimensional map of an irregular cornea due to herpetic keratopathy.

with variable width. The optical zone covers the ideal pupil area as determined by dynamic pupillometry.

CIPTA holds several advantages over wavefront-guided custom treatments. Wavefront, standard, and Placido topographic ablations, even if with different objectives, try to compensate for the refractive error of the eye directly and under the assumption that there is no need to know corneal morphology. However, the refractive process is the natural consequence of the morphology of the corneal surfaces. Keratorefractive surgery, by definition, is focused on the anterior surface of the cornea.

Wavefront, standard, and Placido topographic ablations create a lens over the cornea to compensate for the refractive error. CIPTA, to optimize the quality of vision for the patient, regularizes the anterior surface of the cornea by identifying and locating its ideal shape. CIPTA then ablates the cornea to reveal its ideal shape. This treatment strategy is successful because the refractive correction is the natural consequence of the corneal regularization.

Wavefront-guided techniques suffer from both technical problems and conceptual errors. Custom ablation, to be successful, requires that patient data be precise and repeatable.

Wavefront technology, which is largely used in the optics and telescope field, cannot be applied to the human eye due to the unpredictable level of aberrations. Significant aberrations cause errant locations of area of interest when using lenslet arrays. The use of wavefront technology designed for static lens applications inherits errors when applied to dynamic human optics. CIPTA, through the regularization of the anterior corneal surface, directly compensates for the corneal aberrations. Since the ideal shape is a regularized surface, the quality of vision is not compromised due to the dynamics of the eye. Further, CIPTA defines an ideal regular shape for the anterior corneal surface with specific attention to the transition zone to minimize risk of regression and uncontrolled modifications of the shape.

This technology is also applied to unstable corneas treated with custom lamellar keratoplasty using the software application CLAT. The volume of the patient's ablation is determined by the intersection of the pachymetry map and an ideal, uniform thickness corneal bed for the patient. At the point where the bed has been reduced in thickness, the tissue takes on new elastic properties as a membrane with no cross-sectional rigidity. Only one membrane position will exist along isostatic lines. When the ablation is complete, the membrane bed will have been positioned along the isostatic line that eliminates the deformation induced from the cone.

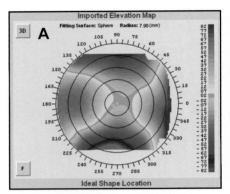

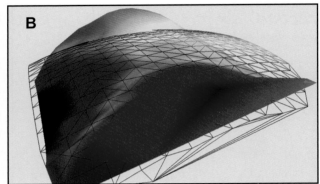

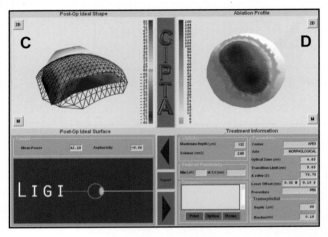

Figure 25-9. A patient suffered 10D of astigmatism S/P LASIK due to misprogramming of the laser. (A) Anterior elevation map; (B) three-dimensional map; (C) the ideal shape and planned ablation; (D) the postoperative three-dimensional simulation.

The volume of the ablation of the donor lamella is obtained by performing a perimetral saddle with depth and width defined by the operator. A trephine is used to cut the cornea of the donor to a diameter equal to the diameter of the patient bed. The donor tissue is positioned on the bed, and a conventional suturing technique is used to secure the donor saddle in place. Future applications may include the use of biomedical glue to reduce or eliminate sutures.

CLINICAL APPLICATIONS

The following are examples illustrating the use of elevation data to guide custom ablation.

Case I

A patient's 5D astigmatism was misprogrammed at an axis 90 degrees away from its true axis for his LASIK surgery. His anterior elevation map is shown in Figure 25-9A. Ten D of astigmatism resulted, with a BCVA of 20/50. Gas permeable correction failed due to discomfort and significant lack of improvement in best correction. The reason for failure of the fitting of the gas permeable lens can be easily seen on the three-dimensional map seen in Figure 25-9B. Using CIPTA, the ideal shape and planned ablation is illustrated in Figure 25-9C, which is seen in three-dimensionally in Figure 25-9D. Two months postoperatively, the patient was 20/25 uncorrected.

Case II

A patient suffered from glare, halos, multiple images, and best corrected vision of 20/40 after myopic PRK. The anterior elevation map suggests a small, decentered optical zone (Figure 25-10A). The planned ablation profile from CIPTA can be seen in Figure 25-10B, and the ideal shape can be seen in two dimensions (Figure 25-10C) and in three dimensions (Figure 25-10D).

Case III

A 45-year-old female presented with decreased vision secondary to LASIK with a PRK enhancement resulting in corneal haze. The slit-scanning maps are shown in Figure 25-11A. The corneal haze resulted in a misrepresentation

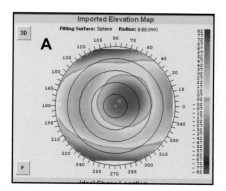

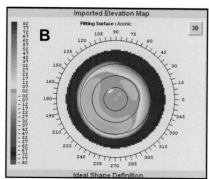

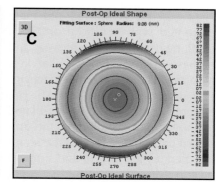

Figure 25-10. The preoperative maps of a patient with a small, decentered optical zone S/P myopic PRK. (A) anterior elevation; (B) the ideal shape based on an iconic reference body; (C) planned ideal shape with a widened zone and improved prolate shape in 2-D and (D) in three-dimensions.

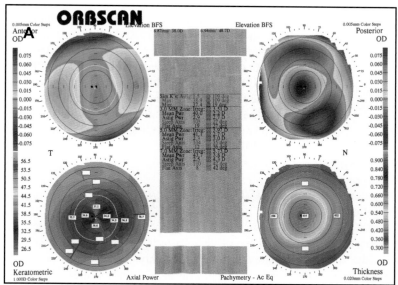

Figure 25-11. (A) Preoperative slit-scanning maps of a patient S/P LASIK and PRK with corneal haze, resulting in a misrepresentation of the posterior surface. (B) The computerized ideal shape map and planned ablation profile as calculated using CIPTA software, and the (C) simulated postoperative elevation map.

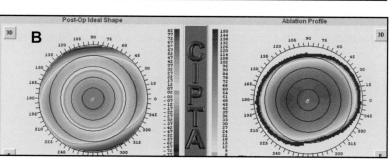

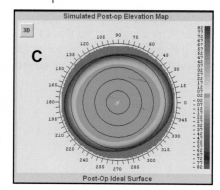

Figure 25-12. A 40 year-old male presented with a history of LASIK resulting in an unstable ectasia, and underwent a custom lamellar keratoplasty. The preoperative pachymetry map is shown in (A). The patient's cornea was custom ablated as shown in (B), resulting in the simulated pachymetry map of the recipient bed (C, left image) and simulated post-operative result (C, right image).

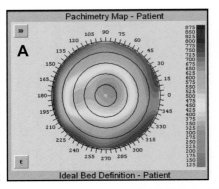

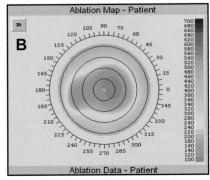

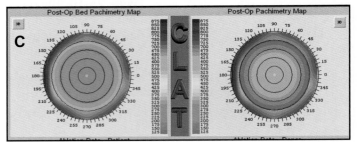

of the posterior surface since her central ultrasound pachymetry was actually 440 µm. Her manifest refraction was −7.75 −2.00 x 100 with 20/100 best-corrected vision. CIPTA was used to regularize the cornea and moderately address the myopia. Figure 25-11B shows the computerized ideal shape map and planned ablation profile. Figure 25-11C shows the simulated postoperative elevation map with a widened optical zone and less aspheric shape.

Case IV

A 40-year-old male presented with a history of LASIK resulting in an unstable ectasia. A custom lamellar keratoplasty was performed using CLAT. The preoperative pachymetry map is shown in Figure 25-12A. The patient's cornea was custom ablated (Figure 25-12B) resulting in the simulated elevation map of the recipient bed (left) and the donor tissue. Note the regularity at the 8 mm edge of the transplanted tissue (seen as a regular blue color). The donor tissue was a lamellar section of 350-µm thickness; therefore, the donor saddle was not ablated in this case because there would not have been enough tissue for transplantation.

Case V

The pachymetric map of a patient suffering from keratoconus is shown in Figure 25-13A. The planned ablation for the recipient and donor are shown in Figure 25-13B. The donor tissue was a lamellar section of 320-µm thickness; therefore, the donor saddle was not ablated in this case because there would not have been enough tissue for transplantation. The simulated ablation maps are shown in two dimensions (Figure 25-13C) and in three dimensions (Figure 25-13D).

Conclusion

The concept of custom topographic ablation based on the ideal shape of the cornea is a revolutionary idea, one that requires precise and highly repeatable information about corneal shape. The high-definition elevation maps produced by the Precisio are the result of an advanced configuration of the two-camera Scheimpflug system engineered to remove multiple sources of error found in other topographic systems.

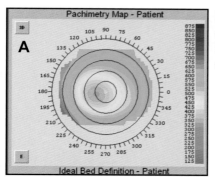

Figure 25-13. (A) The pachymetric map of a patient suffering from kerato-conus. (B) The planned ablation for the recipient and donor. (C) The simulated ablation maps are shown in two dimensions and (D) in three dimensions.

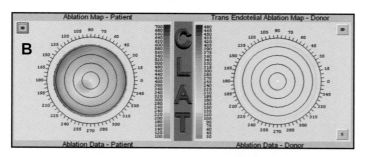

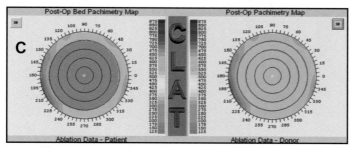

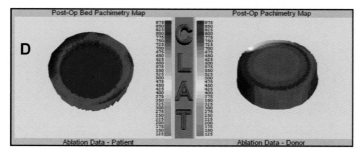

Chapter 26

The Future of Corneal Topography

Arun C. Gulani, MD and Ming Wang, MD, PhD

With the ever-increasing pace of technology, our knowledge base for measuring and surgically altering the cornea for more predictable keratorefractive surgery outcomes continues to expand. Improvements are principally driven by increasing expectations of our patients and our need to reduce surgical complications, particularly visual quality loss following refractive surgery.

The gold standard for analysis of corneal shape and the dominant prerequisite for corneal refractive surgery has been, and will continue to be, corneal topography. In this book, we have seen the evolution of corneal topographic technologies from the traditional Placido disk systems (represented by Humphrey Atlas, Magellean Mapper, Tracey-EyeSys, Optikon, Tomey, and Topcon) and elevational and optical slit scanning systems (represented by Parks and Orbscan), to the newer technologies such as ultrasonic corneal mapper (represented by Artemis), the 3-D checkerboard system (represented by AstraMax), and the more recent Scheimpflug 360 rotational slit-scanning systems (represented by Pentacam and Precisio). Future development of technology may also include OCT used in anterior segment imaging with transverse signal reprocessing for corneal mapping.

With various emerging technologies for keratorefractive surgeries, the challenges of obtaining accurate measurements and translating that information into surgical results remain. Differential subtraction of postsurgical corneal elevation from presurgical elevations reveals the nature of the proposed or obtained surgical lenticule. Comparisons of the desired lenticule to the obtained surgical lenticule contain valuable information that can be used to improve future surgeries.

Customized wavefront-based ablations have gained support, but topography will always have an indispensable place. A symbiotic relationship between wavefront technology and modern corneal topography is emerging. Clinicians realize topography and wavefront can make up for each other's shortcomings. Wavefront is valuable because it provides aberration information of the entire visual pathway while corneal topography only addresses corneal aberrations. The sensitivity of wavefront sensing can help detect earlier situations of corneal pathology in the preoperative evaluations for potential LASIK candidates towards safe and effective outcomes.[1] For example, in cases of forme fruste keratoconus, using wavefront guidance we can detect higher-order aberrations in the form of coma and increased root mean square values,[2] aiding earlier detection of keratoconus and other potential ectatic corneal conditions.

On the other hand, wavefront provides no information as to the location of the aberration and is limited by the size of the pupil and amount of light penetration through the cornea and lens. Whether we focus on corneal subtractive (excimer laser ablative), incisional, or additive (inlays/Intacs) surgeries, topographical knowledge will always be required.

Combining wavefront-sensing and corneal topography will be the mainstay of corneal and wavefront imaging for keratorefractive surgery. What is the best management for a 30-year-old patient having 2.50 D of astigmatism, the majority of it located in the lens? We need to identify such patients prior to refractive surgery. Combined corneal topography and a wavefront imaging system such as what we saw in the Tracey wavefront-topography system (Chapter 17) and the Keratron (Chapter 20) will play an important role in this effort. Once patients having significant amounts of lenticular aberration are identified, should they proceed with keratorefractive surgery knowing that we will be creating a significantly more astigmatic cornea?

Our studies have shown that correcting mostly nonanterior corneal astigmatism with corneal procedures such as LASIK is less effective than correcting anterior corneal astigmatism.[3] Perhaps, a combined and topography-wavefront guided approach can help us identify the optimal solution (Chapter 13) and recognize when the best surgical option is intraocular rather then keratorefractive.

Does the future hold real-time corneal topographic measurement intraoperatively? We can imagine one day performing intraoperative topographically guided excimer treatments. Such technology will be challenging to develop due to the sophisticated optical engineering and imaging technology required. Such developments are complicated by unknown corneal wound healing contribution to the final corneal architecture. Intraoperative, real-time adjustment of certain types of corneal surgeries may lead the way for the development of intraoperative real-time corneal topographic imaging. For example, identifying the exact sectoral location of Intacs ring placement intraoperatively using real-time topographic monitoring would be a significant advancement over the current procedure.

The endpoint of the majority of keratorefractive procedures is affected by healing. We need to combine all pertinent imaging information to help us maximize the predictability of corneal shaping. For example, incorporating the Dynamic Corneal Imaging System (Dynamic corneal imaging: Prof Gunther Grabner et al: University Eye Clinic, Paracelsus Private Medical University, Salzburg, Austria), video-topography for tear film measurement and its contour (Janos Nemeth et al, First Department of Ophthalmology, Semmelweis University, Budapest, Hungary; the Computer and Automation Research Institute, Hungarian Academy of Sciences, Budapest, Hungary; and the Department of Statistics, National Health Insurance Fund Administration, Budapest, Hungary), and wavefront sensing to identify the contribution from internal optical elements would isolate corneal measurements. Confocal visualization of the cornea with posterior corneal analysis offers a full dimension of information about corneal architecture.

It is possible that only through a combined approach using all available technologies, combining components focused on a single structural of the cornea, incorporating biomechanical or optical behavior of cornea such as elasticity modules of the cornea, and using wavefront analysis from the entire visual pathway and cornea, can we ultimately predict the final corneal shape and best protect visual quality after keratorefractive surgery.

REFERENCES

1. Gulani AC, Probst L, Cox I, Veith R. Wavefront in LASIK: the zyoptix platform. *Ophthalmol Clin N Am.* 2004;17: 173–181.

2. Gulani AC. *Wavefront principles: simplified & applied* [instructional course]. Paris, France: ESCRS; 2004.

3. Wang MX. Stereotopography: advancing the state of the diagnostic technology for refractive surgery. *Refractive Eyecare.* 2001;5:1–5.

Index

WAIT
...There's More!

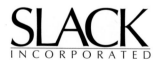